Nystagmus and Vertigo

CLINICAL APPROACHES TO THE PATIENT WITH DIZZINESS

UCLA FORUM IN MEDICAL SCIENCES

UCLA FORUM IN MEDICAL SCIENCES

NUMBER 24

Nystagmus and Vertigo

CLINICAL APPROACHES TO THE PATIENT WITH DIZZINESS

Edited by

VICENTE HONRUBIA

Department of Surgery
School of Medicine
University of California Los Angeles
Los Angeles, California

MARY A. B. BRAZIER

Departments of Anatomy and Physiology
School of Medicine
University of California Los Angeles
Los Angeles, California

1982

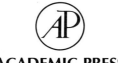

ACADEMIC PRESS

A Subsidiary of Harcourt Brace Jovanovich, Publishers

New York   London

Paris   San Diego   San Francisco   São Paulo   Sydney   Tokyo   Toronto

OPTOMETRY

ACADEMIC PRESS, INC.
111 Fifth Avenue, New York, New York 10003

United Kingdom Edition published by
ACADEMIC PRESS, INC. (LONDON) LTD.
24/28 Oval Road, London NW1 7DX

Library of Congress Cataloging in Publication Data

Main entry under title:

Nystagmus and vertigo.

   (UCLA forum in medical sciences; no. 24)
   Proceedings of a clinical neurotology international
workshop held at the UCLA School of Medicine, Sept. 25-
26, 1980.
   Includes bibliographies and indexes.
   1. Nystagmus--Congresses. 2. Vertigo--Congresses.
I. Honrubia, Vicente. II. Brazier, Mary Agnes Burniston,
Date   . III. University of California, Los Angeles.
School of Medicine. IV. Series. [DNLM: 1. Vestibular
function tests--Congresses. 2. Nystagmus--Congresses.
3. Vertigo--Congresses. 4. Dizziness--Congresses. W3
U17 no. 24 1980 / WV 255 N998 1980]
RE748.N95   616.8'41   82-3906
ISBN 0-12-355080-7   AACR2

PRINTED IN THE UNITED STATES OF AMERICA

82 83 84 85   9 8 7 6 5 4 3 2 1

Contents

List of Contributors and Participants ix
Preface xi
Other Titles in the Series xiii

INTRODUCTORY TOPICS

The Anatomical–Physiological Basis for Vestibular Function

RICHARD R. GACEK 3

Techniques of Anatomical Localization

VICTOR GOODHILL 25

Radiology of Vestibular Disturbances

WILLIAM N. HANAFEE 39

Approach to the Dizzy Patient

ROBERT W. BALOH 49

Evaluation of Rotatory Vestibular Tests in Peripheral Labyrinthine Lesions

VICENTE HONRUBIA, HERMAN A. JENKINS, ROBERT W. BALOH,
AND CLIFFORD G. Y. LAU 57

NEW TRENDS IN CLINICAL TESTING OF THE VESTIBULOOCULAR REFLEX

Technical Problems in Stimulation, Recording, and Analysis of Eye Movements

R. SCHMID 81

Low-Frequency Harmonic Acceleration in the Evaluation of Patients with Peripheral Labyrinthine Disorders

JAMES W. WOLFE, EDWARD J. ENGELKEN, AND JAMES E. OLSON 95

Use of Pseudorandom Angular Accelerations in the Evaluation of Vestibuloocular Function

DENNIS P. O'LEARY, JOSEPH M. FURMAN, AND JAMES W. WOLFE 107

The Correlation between Motion Sensation, Nystagmus, and Activity in the Vestibular Nerve and Nuclei

V. HENN 115

ROUTINE CLINICAL EVALUATION OF PATIENTS WITH PERIPHERAL LABYRINTHINE DISORDERS

A Report from Japan on the Routine Clinical Evaluation of Patients with Vestibular Disorders

JUN-ICHI SUZUKI...127

A Report from Europe

W. J. OOSTERVELD 135

Auditory Evaluation of Vestibular Patients

DOUGLAS NOFFSINGER, DONALD E. MORGAN, AND
DAVID G. HANSON 145

Atypical Cogan's Syndrome: A Case Report

ROBERT D. YEE 157

CLINICAL TESTING OF VESTIBULOSPINAL FUNCTION

Equilibrium Testing of the Disoriented Patient
LEWIS M. NASHNER 165

The Pathophysiology of Postural Imbalance in Cerebellar Patients
JOHANNES DICHGANS AND KARL-HEINZ MAURITZ 179

Diagnostic Implications of Induced Body Sway
ROBERT O. ANDRES 191

TESTING OF VISUAL-VESTIBULAR INTERACTION: CLINICAL APPLICATION

Applied and Clinical Aspects of Visual-Vestibular Interaction
THOMAS BRANDT 207

Illusory Movement of Environment during Head Rotation with Normal Eye Movements
DAVID G. COGAN, FRED C. CHU, AND DOUGLAS B. REINGOLD 225

Quantitative Assessment of Visual-Vestibular Interaction Using Sinusoidal Rotatory Stimuli
ROBERT W. BALOH, ROBERT D. YEE, HERMAN A. JENKINS,
AND VICENTE HONRUBIA 231

Cerebellar Control of Eye Movements
DAVID S. ZEE 241

Pathophysiology of Optokinetic Nystagmus
ROBERT D. YEE, ROBERT W. BALOH, VICENTE HONRUBIA,
AND HERMAN A. JENKINS 251

FREE COMMUNICATIONS

Optokinetic Pattern Asymmetry in Patients with Cerebral Lesions

KIMITAKA KAGA AND JUN-ICHI SUZUKI 279

The Transitions between Saccades and Smooth Eye Movements

DOUGLAS B. REINGOLD 287

Author Index 297
Subject Index 305

List of Contributors and Participants

Names of contributors to this volume are marked with an asterisk.

*__Robert O. Andres,__ Kresge Hearing Research Institute, Ann Arbor, Michigan 48109

*__Robert W. Baloh,__ Department of Neurology, School of Medicine, University of California Los Angeles, Los Angeles, California 90024

*__Thomas Brandt,__ Neurological Clinic with Clinical Neurophysiology, Alfried Krupp Hospital, Essen, Federal Republic of Germany

*__Fred C. Chu,__ Neuro-ophthalmology Section, Clinical Branch, National Eye Institute, National Institutes of Health, Bethesda, Maryland 20205

*__David G. Cogan,__ Neuro-ophthalmology Section, Clinical Branch, National Eye Institute, National Institutes of Health, Bethesda, Maryland 20205

*__Johannes Dichgans,__ Department of Neurology, University of Tübingen, 7400 Tübingen 1, Federal Republic of Germany

*__Edward J. Engelken,__ USAF School of Aerospace Medicine, Brooks Air Force Base, San Antonio, Texas 78235

__George Freyss,__ Hôpital Lariboisière Clinique, ORL, 75010 Paris, France

*__Joseph M. Furman,__ Department of Neurology, School of Medicine, University of California Los Angeles, Los Angeles, California 90024

*__Richard R. Gacek,__ Department of Otorhinolaryngology, Upstate Medical Center, State University of New York, Syracuse, New York 13210

*__Victor Goodhill,__ Division of Head and Neck Surgery (Otology), School of Medicine, University of California Los Angeles, Los Angeles, California 90024

__Ruth Gussen,__ Department of Pathology and Surgery, School of Medicine, University of California Los Angeles, Los Angeles, California 90024

*__William N. Hanafee,__ Department of Radiological Sciences, School of Medicine, University of California Los Angeles, Los Angeles, California 90024

*__David G. Hanson,__ VA Wadsworth Medical Center, Los Angeles, California 90073, and Division of Head and Neck Surgery, School of Medicine, University of California Los Angeles, Los Angeles, California 90024

*__V. Henn,__ Department of Neurology, University of Zürich, 8091 Zürich, Switzerland

*__Vicente Honrubia,__ Department of Surgery, School of Medicine, University of California Los Angeles, Los Angeles, California 90024

Makoto Igarashi, Department of Otorhinolaryngology and Communicative Sciences, Baylor College of Medicine, Texas Medical Center, Houston, Texas 77030

*Herman A. Jenkins, Department of Otorhinolaryngology and Communicative Sciences, Baylor College of Medicine, Houston, Texas 77030

*Kimitaka Kaga, Department of Otolaryngology, Teikyo University School of Medicine, Itabashi-ku, Tokyo 173, Japan

*Clifford G. Y. Lau, Division of Head and Neck Surgery (Otolaryngology), School of Medicine, University of California Los Angeles, Los Angeles, California 90024

Charles H. Markham, Department of Neurology, School of Medicine, University of California Los Angeles, Los Angeles, California 90024

*Karl-Heinz Mauritz, Department of Neurology, University of Freiburg, 7800 Freiburg 1, Federal Republic of Germany

*Donald E. Morgan, Division of Head and Neck Surgery, School of Medicine, University of California Los Angeles, Los Angeles, California 90024

*Lewis M. Nashner, Neurological Sciences Institute, Good Samaritan Hospital and Medical Center, Portland, Oregon 97209

*Douglas Noffsinger, VA Wadsworth Medical Center, Los Angeles, California 90073, and Division of Head and Neck Surgery, School of Medicine, University of California Los Angeles, Los Angeles, California 90024

*Dennis P. O'Leary, Division of Vestibular Disorders, Eye and Ear Hospital, Department of Otolaryngology, University of Pittsburgh School of Medicine, Pittsburgh, Pennsylvania 15213

*James E. Olson, USAF School of Aerospace Medicine, Brooks Air Force Base, San Antonio, Texas 78235

*W. J. Oosterveld, Vestibular Department, E.N.T. Clinic, Wilhelmina Gasthuis, 1054 EG Amsterdam, The Netherlands

*Douglas B. Reingold, Eye Movement Laboratory, Neuro-ophthalmology Section, Clinical Branch, National Eye Institute, National Institutes of Health, Bethesda, Maryland 20205

David Robinson, Department of Ophthalmology, The Wilmer Institute, The Johns Hopkins University, Baltimore, Maryland 21205

Wallace Rubin, Department of Otorhinolaryngology and Biocommunication, School of Medicine, Louisiana State University, Metairie, Louisiana 70002

*R. Schmid, Istituto di Informatica e Sistemistica, Università di Pavia, 27100 Pavia, Italy

*Jun-Ichi Suzuki, Department of Otolaryngology, Teikyo University School of Medicine, Itabashi-ku, Tokyo 173, Japan

*James W. Wolfe, USAF School of Aerospace Medicine, Brooks Air Force Base, San Antonio, Texas 78235

*Robert D. Yee, Department of Ophthalmology, School of Medicine, University of California Los Angeles, Los Angeles, California 90024

*David S. Zee, Department of Neurology and Ophthalmology, School of Medicine, The Johns Hopkins University, Baltimore, Maryland 21205

Preface

This book contains the proceedings of an international workshop on clinical neurotology held at the UCLA School of Medicine on September 25 and 26, 1980. The purpose of the symposium was to share information on new concepts and methods that have been developed for evaluating neurotologic patients.

The vestibular system, in conjunction with visual, auditory, and proprioceptive inputs, is responsible for maintenance of orientation. This basic function, fundamental for animal navigation, depends on the ability of the central nervous system to integrate information from relatively simple reflex arcs into complex brain functions. Understanding of these orienting reflexes is rapidly improving after a long period of empiricism. Crucial to such understanding is our grasp of the workings of the labyrinthine receptor organs, but our knowledge of their anatomy and physiology has lagged behind in comparison to other sensory systems. Indeed, the physical properties of the labyrinthine stimulus are so different from those of other sensory stimuli that the existence of an organ for the control of head motion and position was first suspected less than a century ago when E. Mach, a German biophysicist who was familiar with the laws of mechanics, proposed that a mysterious organ located in the head was responsible for the perception of gravity. Since then, basic principles of vestibular function have been elucidated, including the nature of the physical stimuli (acceleration and gravity), the location and morphology of the end-organs, the primary connections with the central nervous system, and the more prominent symptoms of labyrinthine disorders. New insight into the physiological mechanism of interaction of the various orienting reflexes and their anatomical connections is emerging. The central nervous system is no longer viewed by physiologists as a compartmentalized system, but rather as a complex body of neurons in which many reflexes interact to make possible animal orientation and navigation. Pathological disturbances in any of the system's components lead to the series of symptoms that specialists from different fields are beginning to identify as belonging to a common constellation of disease processes. This new perspective on brain function and, in particular, vestibular pathology has led to renewed interest in the study of patients with neurological disorders and in the development of new tests to evaluate multisensory interactions.

Progress in evaluating the state of the vestibular system has been slow due to the intricacies of its reflex functions, which are not yet well understood, and to inadequacies in instrumentation and techniques. At present, the situation is such that the reader will have no difficulty in appreciating the lack of consensus in approaches to patients by different specialties, both conceptually and in selection of vestibular function tests. This diversity of approaches transcends the boundaries of specialties. Not only does a neurologist approach vestibular patients differently from an ophthalmologist or otolaryngologist, but within an individual specialty there is no agreement as to the value of different tests, and findings are often given different significance.

The trend is clearly toward the use of a common approach based on rigorous pathophysiological principles and quantitative tests of various vestibular reflexes. The basic concept that emerges is that the diagnosis of disorders in the vestibular system is in many ways comparable to that of disorders in the auditory system. It is a complex task that requires information from a variety of sources: the patient's history, the physical examination, and laboratory tests. Because few otological diseases have pathognomic signs that uniquely characterize them, the diagnostic task is first to identify the probable anatomical location of the lesion. In this respect, the visual-vestibulooculomotor system, through measurements of different reflex responses, provides a unique opportunity to evaluate the function of different anatomical parts of the central nervous system.

We wish to thank, first, the National Institutes of Health, whose grant support, NS 16407, made possible the broad representation that was achieved in this workshop. In particular, we appreciate the continuing support of the National Institute of Neurological and Communicative Disorders and Stroke (NINCDS). We also thank the Hope for Hearing Foundation at UCLA, which planned the program and supported the organization and conduct of the meeting. Dean Sherman Mellinkoff and Dean Byron Backlar and the administration of the Division of Head and Neck Surgery made our efforts and those of our colleagues well worthwhile. The editors owe the excellent preparation of manuscripts for publication to Melody Horner.

VICENTE HONRUBIA
MARY A. B. BRAZIER

UCLA FORUM IN MEDICAL SCIENCES

Other Titles in the Series

1. Brain Function. Cortical Excitability and Steady Potentials, Relations of Basic Research to Space Biology. *Edited by Mary A. B. Brazier (1963)*
2. Brain Function: RNA and Brain Function. Memory and Learning. *Edited by Mary A. B. Brazier (1964)*
3. Brain and Behavior: The Brain and Gonadal Function. *Edited by Roger A. Gorski and Richard E. Whalen (1966)*
4. Brain Function: Speech, Language, and Communication. *Edited by Edward C. Carterette (1966)*
5. Gastrin. *Edited by Morton I. Grossman (1966)*
6. Brain Function: Brain Function and Learning. *Edited by Donald B. Lindsley and Arthur A. Lumsdaine (1967)*
7. Brain Function: Aggression and Defense. Neural Mechanisms and Social Patterns. *Edited by Carmine D. Clemente and Donald B. Lindsley (1967)*
8. The Retina: Morphology, Function, and Clinical Characteristics. *Edited by Bradley R. Straatsma, Raymond A. Allen, Frederick Crescitelli, and Michael O. Hall (1969)*
9. Image Processing in Biological Science. *Edited by Diane M. Ramsey (1969)*
10. Pathophysiology of Congenital Heart Disease. *Edited by Forrest H. Adams, H. J. C. Swan, and V. E. Hall (1970)*
11. The Interneuron. *Edited by Mary A. B. Brazier (1969)*
12. The History of Medical Education. *Edited by C. D. O'Malley (1970)*
13. Cardiovascular Beta Adrenergic Responses. *Edited by Albert A. Kattus, Jr., Gordon Ross, and Rex N. MacAlpin (1970)*
14. Cellular Aspects of Neural Growth and Differentiation. *Edited by Daniel C. Pease (1971)*
15. Steroid Hormones and Brain Function. *Edited by Charles Sawyer and Roger A. Gorski (1971)*
16. Multiple Sclerosis: Immunology, Virology, and Ultrastructure. *Edited by Frederick Wolfgram, George Ellison, Jack Stevens, and John Andrews (1972)*
17. Epilepsy: Its Phenomena in Man. *Edited by Mary A. B. Brazier (1973)*
18. Brain Mechanisms in Mental Retardation. *Edited by Nathaniel A. Buchwald and Mary A. B. Brazier (1975)*
19. Amyotrophic Lateral Sclerosis: Recent Research Trends. *Edited by John M. Andrews, Richard T. Johnson, and Mary A. B. Brazier (1976)*
20. Prevention of Neural Tube Defects: The Role of Alpha-Fetoprotein. *Edited by Barbara F. Crandall and Mary A. B. Brazier (1978)*
21. The Evolution of Protein Structure and Function: A Symposium in Honor of Professor Emil L. Smith. *Edited by David S. Sigman and Mary A. B. Brazier (1980)*
22. The Regulation of Muscle Contraction: Excitation-Contraction Coupling. *Edited by Alan D. Grinnell and Mary A. B. Brazier (1981)*

23. Cellular Basis of Chemical Messengers in the Digestive System. *Edited by Morton I. Grossman, Mary A. B. Brazier, and Juan Lechago (1981)*

24. Nystagmus and Vertigo: Clinical Approaches to the Patient with Dizziness. *Edited by Vicente Honrubia and Mary A. B. Brazier*

In preparation:

25. Developmental Immunology: Clinical Problems and Aging. *Edited by Edwin L. Cooper and Mary A. B. Brazier*

INTRODUCTORY TOPICS

The Anatomical–Physiological Basis for Vestibular Function

RICHARD R. GACEK

Department of Otorhinolaryngology
Upstate Medical Center
State University of New York
Syracuse, New York

Introduction

The prime function of the vestibular system is to maintain the body's orientation in space. This orientation is brought about by a series of well-integrated reflexes acting on the body's axial, limb, and extraocular muscles. Although several other modalities interact with the vestibular system, the prime input in maintaining the body's orientation in space is from the labyrinth, where special sensors detect dynamic movements and changes in position. This chapter reviews the salient anatomical and functional characteristics of the vestibular system that are responsible for the maintenance of orientation in space.

Vestibular Sense Organs

Mammals characteristically have two types of vestibular sense organs: the crista ampullaris and the macula utriculi and sacculi (Figure 1). The crista ampullaris is the sense organ of the semicircular canals and is located in the enlarged portion of the membranous canal; each of these canals represents a plane in space. The ridge of neurosensory epithelium that constitutes the crista is covered by a gelatinous cupula composed of mucopolysaccharides. Extending from the surface of the sense organ to the ampullary roof, the cupula serves as an elastic partition that is deformed by movements of endolymph created by the inertial stimulus of angular acceleration or deceleration (19). It is this cupular deflection that bends the rigid cilia protruding from the sensory cells in order to initiate an electrical response in the vestibular nerve. The macula of the utricle and the saccule is a saucer-shaped accumulation of neurosensory cells upon which rests an otoconial membrane with calcium carbonate crystals possessing a specific gravity of 2.71. This arrangement constitutes a structure that is displaced by a stimulus arising from linear acceleration or deceleration or from gravity.

3

NYSTAGMUS AND VERTIGO: CLINICAL
APPROACHES TO THE PATIENT WITH DIZZINESS

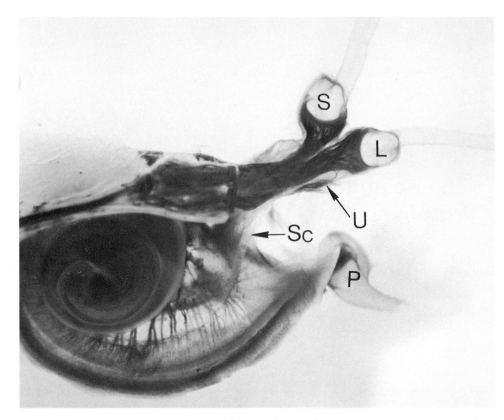

Figure 1.   Dissected specimen of a human labyrinth showing the appearance and arrangement of the vestibular sense organs. S, L, and P, superior, lateral, and posterior canal cristae, respectively; U, utricular macula; Sc, saccular macula.

Although the superstructure and mode of stimulation differ in these two types of sense organ, the hair cells responsible for the initiation of the electrical event are similar. In all mammals two types of such sensory cells, termed Type I and Type II, exist (24,31) (Figure 2). Type I hair cells are characteristically flask-shaped and are almost totally engulfed by a large calyx-like ending supplied by a large-caliber vestibular neuron. Small vesiculated endings contact the nerve ending or the axon. A single large axon usually innervates only one or two Type I hair cells. Innervation of three such hair cells by one nerve fiber is possible but rare. Type II hair cells are cylindrical and are contacted by small bouton-type endings, which are supplied by a small-caliber vestibular axon. Vesiculated bouton-type endings contact the cell surface of the Type II hair cells. Small afferent fibers ramify and innervate a relatively large number of Type II hair cells in the vestibular sense organ. Both types of vestibular hair cells have a special arrangement of cilia protruding from their superior surface. Each cell characteristically has one kinocilium located at one edge of a large number of stereocilia (approximately 70–100+). This arrangement of the kinocilium and stereocilia is important because deflection of the cilia in the direction of the kinocilium decreases the potential difference that exists between the endolymph and the inside of the sensory cell (about 120 mV), causing an intracellular depolarization and an increase in frequency of action potential of the vestibular nerve fibers

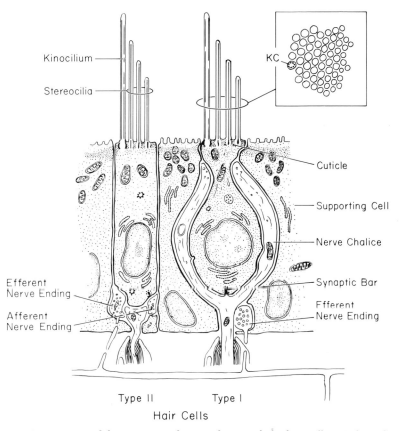

Kinocilium

Stereocilia

KC

Cuticle

Supporting Cell

Nerve Chalice

Synaptic Bar

Efferent
Nerve Ending

Afferent
Nerve Ending

Efferent
Nerve Ending

Type II   Type I

Hair Cells

Figure 2. Drawing of the two types of mammalian vestibular hair cells. KC, kinocilium.

(27,28,32). A deflection of the cilia away from the kinocilium conversely results in intracellular hyperpolarization and a decrease in the vestibular nerve action potentials. It is thought that the transduction of the mechanical stimulus into an electrical impulse at the hair cell–neural junction is produced by two possible mechanisms. As the rather rigid cilia are deflected, they produce a "dimpling" deformation of the cuticular plate of the hair cell because of either a change in electrical resistance or mechanical deformation (6). A second possibility is that as the cilia are deflected they separate from one another, causing a greater exposure of their surface to the ionic currents in the endolymph, and produce an electrical discharge that is transmitted to the hair cell (18). In either case, it is the deflection of the cilia that initiates the transduction of mechanical to electrical energy at the hair cell level.

The distribution of Type I and Type II hair cells in the vestibular sense organs is characteristic for each type of sense organ. In the crista, all hair cells are oriented so that the kinocilium is always on one side of the stereocilia. In the crista of the lateral canal, this organization is such that the kinocilia are located closest to the utricle, whereas in the vertical canals the kinocilia are located away from the utricular end of the membranous canal (25). This organization is referred to as the polarization of the vestibular hair cells (Figure 3). In the macula of the utricle and the saccule, the vestibular hair cells are oriented in opposite directions. In the utricular macula, the

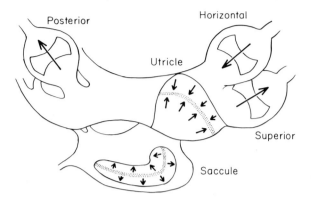

Figure 3.   Schema showing the direction of polarization of vestibular hair cells in the sense organs.

polarization of the hair cells is toward a line that more or less bisects the macula itself. This line is referred to as the striola line. In the saccular macula, the polarization of the hair cells of the two halves of the macula is away from the striola line. This arrangement of hair cells in the maculae makes it possible for opposite effects to occur in hair cells of each half of the macula when stimulation occurs. In the cristae, the movement of endolymph in a particular canal can only produce either an increase or a decrease in the resting potentials, and all the hair cells are stimulated in the same fashion. However, it should be remembered that, when angular acceleration occurs, one canal from each labyrinth is stimulated by endolymph movement in the opposite direction, and the two canals are therefore said to be complementary. The canals are so arranged that the movement of endolymph in the particular plane produces an increase in the resting potential of hair cells of one canal and a corresponding decrease in the potential of hair cells of the other canal. The canals are different from the maculae in which excitation and inhibition of hair cells occur within each half of the sense organ during stimulation.

The location of the two types of hair cells is different in the cristae and the maculae. In the cristae, the Type I hair cells are more concentrated at the top of the crista, whereas the Type II hair cells predominate along the slopes (25). However, in the maculae, no clear-cut arrangement exists, and Type I hair cells seem to be more prevalent near the striola line (17).

Vestibular Nerve (First-Order Vestibular Neuron)

The vestibular nerve, which innervates the five vestibular sense organs, is composed of true bipolar neurons with myelinated peripheral and central processes. The ganglion cells of these bipolar neurons are located in the internal auditory canal and are arranged in a fairly compact, but linear fashion. In the human, the vestibular nerve is composed of approximately 18,000 neurons (20). The monkey has a similar number of first-order vestibular neurons; the cat has 12,000, and the guinea pig and chinchilla each have approximately 7000 (10). In each species, the sense organs located in each of the semicircular canals and the utricle receive an approximately equal number of nerve fibers, whereas the saccule receives slightly fewer. Figure 4 shows the location and organization of neurons supplying each vestibular sense organ in the cat. It can be seen that, although the neurons supplying the cristae are

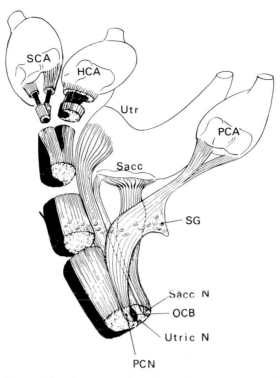

Figure 4.   Drawing of the peripheral nerve supply to the vestibular sense organs of the cat. The dark area indicates the location of large-caliber neurons supplying the cristae of the superior vestibular division. SCA, HCA, and PCA, superior, horizontal, and posterior canal ampullae, respectively; Utr, utricle; Sacc, saccule; SG, Scarpa's ganglion; Sacc N, saccular nerve; OCB, olivocochlear bundle; Utric N, utricular nerve; PCN, posterior canal nerve.

associated with both the inferior and the superior vestibular divisions, they gather together as they course central to the ganglion and project their axons in the rostral one-half of the vestibular nerve as it enters the brainstem. Conversely, the neurons supplying both the utricular and the saccular maculae converge into the caudal half of the vestibular nerve before entering the brainstem (8). It is probable that this rearrangement of first-order neurons from the diversely located sense organs correlates with a difference of termination in the brainstem vestibular nuclei.

It has been demonstrated that vestibular neurons have a wide spectrum of fibers, including a large population of smaller-sized nerve fibers and a smaller population of very large caliber fibers (10). In the peripheral ampullary nerves, the arrangement of these two types of nerve fibers is characteristic, with the large fibers located in the center of the nerve and smaller ones located at the periphery (Figure 5). Undoubtedly, this arrangement in the nerve branch is a reflection of the peripheral termination of these fibers, the large fibers supplying the Type I hair cells at the crest of the sense organ and the smaller fibers richly supplying the Type II cells at the slopes. In the superior vestibular division, the large fibers from the lateral and superior cristae come together as they reach the ganglion and travel in the most rostral and ventral portion of the vestibular nerve at the root entry zone (Figures 4 and 6). Smaller fibers

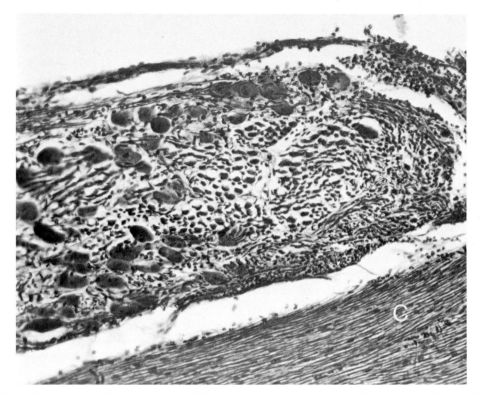

Figure 5. Protargol silver preparation of the posterior canal nerve of the cat demonstrating the central location of large axons with smaller axons at the periphery. C, cochlear nerve.

from these sense organs are located slightly caudal and dorsal to the large fibers at this point. The small- and large-fiber components supplying the utricular and saccular maculae occur as large fibers scattered among the small ones both in the peripheral branches and the vestibular nerve trunk.

Functional studies have shown that the spontaneous electrical activity in the large and small fibers is different, the large fibers showing an irregular discharge pattern and the small fibers, a regular discharge pattern (4,11,29). It is possible that these patterns relate to the morphology of the nerve terminals at the hair cell level. These functional and morphological descriptions present strong evidence that two types of functional units exist within the vestibular sense organs. The significance of this difference, however, is not known. A third, or intermediate, type of nerve discharge pattern has also been described but occurs infrequently. Intermediate types of hair cell innervation are also infrequently seen and may constitute a third functional unit.

The vestibular nerve fibers are spontaneously active, with discharge rates ranging from 10 or fewer spikes per second to over 100 spikes per second. The mean spontaneous discharge rates in the nerves supplying the cristae are somewhat higher than in those supplying the maculae (cristae, 90 spikes per second; maculae, 60 spikes per second) (4,11). This spontaneous discharge in the vestibular nerve fibers allows for a bidirectional change in their mean firing rate, depending on the deflection of the hair cell cilia in the sense organ.

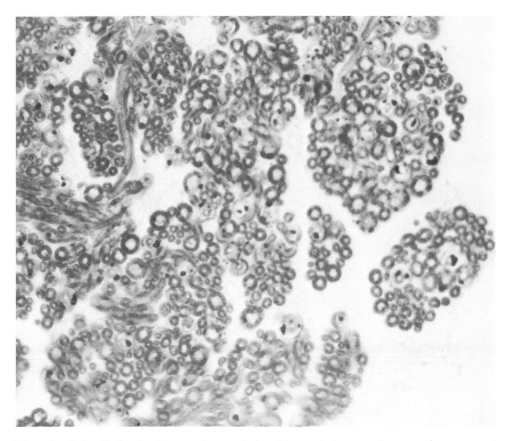

Figure 6. Sudan black stain of axons at the rostral edge of the vestibular nerve showing a concentration of large axons with a transition to smaller axons at the left.

VESTIBULAR NUCLEI

The incoming first-order vestibular neurons terminate in all four major vestibular nuclei and in three minor ones. The main vestibular nuclei are called the superior, lateral, medial, and descending; the minor vestibular nuclei receiving peripheral input are groups Y and L (Brodal) and the interstitial nucleus of the vestibular nerve (Figures 7, 8, and 9). It has been shown that all regions of the four vestibular nuclei, except for the dorsal part of the lateral nucleus, receive input from the vestibular nerve. However, the two types of sense organ project differentially in the vestibular nuclei, thus distinguishing the reflex projections activated by their stimulation. The first-order neurons supplying the cristae bifurcate upon entering the brainstem and terminate primarily in the superior vestibular nucleus and the rostral portion of the medial vestibular nucleus (Figure 10). A small collateral branch does leave the descending ramus to terminate in the ventral portion of the lateral vestibular nucleus. Rich collateral termination from the primary canal axons is present in the interstitial nucleus of the vestibular nerve. The ascending rami of canal afferents, after giving off terminals within the superior nucleus, continue onto the vestibular portion of the cerebellum, namely, the nodulus, the uvula, the flocculus, and the paraflocculus.

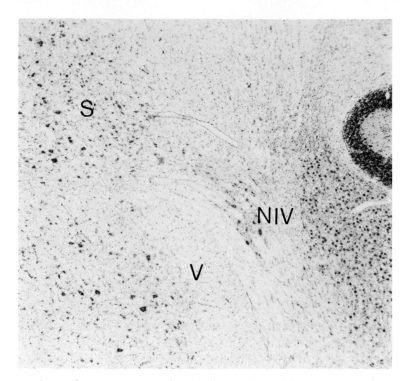

Figure 7.   Nissl-stained transverse section through the rostral part of the incoming vestibular nerve root where the interstitial nucleus (NIV) of the nerve is located. S, superior vestibular nucleus; V, descending trigeminal root.

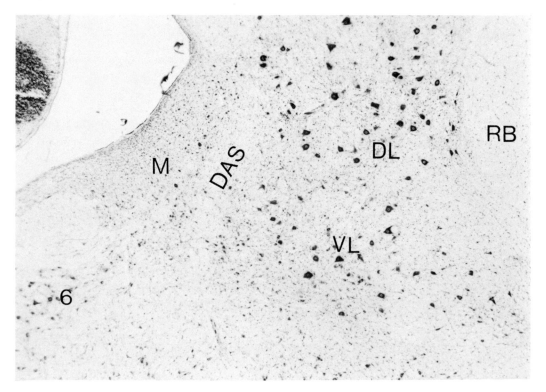

Figure 8.

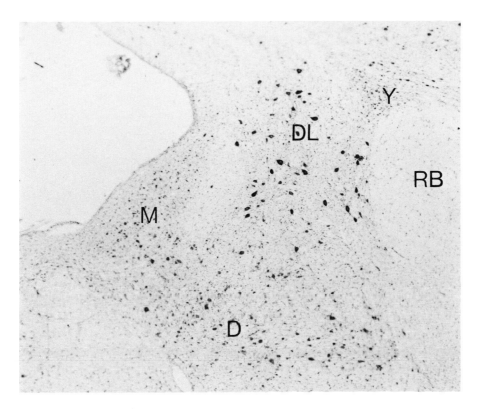

Figure 9. Transverse section through the caudal part of the lateral nucleus (DL) where the descending nucleus (D) begins. M, medial nucleus; Y, group Y nucleus; RB, restiform body.

Furthermore, there is a differential localization for the canal sense organs innervated by the superior vestibular division and the one innervated by the inferior vestibular division, that is, the posterior canal crista. This difference is emphasized in the superior vestibular nucleus and the interstitial nucleus of the vestibular nerve. In the superior nucleus, the posterior canal neurons terminate on large neurons located in the medial and caudal portion of the nucleus, whereas those neurons innervating the cristae of the superior division terminate rostrally and laterally. However, although these two groups of canal afferents end on different groups of second-order neurons, they also send off long collaterals that converge on neurons in the medial portion of the nucleus. Convergence of the canals of both divisions also can be seen in the rostral portion of the medial nucleus, particularly on the large and medium neurons.

On the basis of selective lesions involving superior division ganglion cells supplying large and small nerve fibers to the cristae, it seems that the large fibers terminate in central regions of the superior nucleus where the large vestibuloocular neurons predominate, whereas small fibers end peripherally where small neurons are concen-

Figure 8. Transverse section through the middle of the vestibular nuclei demonstrating the large multipolar neurons of the dorsal (DL) and ventral (VL) divisions of the lateral vestibular nucleus. The rostral extension of the medial nucleus (M) has medium and small cells. RB, restiform body; DAS, dorsal acoustic stria.

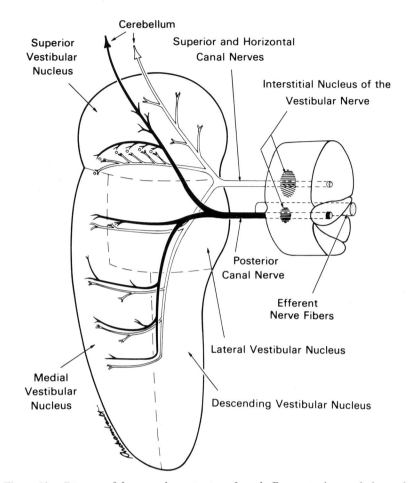

Figure 10.   Diagram of the central termination of canal afferents in the vestibular nuclei.

trated. This differential location of large and small fibers adds more data to the concept of separate units from the two types of hair cells conveying different information.

The macula of the utricle provides input primarily to the ventral portion of the lateral vestibular nucleus and the adjacent rostral part of the medial nucleus (Figure 11). Its descending ramus terminates more caudally in the medial and descending vestibular nuclei, where canal afferents are also known to terminate. This represents an area of convergence between the canals and the maculae of the utricle and saccule. First-order macular afferents do not terminate in the cerebellum or in the interstitial nucleus of the vestibular nerve. Saccular afferents are much fewer in number than are the utricular afferents, but they also end in the ventral portion of the lateral vestibular nucleus and in the medial and descending vestibular nuclei. They are differentiated from all of the sense organs by their termination in the group Y nucleus, which is located between the restiform body and the dorsal half of the lateral nucleus (Figure 9). Although the macular afferents do not terminate directly in the vestibulocerebellum as the canals do, their activity can be projected to the cerebellum polysynaptically over the second-order neurons in the medial and descending nuclei or the reticular formation.

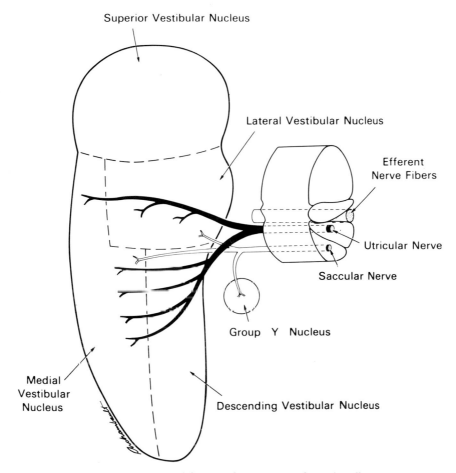

Figure 11. Diagram of the central termination of macular afferents.

Four types of second-order vestibular neurons have been described in the vestibular nuclei (2,22). Type I neurons are the most numerous, comprising approximately 80 or 90% of the active second-order neurons. Type I neurons are those that respond the same directionally as first-order afferents. Type II neurons exhibit an opposite directional response and are next in number. Type III and IV neurons show increased and decreased activity during rotation in both directions. The vast majority of Type I and II second-order neurons are located in the rostral portion of the medial vestibular nucleus and the superior nucleus. These two nuclei receive the bulk of the first-order input.

In addition to primary termination in the vestibulocerebellum by canal afferents, first-order termination to extranuclear areas includes that to the reticular formation to a very small degree, and to the ipsilateral abducens nucleus. It is possible that the first-order ganglion cells projecting to the abducens nucleus represent those afferents supplying the utricular macula.

CEREBELLAR AND COMMISSURAL PROJECTIONS

The cerebellovestibular and commissural projections can be regarded as efferent projections of the vestibular nuclei that modify or influence the activity of the vestibular nuclei themselves. These two projections do not directly result in activation of an effector organ, that is, a muscle which brings about stabilization of the body's orientation.

CEREBELLOVESTIBULAR CONNECTIONS

Connections between the cerebellum and the vestibular nuclei are very prominent. The magnitude of this prominence emphasizes the influence that the cerebellum has on vestibular nuclear activity. All four major vestibular nuclei, especially the medial and the descending, project second-order neurons to the anterior and posterior lobes of the vermis and to the vestibulocerebellum. We have already mentioned that the labyrinth projects to the vestibular part of the cerebellum by way of first-order afferents from the canals, over second-order neurons in the caudal vestibular nuclei, and over the reticular formation. Reciprocating cerebellovestibular projections terminate in all four vestibular nuclei as well. The major part of this activity represents that of the Purkinje cells in both the vestibulocerebellar cortex and the vermis. This activity is inhibitory and modifies the vestibular nuclear activity, which gives rise to effector reflexes (15). Input to the ventral half of the lateral nucleus and to the medial and descending nuclei also arrives by way of the deep cerebellar nuclei, particularly the fastigial. This relay through the fastigial nucleus orginates in the vermal cortex and has an excitatory effect on the vestibular nuclei. Clearly, cerebellar connections with the vestibular nuclei are important for the smooth and efficient activation of vestibular reflexes.

COMMISSURAL PROJECTIONS

Commissural projections are also quite prominent and have been shown by means of retrograde tracer techniques to be located primarily in the superior and medial vestibular nuclei (Figure 12). In these nuclei, the commissural projections are formed by small neurons that populate the nuclei (Figures 7 and 8). Larger neurons in the medial and superior vestibular nuclei are characteristically those that project to extraocular muscle neurons. A smaller commissural projection also extends from the descending vestibular nucleus, and a small but consistent commissural projection arises from the group Y nucleus. The action of the commissural projections is almost without exception inhibitory and is activated mainly by canal input (23). Except for the saccular group Y projection, it does not appear to be activated by macular input. The significance of commissural inhibitory activity may be that it potentiates the inhibition of the contralateral complementary canal when the ipsilateral canal is excited. Therefore, the opposite polarization of hair cells in complementary canals as

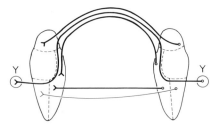

Figure 12.   Diagram summarizing commissural vestibular projections. Y, group Y nucleus.

well as commissural inhibition may be responsible for the differential electrical response when stimulation in a given plane of rotation occurs. Since the maculae have an opposite polarization of hair cells in the two halves of the sense organ, commissural projections may not be necessary to produce the differential effect from sense organ activation.

VESTIBULOSPINAL PROJECTIONS

Vestibulospinal projections and reflexes are among the most important activities of the vestibular system. Vestibulospinal projections can be divided into the lateral vestibulospinal tract (LVST) and the medial vestibulospinal tract (MVST). The LVST is an entirely ipsilateral projection that originates solely from the neurons of the lateral vestibular nucleus (Figure 13). The dorsal division of the lateral vestibular nucleus (which has a closer relationship to the cerebellum since it receives direct Purkinje cell input, whereas the ventral division does not) gives rise to the LVST projecting to the lower part of the spinal cord (33). This projection ends at the lumbar and sacral levels of the cord, where it terminates either directly or by way of interneurons on anterior horn cells and supplies limb muscles primarily. The ventral half of the lateral vestibular nucleus projects through the LVST to cervical and thoracic levels, where again the anterior horn cells to upper limb muscles are supplied. The activity of the LVST is excitatory. It activates extensor muscles and inhibits flexors in the limbs. It should be noted that the lateral vestibular nucleus, which gives rise to this tract, is activated by input from the proprioceptive impulses in the somatosensory system. These inputs from joints, muscle tendons, etc., arrive via spinal vestibular tracts. The peripheral input to the ventral part of the lateral nucleus is from all the sense organs, but particularly from the utricular and saccular maculae (Figures 14 and

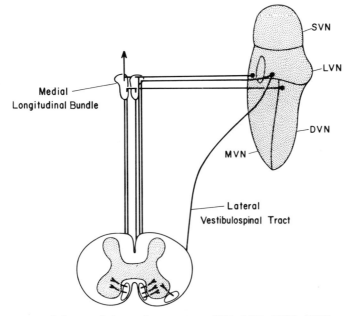

Figure 13. Diagram of the vestibulospinal projections. SVN, LVN, DVN, MVN, superior, lateral, descending, and medial vestibular nucleus, respectively.

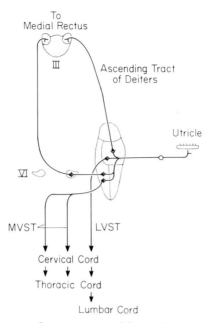

Figure 14. Diagram summarizing reflex connections of the utricle. MVST, medial vestibulospinal tract; LVST, lateral vestibulospinal tract.

15, respectively). Therefore, the LVST to the cervical and thoracic level upper limb musculature is activated by these sense organs.

The MVST is shorter and projects bilaterally by way of the medial longitudinal fasciculus (MLF) to the cervical and upper thoracic cord levels. The MVST originates from the medial, lateral, and descending vestibular nuclei (33). The action of this

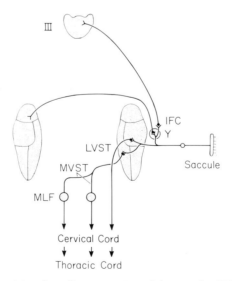

Figure 15. Diagram summarizing the reflex connection of the saccule. IFC, infracerebellar nucleus; LVST, lateral vestibulospinal tract; MVST, medial vestibulospinal tract; MLF, medial longitudinal fasciculus.

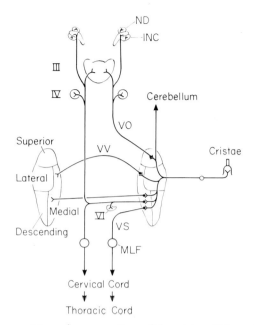

Figure 16. Diagram summarizing reflex connections of the cristae. ND, nucleus of Darkeschewitsch; INC, interstitial nucleus of Cajal; VO, vestibuloocular; VV, commissural; VS, vestibulospinal; MLF, medial longitudinal fasciculus.

tract is both excitatory and inhibitory. Its peripheral input is largely from the canals and to a lesser extent from the utricle.

Clearly, the vestibulospinal tracts arising from the caudal levels of the vestibular nuclei are primarily activated by gravity receptors, that is, the utricle and saccule. Nevertheless, cervical reflexes, in particular, are also initiated by the canals because of their connections in the caudal levels of the vestibular nuclear complex (Figure 16).

Vestibuloocular Reflexes

By means of both anterograde degeneration techniques (26) and retrograde tracer methods, the vestibuloocular second-order neurons have been located in the superior and medial vestibular nuclei, in the ventral portion of the lateral vestibular nucleus, in a portion of the group Y nucleus, and even from first-order vestibular neurons probably supplying the utricle. The projection pathways of these vestibuloocular neurons are the MLF, the ascending tract of Deiters, the reticular formation, and the brachium conjunctivum.

It may be useful to divide the vestibuloocular projections into those that bring about horizontal eye movements (in other words, those that activate the medial rectus and the lateral rectus muscles) and those that bring about vertical or oblique eye movements. The latter pathways innervate the remaining divisions of the oculomotor nucleus (that is, the superior rectus, inferior rectus, and inferior oblique) and the trochlear nucleus, which serves the superior oblique eye muscle.

The vestibuloocular neurons supplying vertical and oblique eye muscle motor neurons arise from the superior nucleus and rostral portions of the medial vestibular nucleus (Figure 17). They project in a parallel way, with the superior nucleus projecting ipsilaterally and the medial nucleus, contralaterally in the MLF. Their pro-

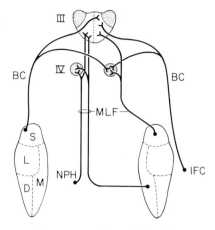

Figure 17. Diagram of location and projection of vestibuloocular neurons for vertical and oblique eye movements. BC, brachium conjunctivum; NPH, nucleus praepositus hypoglossi; MLF, medial longitudinal fasciculus; IFC, infracerebellar nucleus; S, L, M, D, superior, lateral, medial, and descending vestibular nucleus, respectively.

jections to the fourth and subgroups of the third nucleus are approximately equal and symmetric. Some neurons in the dorsal part of the superior nucleus project by way of the brachium conjunctivum to reach both the fourth and the third nuclei. Cells near the group Y nucleus (infracerebellar) also project to the fourth and subgroups of the third nuclei. Since the saccule projects to this nucleus, it provides a pathway for vertical eye movements from saccular activity (Figure 15). The vestibuloocular pathway arising from the superior nucleus is inhibitory, whereas that projecting contralaterally from the medial nucleus is excitatory (13,14). The opposite activities of these two parallel vestibuloocular pathways make possible a synchronized directional eye movement.

The vestibuloocular projections serving horizontal eye movements innervate the

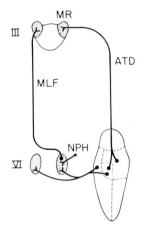

Figure 18. Diagram of vestibuloocular neurons for horizontal eye movements. MR, medial rectus subnucleus; ATD, ascending tract of Deiters; MLF, medial longitudinal fasciculus; NPH, nucleus praepositus hypoglossi.

lateral rectus and medial rectus motor neuron pools (Figure 18). It has been shown that the second-order neurons projecting to both the ipsilateral and contralateral abducens nuclei are located almost entirely within the medial vestibular nucleus, particularly in the portion adjacent to the dorsal acoustic stria. The excitation exerted on the ipsilateral abducens nucleus and inhibition on the contralateral abducens nucleus again provide evidence for reciprocal actions of the vestibuloocular system that result in synchronous movement. Some of these neurons projecting to the abducens nucleus, however, are located far enough rostrally that they can be reached by collaterals of afferents entering the superior nucleus. An interneuron in the abducens nucleus has also been demonstrated that projects contralaterally through the MLF to the medial rectus subnucleus, therefore connecting the lateral rectus and contralateral medial rectus motor neurons. Neurons in the medial nucleus adjacent to the part that contains the abducens vestibuloocular neurons, together with some second-order neurons in the ventral half of the lateral nucleus, give rise to the ascending tract of Deiters, which supplies the ipsilateral medial rectus subnucleus, providing it with an excitatory input. Therefore, the set of vestibuloocular projections to the abducens and medial rectus motor neurons can be activated by both utricular (Figure 14) and canal afferents (Figure 16)

Although vestibuloocular projections do occur through the reticular formation, the anatomy of this part of the vestibuloocular reflex has not been thoroughly documented.

In conjunction with ascending vestibuloocular pathways, it should be noted that definite descending projections from the oculomotor nucleus, particularly from the Edinger–Westphal component and from the third nerve nucleus itself, project caudally to the vestibular nuclei, especially the medial nucleus, where they may modify vestibular activity. The interstitial nucleus of Cajal located near the oculomotor nucleus has been shown by both anterograde and retrograde methods to project to the MLF in a descending direction. Other avenues of interface between the vestibular and visual systems occur through the cerebellum.

The vestibular cerebellum (flocculus, nodules, and uvula) plays an important role in the control of visual-vestibular reflexes and interactions. One of the most significant inputs to the cerebellum is mediated by climbing fibers arriving from the contralateral inferior olive. Another input consists of mossy fibers arriving from the brainstem reticular formation. Neural activity in Purkinje cells of the vestibular cerebellum is modulated by a range of visual or vestibular physiological stimulation. In the rabbit, with which most studies have been made, it has been shown that the visual information to the cerebellum is conveyed by neurons of the accessory optic tract, with relay in the tectum and midbrain. Cerebellar afferent signals are sent to the vestibular nuclei and reticular formation in the brainstem through Purkinje cell axons. Hence, vestibular nuclei neurons are influenced by both primary vestibular afferent inputs and visual signals. [For a review of the current status of the organization of these connections see Barmack (1).]

Efferent Vestibular Pathway

A detailed description of the efferent component of the vestibular nerve projecting to the vestibular sense organs is now available (Figure 19). The cells of origin of the efferent pathway are small neurons located immediately lateral to the abducens

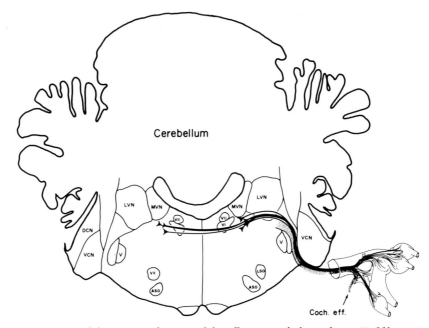

Figure 19. Diagram of the origin and course of the efferent vestibular pathway. V, fifth nerve; DCN, dorsal cochlear nucleus; VCN, ventral cochlear nucleus; MVN, medial vestibular nucleus; LVN, lateral vestibular nucleus; ASO, accessory superior olive; LSO, lateral superior olive.

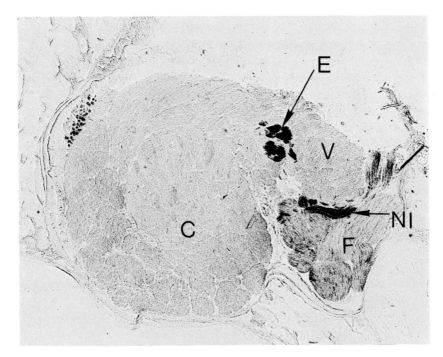

Figure 20. Transverse section of the facial (F), cochlear (C), and vestibular (V) nerves in the internal auditory canal showing the high acetylcholinesterase activity (E) in the efferent vestibular and cochlear bundles. NI, nervus intermedius.

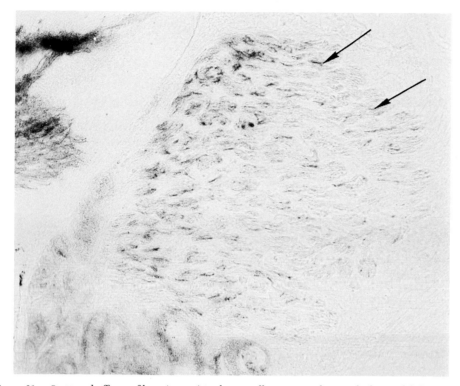

Figure 21. Scattered efferent fibers (arrows) in the ampullary nerves showing high acetylcholinesterase activity.

nucleus, where they can be contacted by either incoming first-order neurons or second-order vestibular neurons (9,30). Approximately 300 to 400 such efferent neurons are located in this region in the cat and are approximately evenly divided in their projections. In other words, they contribute approximately the same number of nerve fibers to the efferent component supplying one labyrinth. As they travel together with the efferent cochlear fibers in the vestibular nerve, they can be shown, either by histochemical staining methods (Figure 20) or by anatomical degeneration techniques, to be a rather compact bundle. These fibers branch both within the vestibular nerve trunks (Figure 21) and near the neuroepithelium. They terminate in all sense organs as small vesiculated endings on both Type I and Type II hair cells. However, their mode of termination on the two types of hair cells is different. The terminals contact the afferent endings on Type I hair cells and make direct contact with the hair cell membrane on Type II hair cells. It is possible that activation of this efferent component may produce different effects at the periphery. Depending on the species studied, the effect of excitation of the efferent component has been inhibition of the neural response (7,16,21), facilitation of the neural response (12), or both excitation and inhibition (3). It has been postulated (3) that these various affects are related to the morphology at the periphery, with the direct termination on Type II hair cells providing an excitatory mode and the contact on the ending supplying Type I hair cells inhibiting the action potentials that originate from these hair cells.

REFERENCES

1. Barmack, N. H., Immediate and sustained influences of visual olivocerebellar activity on eye movements. In: *Posture and Movement* (R. E. Talbot and D. R. Humphrey, eds.). Raven, New York, 1979:123–168.

2. Curthoys, I. S., and Markham, C. H., Convergence of labyrinthine influences on units in the vestibular nuclei of the cat. I. Natural stimulation. *Brain Res.*, 1971, **35**:469–490.

3. Dechesne, C., and Sans, A., Control of the vestibular nerve activity by the efferent system in the cat. *Acta Oto-Laryngol.*, 1980, **90**:82–85.

4. Estes, M. S., Blanks, R. H. I., and Markham, C. H., Physiologic characteristics of vestibular first-order canal neurons in the cat. I. Response plane determination and resting discharge characteristics. *J. Neurophysiol.*, 1975, **38**:1232–1249.

5. Fernandez, C., and Goldberg, J. M., Physiology of peripheral neurons innervating otolith organs of the squirrel monkey. I. Response to static tilts and to long-duration centrifugal force. *J. Neurophysiol.*, 1976, **39**:970–984.

6. Flock, A., Flock, B., and Murray, E., Studies on the sensory hairs of receptor cells in the inner ear. *Acta Oto-Laryngol.*, 1977, **83**:85–91.

7. Flock, A., and Russell, I. J., Inhibition by efferent nerve fibres: Action on haircells and afferent synaptic transmission in the lateral line canal organ of the burbot *Lota lota. J. Physiol. (London)*, 1976, **257**:45–62.

8. Gacek, R. R., The course and central termination of first order neurons supplying vestibular end organs in the cat. *Acta Oto-Laryngol., Suppl.*, 1969, **254**:1–66.

9. Gacek, R. R., and Lyon, M., Localisation of vestibular efferent neurons in the kitten with horseradish peroxidase. *Acta Oto-Laryngol.*, 1974, **77**:92–101.

10. Gacek, R. R., and Rasmussen, G. L., Fiber analysis of the stato-acoustic nerve of guinea pig, cat and monkey. *Anat. Rec.*, 1961, **139**:455–463.

11. Goldberg, J. M., and Fernández, C., Physiology of peripheral neurons innervating semi-circular canals of the squirrel monkey. I. Resting discharge and response to constant angular accelerations. *J. Neurophysiol.*, 1971, **34**:635–660.

12. Goldberg, J. M., and Fernández, C., Efferent vestibular system in the squirrel monkey. *Soc. Neurosci. Abstr.*, 1977, **3**:543, No. 1723.

13. Highstein, S. M., The organization of the vestibulo-oculomotor and trochlear reflex pathways in the rabbit. *Exp. Brain Res.*, 1973, **17**:285–300.

14. Ito, M., Inhibitory and excitatory relay neurons for the vestibuloocular reflexes. *Prog. Brain Res.* 1972, **37**:543–544.

15. Ito, M., and Yoshida, M., The origin of cerebellar-induced inhibition of Deiters' neurones. I. Monosynaptic initiation of the synaptic potentials. *Exp. Brain Res.*, 1966, **2**:330–349.

16. Klinke, R., and Schmidt, C. L., Efferent influence on the vestibular organ during active movements of the body. *Pfluegers Arch.* 1970, **318**:352–353.

17. Lindeman, H. H., Anatomy of the otolith organs. *Adv. Oto-Rhino-Laryngol.*, 1973, **20**:405–433.

18. Malcolm, R., A mechanism by which haircells of the inner ear transduce mechanical energy into a modulated train of action potentials. *J. Gen. Physiol.*, 1974, **63**:757–772.

19. McLaren, J. W., and Hillman, D. E., Displacement of the semicircular canal cupula during sinusoidal rotation. *Soc. Neurosci. Abstr.*, 1977, **3**:544, No. 1730.

20. Rasmussen, A. T., Studies of the eighth cranial nerve of man. *Laryngoscope*, 1940, **50**:67–83.

21. Sala, O., The efferent vestibular system. Electrophysiological research. *Acta Oto-Laryngol., Suppl.*, 1965, **197**:1–34.

22. Shimazu, H., and Precht, W., Tonic and kinetic responses of cat's vestibular neurons to horizontal angular acceleration. *J. Neurophysiol.*, 1965, **28**:989–1013.

23. Shimazu, H., and Precht, W., Inhibition of central vestibular neurons from the contralateral labyrinth and its mediating pathway. *J. Neurophysiol.*, 1966, **29**:467–492.

24. Spoendlin, H. H., Ultrastructural studies of the labyrinth in squirrel monkeys. *NASA [Spec. Publ.] SP*, 1965, **NASA SP-77**:7–22.

25. Spoendlin, H. H., The ultrastructure of the vestibular sense organ. In: *The Vestibular System and Its Diseases* (R. J. Wolfson, ed.). Univ. of Pennsylvania Press, Philadelphia, 1966:39–68.

26. Tarlov, E., Organization of vestibulo-oculomotor connections in the cat. *Brain Res.*, 1970, **20**:159–179.

27. Trincker, D., Electrophysiological studies of the labyrinth of the guinea pig. *Ann. Otol., Rhinol., Laryngol.*, 1959, **68**:145–152.

28. Trincker, D., The transformation of mechanical stimulus into nervous excitation by the labyrinthine receptors. *Symp. Soc. Exp. Biol.*, 1962, **16**:289–316.

29. Walsh, B. T., Miller, J. B., Gacek, R. R., and Kiang, N. Y. S., Spontaneous activity in the eighth cranial nerve of the cat. *Int. J. Neurosci.*, 1972, **3**:221–236.

30. Warr, W. B., Olivocochlear and vestibular efferent neurons of the feline brainstem; their location, morphology and number determined by retrograde axonal transport and acetylcholinesterase histochemistry. *J. Comp. Neurol.*, 1975, **161**:159–182.

31. Wersäll, J., Studies on the structure and innervation of the sensory epithelium of the cristae ampullares in the guinea pig. A light and electron-microscopic investigation. *Acta Oto-Laryngol., Suppl.*, 1956, **126**:1–85.

32. Wersäll, J., Flock, A., and Lundquist, P. G., Structural basis for directional sensitivity in cochlear and vestibular sensory receptors. *Cold Spring Harbor Symp. Quant. Biol.*, 1965, **30**:115–132.

33. Wilson, V. J., Wylie, R. M., and Marco, L. A., Projection to the spinal cord from the medial and descending vestibular nuclei of the cat. *Nature (London)*, 1976, **215**:429–430.

Techniques of Anatomical Localization

VICTOR GOODHILL

Division of Head and Neck Surgery (Otology)
School of Medicine, University of California Los Angeles
Los Angeles, California

INTRODUCTION

The role of the otologist in localizing vestibular pathology involves careful listening to and examination of the patient. The first physician who sees a "dizzy" patient is usually neither an otologist nor a neurologist. Regardless of his or her specialty, the primary physician who accepts the responsibility of examining the patient must have a broad view of the entire spectrum of the potential lesions and their anatomical locations involved in the complex clinical term "dizziness."

TERMINOLOGY

"Dizziness" is one of the most common symptoms in medicine. Such terms as "giddiness," "motion sickness," "imbalance," "wooziness," "faintness," and "passing out" frequently are loosely equated with disorders of equilibrium. Thus, the word "dizziness" may be used to describe cortical or visual disorientations, altered states of consciousness, and limb incoordination in addition to equilibrium disorders.

I use three conceptual terms for "dizziness": vertigo, dysequilibrium, and motion sickness. These can be defined arbitrarily as follows. The term *vertigo* describes symptoms arising from the vestibular (equilibrium) system, i.e., disorders in the peripheral labyrinth, disorders in the retrolabyrinth, and/or central nervous system (CNS) vestibular system disorders. The term *dysequilibrium* describes symptoms of spatial disorientations. It includes ataxia (CNS limb incoordinations). The term *motion sickness* refers to the vestibular, proprioceptive, and visual systems and can be considered a maladaptation syndrome related to motion.

VERTIGO

"Vertigo" denotes specific illusions of motion, such as sensations of turning or falling, that result from asymmetric neuronal firing patterns between the right and left vestibular systems. Nystagmus is the accompanying involuntary eye movement

NYSTAGMUS AND VERTIGO: CLINICAL
APPROACHES TO THE PATIENT WITH DIZZINESS

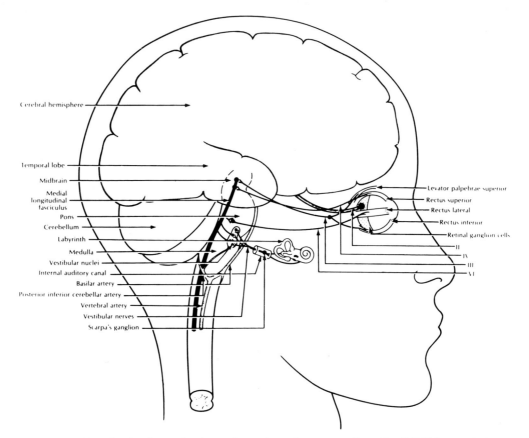

Figure 1.   Peripheral and central pathways for vertigo and nystagmus. From Goodhill (7) by permission.

that is the major subject of this volume. Vertigo and nystagmus can be produced either by peripheral (labyrinthine) or by CNS disorders of the vestibular system and occasionally by combined lesions (Figure 1).

Peripheral Vertigo

Peripheral vertigo is due to either intralabyrinthine or extralabyrinthine lesions. Both types of lesion may involve either cochlear and vestibular sense organs (cochleovestibular) or vestibular sense organs alone.

Cochleovestibular disorders usually produce auditory symptoms and findings (hearing loss and tinnitus), as well as vestibular symptoms and findings (vertigo and nystagmus). Cochleovestibular lesions occur in the labyrinth, in the internal auditory canal and the internal auditory meatus, or in the cerebellopontine angle (Table 1).

Vestibular disorders produce only vertigo and nystagmus and can occur in the labyrinth, in the eighth nerve (auditory-vestibular nerve) throughout its internal auditory canal and internal auditory meatus, or in the cerebellopontine angle.

Because the seventh nerve (facial nerve) accompanies the eighth nerve throughout its internal auditory canal course from the temporal bone petrosa through the internal auditory meatus to the cerebellopontine angle, and since the seventh nerve courses through the temporal bone into the neck, seventh nerve symptoms and findings may

TABLE 1
COCHLEOVESTIBULAR DISORDERS THAT PRODUCE HEARING LOSS, TINNITUS, VERTIGO, AND NYSTAGMUS

Intralabyrinthine
    Ménière's disease
    Otosclerosis and sequelae of otosclerosis surgery
    Otomastoiditis with complications including labyrinthitis and labyrinthine fistula
    Heredity of acquired congenital or delayed cochleovestibular syndromes
    Trauma of middle ear, inner ear
    Osteodystrophies
    Viropathies
    Syphilis
    Ototoxic drugs
    Tumors
Extralabyrinthine
    Intracanalicular tumors and anomalies
    Cerebellopontine angle tumors and anomalies of blood vessels

accompany either intralabyrinthine or extralabyrinthine lesions, causing vertigo (Table 2).

Central Nervous System Vertigo and Nystagmus

Central nervous system vertigo and nystagmus come from lesions in the four vestibular nuclei in the brainstem or from midbrain, cerebellum, and higher CNS vestibular pathway lesions.

Both vascular lesions and nonvascular lesions in the CNS produce vertigo, nystagmus, occasionally hearing loss, and occasionally tinnitus. The types of lesions that may produce CNS vertigo and nystagmus are listed in Table 3.

IMPORTANCE OF HISTORY IN LOCALIZATION

The history is crucial in anatomical localization. Therefore, I use a questionnaire dealing with the chronology of the dizziness, its general patterns, hearing loss, tinnitus, specific ear diseases, specific ocular questions, and a number of CNS ataxia and dysequilibrium questions (see Table 4).

GENERAL MEDICAL EXAMINATION OF THE DIZZY PATIENT

A patient who complains of dizziness requires a careful general medical examination. It may seem simplistic to state that a patient complaining of dizziness should not be approached primarily as an individual having an otological, ophthalmological, or neurological problem. However, such approaches are frequently taken, leading to

TABLE 2
VESTIBULAR DISORDERS THAT PRODUCE VERTIGO AND NYSTAGMUS ONLY

Intralabyrinthine
    Motion sickness, congenital vestibular end organ asymmetry associated with sensory maladaptation
    Benign paroxysmal positional vertigo, otolithic vertigo
    Vestibular viral neuronitis
Extralabyrinthine (retrolabyrinthine)
    "Toxic" vestibular neuronitis

TABLE 3
LESIONS THAT PRODUCE VERTIGO

Vascular lesions
    Subclavian and other "steal" syndromes
    Cervical spondylosis
    Intermittent vertebral-basilar insufficiency
    Vertebral-basilar "migraine"
    Posterior inferior cerebellar artery syndromes
    Anterior inferior cerebellar artery syndromes
    Internal auditory vestibular branch syndromes
Degenerative, neoplastic, or traumatic lesions
    Multiple sclerosis
    Vertiginous epilepsy
    Cerebellar lesions (degeneration and tumors)
    Head injury

TABLE 4
DIZZINESS QUESTIONNAIRE

Chronology
    When did your dizziness start?
    Is your dizziness constant?
    If your dizziness comes in attacks, how often?
    Give dates (approximate) of most recent attacks.
    How long does an attack last?
    What kind of "warning" do you have before an attack?
    Are you free of dizziness between attacks?
    Does your dizziness start when you awaken in the morning?
    Do you get airsick or seasick?
    Do you get car sick, especially in the back seat?
    Did your dizziness come on after a severe flu?
    Did your dizziness follow a recent airplane trip?
    Did your dizziness follow swimming or diving or physical exertion?
General pattern
    When you have an attack, do you feel as if you are falling?
        To the right _____To the left _____.
        Forward _____Backward _____.
        Do you have nausea during an attack? Vomiting?
        What position provokes an attack?
        What do you think brings on an attack?
        When you are dizzy, must you support yourself when you are standing?
    Do you have a sensation of objects spinning or turning around you?
    Do you have a sensation that you are turning or spinning inside?
    Do you have "loss of balance" when walking?
    Do you know anything that will stop your dizziness? Or make it feel better? Or make it worse?
    Do you feel better if you sit or lie down when you become dizzy?
    Has there been any dizziness in any member of your family?
Hearing loss, tinnitus, or ear disease
    Do you have a draining ear?
    Have you ever had any kind of ear surgery?
    Do you have a feeling of stuffiness in your ears when you have a dizzy spell?
    Does your hearing seem to change at times?
    Do you have any buzzing, ringing, or hissing in either ear?
    Do you have any increase in ringing or buzzing before a dizzy attack? After a dizzy attack?
    Do you have a hearing loss in either ear?
    Do you have earaches?

TABLE 4 (*Continued*)

Ocular problems
   Do you ever have double vision?
   Do you have trouble walking in the dark?
   Do you have periods of blurred vision?
   Do you ever have spots before your eyes?
   Did you get new glasses recently?
CNS ataxia problems
   Do you ever have numbness of the face, arms, or legs?
   Do you have a weakness in your arms or legs?
   Do you have a feeling of clumsiness in your arms or legs?
   Do you drop books or dishes unintentionally?
   Do you have difficulty in speaking?
   Is it hard for you to get words out, even though you know what you want to say?
   Do you have difficulty with swallowing?
   Do you ever have any tingling around your mouth?
   Have you ever had a head injury? Were you unconscious?
Dysequilibrium
   When you are dizzy, are you light-headed?
   When you are dizzy, do you have a swimming sensation in the head?
   When you are dizzy, do you feel as if you are going to black out?
   When you are dizzy, do you lose consciousness?
   When you are dizzy, do you also have a headache?
   When you are dizzy, do you have a feeling of pressure in the head?
   When you are dizzy, do you feel faint?
   Do you get dizzy after overwork or exertion?
   Do you get dizzy when you are hungry?
   Do you have dizziness related to your menstrual cycle?
   Do you use the "pill" (oral contraceptive)?
   Do you get upset easily and cry easily?
   Have you been under great emotional stress?
   Do you smoke?
   Do you drink alcohol?
   What medications are you taking?
   Do you have high blood pressure? Low blood pressure?
   Are you anemic?
   Are you on thyroid medication?
   Do you feel dizzy when you turn over in bed or when you first get up out of bed?

incorrect diagnoses. Before the basic medical examination, a careful general medical history should be taken, and fundamental laboratory studies including urine, blood, chest x-rays, electrocardiogram, and other indicated procedures should be performed.

Positive findings, after the initial tests, indicate that the dizziness is a dysequilibrium caused by any one of a number of medical conditions, including postural hypotension, hyperventilation, arteriosclerosis, hypertension, hematological disorders, or metabolic problems.

OTOLOGICAL EXAMINATION OF THE DIZZY PATIENT

The basic otological examination includes basic ear, nose, and throat, audiometric, radiological, vestibular, and screening neurological examinations.

The ear examination is preceded by an examination of the nose, paranasal sinuses, pharynx, oral structures, and larynx. The neck is examined for masses and auscultated for bruits. The maxillas and mandible are palpated. A preliminary examination for ocular paralysis or manifest spontaneous nystagmus is made.

An examination of the postauricular area and auricle precedes otoscopic study. Adequate visualization of the external auditory canal and tympanic membrane may require preliminary careful removal of cerumen and epithelial debris, as well as laboratory studies of material from a discharging ear that should be examined by appropriate smears and cultures.

Examination of the tympanic membrane includes a careful search for perforations, especially small ones in the epitympanic area, granuloma, or tumors, evaluation of tympanic membrane mobility by pneumatic otoscopy, and observation of mobility following simple Valsalva inflation and air insufflation by politzerization. In the presence of a perforation, pneumatic compression may elicit a possible fistula response in terms of definitive nystagmus or atypical nystagmoid eye deviations, which may or may not be accompanied by a sudden sensation of vertigo and/or nausea. A positive fistula test with nystagmus or ocular deviation may occur with an intact tympanic membrane (12). In addition to classic otoscopic fistula test performance, we have recently combined the use of such a "Hennebert" sign while an electronystagmographic (ENG) tracing is being made. Compression and rarefaction of the canal with a pneumatic otoscope during ENG tracings may be accompanied by definitive changes in the tracing, indicating the possibility of a labyrinthine fistula. Similarly, we ask patients during the performance of Békésy audiometry to signal the audiologist if there is a sudden feeling of dizziness at a particular region of pitch.

CAUSES OF DIZZINESS

COCHLEOVESTIBULAR DISORDERS

Cochleovestibular disorders that usually produce auditory symptoms and findings (hearing loss and tinnitus), in addition to vestibular symptoms and findings (vertigo and nystagmus), may occur in the labyrinth (intralabyrinthine) or medial to the labyrinth (extralabyrinthine, retrolabyrinthine).

Intralabyrinthine Lesions

Ménière's Disease.   This is a very common cause of peripheral labyrinthine vertigo. It is an acquired deformation of the endolymphatic vestibular viscera that is accompanied by endolymphatic hydrops of the scala media and very frequently of the saccule, utricle, and semicircular canal systems. It is characterized by episodic attacks of vertigo, fluctuating cochlear hearing loss, and fluctuating tinnitus.

Otosclerosis and Complications of Otosclerosis Surgery.   These conditions may produce cochleovestibular syndromes comparable to those of Ménière's disease. In the early stage of otosclerosis, the two most common symptoms are tinnitus and slowly developing hearing loss. However, in some patients, vertigo is also present. Occasional vestibular abnormalities will be demonstrated on ENG examination. As the disease matures in time and in severity, vertigo usually disappears.

Fenestration surgery, the earliest for otosclerosis, is rarely performed now, but many postfenestration patients still require care. Since the procedure involves deliberate fistulization of the horizontal semicircular canal, operative cavity problems can produce vertigo and nystagmus.

The primary surgery for otosclerosis is now stapedectomy, which may be accompanied by preoperative and postoperative vertigo. In most instances, however, such vertigo is transitory. A persistent oval window fistula following otosclerosis surgery can result in positional vertigo. Delayed, sudden vertigo occurring at any time after otosclerosis surgery is almost always a sign of a labyrinthine fistula or a granuloma. This calls for consideration of immediate exploratory surgery since the retention of cochlear function may well depend on prompt surgical intervention.

Infrequently, a postoperative middle ear granuloma can form with vestibular extension and vertigo.

Otomastoiditis and Labyrinthine Complications. The following conditions may be involved:

1. Tubotympanitis. The acute tubotympanitis accompanying an upper respiratory infection usually causes only fullness and conductive hearing loss but can cause vertigo, probably due to vestibular response asymmetry. Such vertigo subsides promptly upon treatment of the eustachian tube blockade.

2. Secretory otitis media. This relatively common disease only occasionally produces mild vertigo.

3. Otitis perforata. Whether quiescent or draining, otitis perforata can cause vertigo as a result of the caloric effect of cool air on the exposed oval and round window regions. Such vertigo usually stops when the ear canal is occluded. If it persists, labyrinthitis must be considered.

4. Otomastoiditis and labyrinthitis. Labyrinthine vertigo can follow either acute or chronic otomastoiditis. Invasion of the labyrinth can occur directly through the oval or round windows, through erosion of the bony otic capsule of the semicircular canal, or via retrograde thrombophlebitis routes. Diffuse or circumscribed types of labyrinthitis can occur, with various vertiginous symptoms.

A labyrinthine fistula due to erosion of the bony capsule presents the characteristic findings of a positive fistula sign, an evoked nystagmus induced by pressure change as transmitted through the external auditory canal to the middle ear. It can be produced with positive or negative pneumatic pressures.

Congenital Cochleovestibular Syndromes (Hereditary or Acquired). A number of congenital (with birth), hereditary, or acquired cochleovestibular lesions can produce various degrees of hearing loss, tinnitus, and vertigo. The vertigo may be due to a tullio-like effect produced by high-level hearing aid amplification in some instances. Vertiginous episodes may be accompanied by spontaneous nystagmus and can occur sporadically without hearing aid use in both pediatric and adult cases. The vertigo, which may simulate Ménière's disease, is due either to progression of the endolabyrinthine lesion (e.g., hydrops, vascular occlusions, or hemorrhages) or to associated otitis media.

Trauma. The following are some significant examples of traumatic causations of dizziness:

1. Barotrauma. Airplane flight or underwater stresses produce labyrinthine symptoms. Nitrogen embolization caused by scuba diving produces auditory and vestibular labyrinthine symptoms that are usually temporary but occasionally permanent.

2. Labyrinthine membrane ruptures. Both implosive (aerodynamic) and explosive (hydrodynamic) ruptures due to cerebrospinal fluid pressure transmission and to intranasal forces constitute physically induced intralabyrinthine membrane ruptures (5,6,8–10). Hearing loss and vertigo may occur simultaneously or separately. The vertigo may be as severe as that seen in acute episodic Ménière's disease and accom-

panied by nausea, vomiting, and brisk manifest nystagmus. Spontaneous healing of membranes may occur with bed rest. In some instances, prompt surgical intervention and repair of an oval and/or round window fistula is effective in controlling the vertigo. Hearing improvements are variable.

3. Temporal bone fractures. In transverse fractures of the temporal bone, the labyrinth is usually involved (Figure 2). Severe vertigo with hearing loss is common. In milder injuries without fractures, labyrinthine "concussion" may occur with transitory and auditory vestibular symptoms.

4. Skull injuries. Various types of head injuries without fractures can produce labyrinthine window membrane ruptures with or without internal labyrinthine membrane damage and various symptoms of hearing loss, tinnitus, and vertigo.

5. Traumatic lesions through tympanic membrane. Tympanic membrane ruptures produced by self-inflicted manipulation of cotton-tipped wooden applicators, hairpins, and other foreign bodies, or trauma produce hearing loss and vertigo in many cases. The severity of the vertigo is related to the extent of middle ear and inner ear damage in addition to the tympanic membrane defect itself.

6. Acute acoustic trauma and chronic-noise-induced hearing loss. Gunfire close to the external auditory canal can cause major hearing loss, frequently accompanied by severe vertigo. Chronic-noise-induced hearing loss may occur as a result of either industrial or community environmental noise, and in some patients various degrees of vertigo may be present.

Labyrinthine Osteodystrophies and Granulomas. A number of granulomas and bony dystrophies can invade any portion of the temporal bone. Paget's disease,

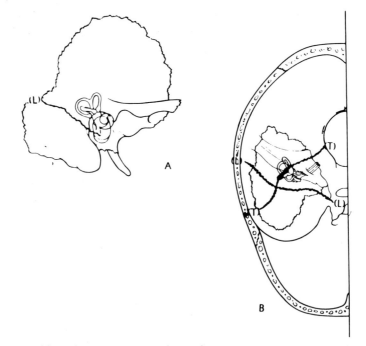

Figure 2. Temporal bone fractures. (A) Lateral view demonstrating course of longitudinal fracture (L). (B) View of skull base showing longitudinal (L) and transverse (T) fracture lines. From Goodhill (7) by permission.

histiocytosis X, osteogenesis imperfecta, and other granulomatous and osteolytic lesions involving the middle ear, labyrinthine windows, or the labyrinth itself can produce the triad of hearing loss, tinnitus, and vertigo. Acute vertigo is not common, but ENG responses to caloric tests may be abnormal.

Viropathies. Post-mumps labyrinthitis is the prototype of all other labyrinthine viropathies. Hearing loss, tinnitus, and vertigo in various degrees accompany minor and major viral invasions of the labyrinth.

A nonspecific "viral labyrinthitis" is frequently described clinically and is often confused with viral vestibular neuronitis or with benign paroxysmal positional vertigo. It is possible, however, that true viral "serous" labyrinthitis may accompany certain upper respiratory infections. There is scant histopathological confirmation for such a diagnosis. Clinically, however, episodic vertigo may occur in the course of a viral upper respiratory infection or shortly thereafter. Most commonly, the symptoms are confined to vertigo; hearing loss and tinnitus are relatively uncommon. It is quite likely that most of these "viral labyrinthitis" cases are probably not true labyrinthine lesions but represent inflammatory lesions related either to tubotympanic and asymmetric middle ear intratympanic pressures or to viral vestibular neuronitis.

Herpes zoster oticus (the Ramsay Hunt syndrome) is an intrapetrosal lesion involving a viropathy of the geniculate ganglion, its neural distribution, and its spread into neighboring auditory and vestibular nerve fibers. The usual symptoms of herpes zoster oticus are severe otalgia and seventh nerve paralysis. In addition, herpetic auricular and periauricular lesions, vertigo, hearing loss, and tinnitus can also be present.

Syphilis. Congenital and acquired syphilis continue to be problems and can produce vertigo with hearing loss and tinnitus similar to those seen in Ménière's disease (Figure 3). However, acute attacks are not common. Subacute dysequilibrium is more common. Bilateral peripheral vestibular end organ paralysis can be found on ENG studies in temporal bone syphilis, in spite of the fact that vertigo may be completely absent.

Drug Ototoxicity. A number of antibiotics, diuretics, and antioncological chemicals have ototoxic properties, frequently with accompanying renal sequelae. Aminoglycosides can act on vestibular and cochlear sensory cells. Toxicity is related to high concentration and long half-life in perilymph as compared with blood. The antibiotic drugs that may cause ototoxicity when given parentally include streptomycin, dihydrostreptomycin, gentamicin, neomycin, of the aminoglycoside group. Vancomycin, chemically similar to the aminoglycosides, viomycin, and capreomycin may be ototoxic. Vertigo may occur alone or accompany hearing loss and tinnitus.

Tumors. Tympanic glomus tumors usually produce pulsating tinnitus, hearing loss, occasional pain, and vertigo. An acute hemorrhage into a glomus tumor can be accompanied by sudden episodic vertigo (Figure 4). External and middle ear carcinoma produces vertigo in addition to otorrhea, pain, and hearing loss only if there is invasion of the labyrinthine windows or canal fistulization. Extralabyrinthine (internal auditory meatus) tumors, such as neurolemmoma (schwannoma) meningioma, cause hearing loss, but only occasionally does vertigo occur. The common "acoustic (eighth nerve) neurinoma" (vestibular schwannoma) produces vestibular findings but rarely produces severe vertigo. It can produce symptoms clinically similar to those of labyrinthitis or Ménière's disease.

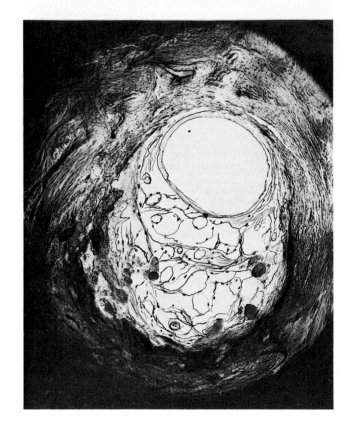

Figure 3. Medial limb of superior semicircular canal showing early fibrosis and bony irregularity of perilymphatic lumen. From Goodhill (4) by permission.

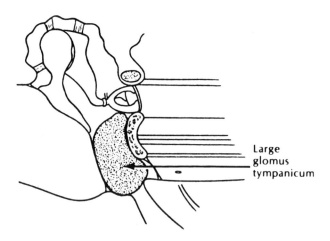

Large
glomus
tympanicum

Figure 4. Tympanic glomus. From Goodhill (7) by permission.

Extralabyrinthine Lesions

Intracanalicular Tumors and Anomalies. The most common intracanalicular eighth nerve tumor is the "acoustic neurinoma," which usually starts in the vestibular nerve within the internal auditory canal as a vestibular schwannoma. Because the tumor grows slowly, vertigo is not a common finding, although hearing loss and vertigo may both be present and may mimic Ménière's disease. Acute vertigo may be superimposed on a mild dysequilibrium with a sudden change in blood supply to the tumor. Similarly, vascular anomalies without tumors in the internal auditory meatus are responsible for episodic vertigo in some patients. Electronystagmographic findings usually demonstrate canal paresis.

Cerebellopontine Angle Tumors and Vascular Anomalies. Cerebellopontine angle (CPA) tumors (meningioma, congenital keratomas, neurilemmoma) and vascular anomalies produce both hearing loss and vertigo along with seventh, fifth, and other cranial nerve symptoms. Episodic severe vertigo is not a common symptom of CPA lesions. Vestibular asymmetry or canal paresis is noted upon ENG studies.

PERIPHERAL VESTIBULAR DISORDERS (VERTIGO AND NYSTAGMUS ONLY)

Intralabyrinthine Lesions

Motion Sickness: Congenital Vestibular End Organ Asymmetry. The term "motion sickness" is frequently used as a synonym for dizziness or vertigo, but it should be reserved for symptoms definitely related to motion. The most common varieties of motion sickness are seasickness, airsickness, and car sickness. Car sickness is usually increased when the passenger is not the driver and is in the back seat. In patients complaining of any one or all three of these types of motion sickness, spontaneous or positional nystagmus may occasionally be elicited. Vestibular asymmetry is frequently found on caloric studies. Hearing is usually normal. Asymmetric congenital vestibular responses are probably enhanced by constitutional or psychogenic factors. It may be a maladaptation syndrome.

Benign Paroxysmal Positional Vertigo: Otolithic Vertigo. Benign paroxysmal positional vertigo is paroxysmal vertigo that occurs only on positional change. The self-limited vertigo is unaccompanied by hearing loss or tinnitus. It has variously been attributed to labyrinthine anomalies or to metabolic or psychogenic problems.

Bárány drew attention to this type of positional vertigo in 1921 (1) when he described the symptoms of a 27-year-old woman, stating, "The attacks only appeared when she lay on her right side. When she did this there appeared a strong rotatory nystagmus to the right. The attack lasted about 30 seconds and was accompanied by violent vertigo and nausea. If immediately after the cessation of the symptoms the head was immediately turned to the right, no attack occurred, and in order to evoke a new attack in this way the patient had to lie for some time on her back or on her left side."

Thus, benign paroxysmal positional vertigo is characterized by the following syndrome. (a) The attack occurs when the patient assumes a supine position with the head turned so that the involved ear is undermost. (b) There is almost always a latent period, 5 or 6 sec, before the onset of symptoms. (c) The nystagmus is chiefly rotatory, the direction being toward the undermost ear.

Schuknecht (13,14) attributed benign paroxysmal positional vertigo to cupulolithiasis. Gacek (3) demonstrated temporal bone evidence of otolith displacement in severe cases of the vertigo. Degenerative otoliths from the utricular macula gravitate down and become embedded in the cupula of the posterior canal crista. Benign paroxysmal positional vertigo occurs at infrequent intervals in most patients, and in most instances the condition is self-limited. However, in some patients it is a handicapping vertigo lesion. In such cases Gacek (3) recommends surgical section of the posterior ampullary (singular) nerve by transsection via the round window niche.

In addition to the cupulolithiasis theory, it must be pointed out that benign paroxysmal positional vertigo accompanied by positional nystagmus can be something other than "benign." It is sometimes found in association with CNS lesions. Consequently, repetitive neurological studies should be considered in such cases.

Vestibular Viral Neuronitis. Dix and Hallpike (2) described the viral vestibular neuronitis syndrome. An acute lesion unaccompanied by hearing loss, it frequently occurs following a viral upper respiratory infection and is characterized by severe episodic vertigo with spontaneous nystagmus. Moderate or severe canal paresis can be found on ENG studies, and auditory tests usually show normal hearing.

The disease is usually self-limited. The episodic attacks decrease in frequency, and in most instances the symptoms disappear in 6 to 9 months. In some patients there is a return to normal caloric vestibular function following subsidence. The clinical picture closely resembles that of benign paroxysmal positional vertigo.

Morgenstein and Seung (11) described the histopathological changes in a case of vestibular neuronitis that showed degeneration of Scarpa's ganglion and its central and peripheral neurons, as well as semicircular canal and utricle changes.

A problem with the presumptive diagnosis of vestibular neuronitis is nonspecificity. The clinical findings may represent early signs of undetected labyrinthine or CNS lesions. Long-term follow-up is advisable.

Extralabyrinthine (Retrolabyrinthine) Lesions: "Toxic" Vestibular Neuronitis

Episodic vertigo without auditory symptoms, with variable caloric ENG findings, without the positional features of benign paroxysmal positional vertigo, and without a history of viral infection has been termed "toxic" vestibular neuronitis in some texts. This designation is purely a clinical concept that has not been confirmed by current neurootological studies.

SUMMARY

The otologist facing a dizzy patient who staggers into his examining room must consider systemic diseases as well as peripheral and central vestibular diseases. The details of vestibular testing, especially those involved in anatomical localization, form the substance of this volume.

REFERENCES

1. Bárány, R., Diagnose von Krankheitser-Scheinungen im Pereische des Otolithenapparates. *Acta Otolaryngol.*, 1971, **2**:434–437.
2. Dix, R., and Hallpike, C. S., The pathology, symptomatology and diagnosis of certain common disorders of the vestibular system. *Ann. Otol., Rhinol., Laryngol.*, 1952, **61**:987–1016.

3. Gacek, R. R., Transection of the posterior ampullary nerve for the relief of benign paroxysmal positional vertigo. *Ann. Otol., Rhinol., Laryngol.*, 1974, **83:**596–605.

4. Goodhill, V., Syphilis of the ear: A histopathologic study. *Ann. Otol., Rhinol., Laryngol.*, 1939, **48:**676–707.

5. Goodhill, V., Sudden deafness and round window rupture. *Laryngoscope*, 1971, **81:**1462–1474.

6. Goodhill, V., Labyrinthine membrane ruptures in sudden sensorineural hearing loss. *Proc. R. Soc. Med.*, 1976, **69:**565–572.

7. Goodhill, V., *Ear Diseases, Deafness and Dizziness.* Harper & Row, Hagerstown, Maryland, 1979.

8. Goodhill, V., The idiopathic group and the labyrinthine membrane rupture group approaches to sudden sensorineural hearing loss. In: *Controversy in Otolaryngology* (J. Snow, Ed.). Saunders, Philadelphia, Pennsylvania, 1980.

9. Goodhill, V., Traumatic fistulae. *J. Laryngol. Otol.*, 1980, **94:**123–128.

10. Goodhill, V., Harris, I., Brockman, S. J., and Hantz, I., Sudden deafness and labyrinthine window ruptures. *Ann. Otol., Rhinol., Laryngol.*, 1973, **82:**2–12.

11. Morgenstein, K. M., and Seung, H. I., Vestibular neuronitis. *Laryngoscope*, 1971. **81:**131–139.

12. Nadol, J. B., Positive fistula sign with an intact tympanic membrane. Clinical report of three cases and histopathological description of vestibulofibrosis as the probable cause. *Arch. Otolaryngol.*, 1974, **100:**273–278.

13. Schuknecht, H. F., Positional vertigo: Clinical and experimental observations. *Trans. Am. Acad. Ophthalmol. Otolaryngol.*, 1962, **66:**319–331.

14. Schuknecht, H. F., Cupulolithiasis. *Arch. Otolaryngol.*, 1969, **90:**765–778.

Radiology of Vestibular Disturbances

WILLIAM N. HANAFEE

Department of Radiological Sciences
School of Medicine, University of California Los Angeles
Los Angeles, California

The diagnosis of vestibular disturbances is best studied by clinical examination and physiological testing. Some specific areas of difficulties still require radiological techniques to rule out such diagnoses as acoustic neuroma, fistulas of the horizontal semicircular canal, miscellaneous tumors of the petrous apex and pontocerebellar angle, and some systemic bone diseases that can affect temporal bone. In this chapter we attempt to discuss these problems as concisely as possible. More details are available in the works of Vignaud (7), Valvassori (9), and others (2–6).

ACOUSTIC NEUROMA

The internal auditory canal (IAC) lies on the plane that is parallel to a piece of film placed behind the patient's head when the patient is in a supine position. A well-penetrated anteroposterior view taken at about 68 to 80 kV using one-tenth of a second and 100 mA usually produces diagnostic films of the IAC, provided that the canal is projected midway in the orbit. In approximately 40% of patients some air cells or overlapping bony structures may cause obscuration of a sufficient degree to prevent an absolute diagnosis from being made. Tomography of the IAC in the anteroposterior projection aids in resolving the diagnostic dilemma. One to 1.5 mm of difference in vertical height between the two IAC's at the level of the porus acousticus should be viewed with suspicion but can be within normal limits. Such a finding must be evaluated in the light of clinical examination. A difference of 2 mm or more is almost pathonomonic of an acoustic neuroma. One must remember that the IAC stops at the level of the posterior wall which delineates the porus acousticus. Measurements should not be made medial to the posterior wall since this is merely a groove on the posterior surface of the temporal bone and may give spurious impressions of constriction or dilatation. At times, lateral or axial projections can be used to good advantage to show the relationships of the anteroposterior walls of the IAC's. Computerized tomography (CT) in the axial projection also provides an alternative to conventional tomography, provided that bone window settings are used.

NYSTAGMUS AND VERTIGO: CLINICAL
APPROACHES TO THE PATIENT WITH DIZZINESS

In the past, pneumoencephalography and vertebral angiography played major roles in the diagnosis of acoustic neuroma. The current procedure of choice for directly visualizing acoustic neuroma is CT scanning. Intravenous contrast agents increase the reliability of CT diagnosis from approximately 50 to 90%, provided that the tumor mass bulges more than 1.5 cm into the pontocerebellar angle (1). More advanced scanners reduce the size of demonstrable tumors to 5 mm or less and in the future may even be able to demonstrate the smaller intracanalicular tumors (8).

At present, the diagnosis of intracanalicular tumors requires some type of intrathecally administered contrast agents. Metrizamide has been tried with limited success, but small amounts of air injected into the lumbar cistern and maneuvered into the IAC offer the most reliable technique. These procedures are followed if indicated by careful evaluation of symptoms and auditory and vestibular test results (Figure 1).

The technique for CT air studies of the pontocerebellar angle is as follows. On an outpatient basis and without premedication, the patient is taken to a conventional fluoroscopic room, where lumbar puncture is performed under fluoroscopic control. Approximately 5 cc of air is instilled into the lumbar cistern, and the patient is transferred on a gurney in the recumbent position. During all maneuvers the sus-

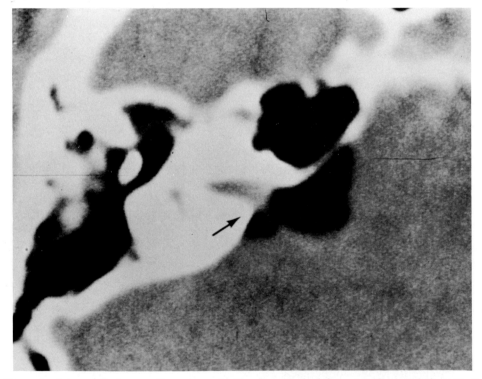

Figure 1. Intracanalicular acoustic neuroma. Looking down on the left temporal bone with the patient's face to the top of the page. Five cubic centimeters of air injected into the lumbar cistern has been maneuvered into the left pontocerebellar angle. Air outlines the porus acousticus, and a tumor mass can be seen arising from the internal auditory canal and bulging into the air shadow (→). The normal nerve proximal to the tumor within the angle is clearly seen.

pected temporal bone is kept uppermost in case any air leaks from the lumbar cistern. The needle is removed, and there is no hurry to complete the CT scanning since the air will remain in the lumbar cistern for "hours." When the scanner becomes available, the patient is tranferred from the gurney to the examining couch while the sagittal plane of the skull is kept approximately parallel to the floor. The patient is asked to rise up on the dependent elbow for a period of 3 to 5 min to allow the air to rise from the lumbar cistern into the intracranial cavity. The patient is then placed in a lateral recumbent position with the suspected side high into the head holder for scanning.

Scans are begun 1 cm above the external auditory canal and are taken proceeding caudad at 2-mm intervals until the entire IAC has been covered. The scans are viewed, and if there is any doubt regarding the presence of air in the IAC the 1-mm intervals between scans are taken and processed for viewing. By this overlapping technique, air can be identified within the IAC in most normal patients.

If additional information is required regarding the nerves, a computer maneuver

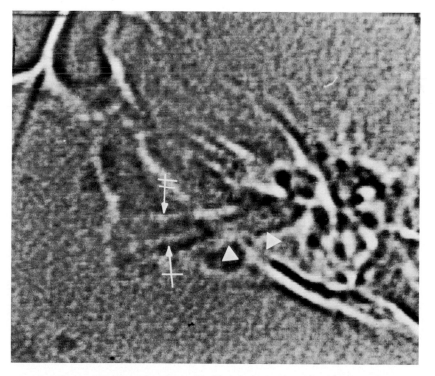

Figure 2. Normal internal auditory canal visualized by edge enhancement technique. The scan was taken while the patient was lying with the normal ear uppermost, but by convention the reader is viewing the scan with the patient's face to the top of the page and looking down on top of the temporal bone. Four cubic centimeters of air is present in the pontocerebellar angle. The most anterior structure in the angle is the auditory artery (↦) entering the internal auditory canal. Slightly more posterior is the facial nerve (↔), which can be seen as a separate structure in the pontocerebellar angle, but it joins the eighth nerve (▶) in the internal auditory canal. In the lateral portion of the internal auditory canal, the cochlear nerve can be seen to separate and enter the modiolus nucleus.

can be performed to create contrast enhancement of the nerves within the canal. Edges are enhanced by mathematically taking the second derivative of the raw data after digitalizing the data by the CT scanner. The procedure is performed by taking the original scan and using a "coarse filter" within the computer. This means that the computer will average adjacent pictures to develop a "fuzzy" image. The densities of the fuzzy image are reversed by the computer, and the two images (the fuzzy and the original) are added, thus giving a great reduction in the gray scale but good edge enhancement. This technique is similar to an old photographic technique of edge enhancement called "unsharp masking." The resultant image is noisy, but by the proper selection of gray scale and edge enhancement the eighth and seventh nerves can be traced through the pontocerebellar cistern and visualized within the IAC (Figure 2). In most cases the bifurcation of the eighth nerve into its cochlear and vestibular components can be seen in the lateral portion of the canal.

Acoustic neuromas are seen by the air technique as rounded masses within the pontocerebellar angle or within the IAC. Air does not pass laterally to an intracanalicular neuroma.

Complications occur when air is injected into the subdural space and will not pass intracranially or when a mistake has been made and the patient comes for an air study with a very large acoustic neuroma. Performing a lumbar puncture on a patient with increased intracranial pressure and a large posterior fossa mass can be hazardous because of brain shifts and herniations. All suspected patients should be screened by conventional CT with intravenous contrast and neurological evaluation.

Semicircular Canal Fistula

Fistula may be related to cholesteatoma, trauma, or extensions of tumors. Most diagnostic problems arise from fistula of the horizontal semicircular canal due to cholesteatoma. The other lesions are usually readily demonstrated on pluridirectional tomography or even routine views.

Cholesteatomas cause bony sclerotic reactions and increased densities within the middle ear cavity and epitympanic recess that partially obscure the bony coverings of the semicircular canals. A factor in diagnosis is a basic law of the physics of tomography called the "law of tangents." This principle states that an x-ray beam must pass tangent to a cortical surface sometime during the sweep of the x-ray tube and film in order to be visualized (10). The anterolateral margin of the horizontal semicircular canal is so situated that it cannot be seen with a high degree of certainty in the anteroposterior, Guillen, or lateral projection. The base projection (axial projection; terminology used in CT) is the best view to see the lateral wall of the horizontal semicircular canal (4). Computerized tomography is extremely sensitive to the calcium content of tissues so that this modality will undoubtedly play the major role in

Figure 3. (A) Horizontal semicircular canal and middle ear cavity. Looking down on top of the right temporal bone with the patient's face to the top of the page and external ear to the right of the page. The internal auditory canal (IAC) is seen to open through the posterior surface of the temporal bone. The horizontal semicircular canal (HSC) is viewed from above, and a thick cortical margin is present all along this lateral border. The epitympanic recess (small arrowhead) contains the head of the malleus and body of the incus. The epitympanic recess communicates by the additus ad antrum to the posteriorly placed mastoid antrum (large arrowhead) and the surrounding periantral air cells. (B) Cholesteatoma destroying the additus ad antrum and causing demineralization of the lateral wall of the horizontal semicircular canal (→). There is still some covering over the horizontal semicircular canal, but the bone has become demineralized.

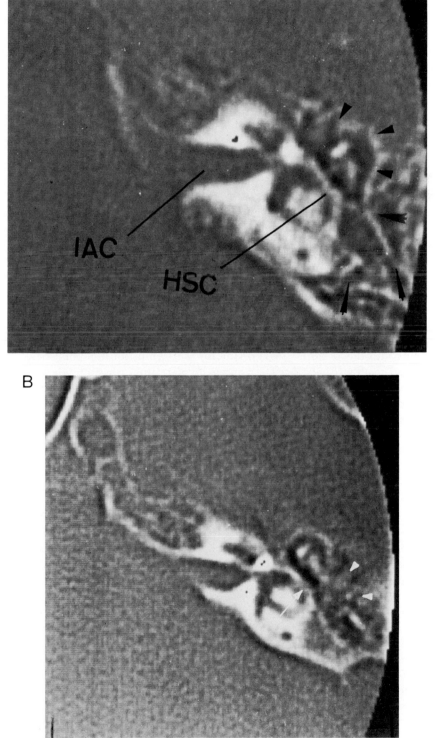

Figure 3

the diagnosis of horizontal semicircular canal fistula. The same techniques described in the section on acoustic neuroma are used for the CT examination and demonstration of horizontal semicircular canal fistula. The scans should be obtained at 1-mm intervals and edge enhancement techniques performed for accurate delineation of the thin bony covering of the horizontal semicircular canal. At times, osteitis with demineralization may be present. The osteitis may cause loss of mineral or a surrounding area of sclerosis. Regardless of the total reaction, CT can demonstrate the true status of the otic capsule overlying the horizontal semicircular canal (Figure 3).

Miscellaneous Tumors

Primary cholesteatomas, metastases to the temporal bone, squamous cell carcinomas of the middle ear, and meningiomas of the geniculate ganglion are but a few of the lesions that affect the adult temporal bone. In children, histiocytosis and rhabdomyosarcomas may produce destructive or productive lesions within the temporal bone. All require extensive plain film and tomographic examinations to demonstrate the extent of their destruction or bony expansions. The primary cholesteatomas may be in the middle ear or near the petrous apex. Bone expansion and widespread destruction are the clues to diagnosis (Figure 4).

Although a rare cause of vertigo, glomus tumors of either the jugular fossa or tympanic region offer an opportunity for definitive diagnosis by CT scanning. These lesions should be examined with and without intravenous contrast enhancement. Because of their very vascular nature they stain intensely on CT scanning, and any extensions into the posterior fossa or inferior surface of the temporal bone can be determined readily (Figure 5). The glomus jugulare tumor has a tendency to follow blood vessels either intracranially or into the neck around the internal jugular vein. If the tumor has spread intracranially, it may pass laterally along the sigmoid sinus to the region of the transverse sinus or medially in the groove between the petrous apex and clivus to follow the inferior petrosal sinus. Erosions into the otic capsule are unusual and are found only in more aggressive lesions.

Pontocerebellar Angle Tumors Other Than Acoustic Tumors

In addition to the intracranial extensions of glomus tumors, one may encounter meningiomas, epidermoid tumors, metastatic tumors, or lobular extensions of pontine gliomas into the pontocerebellar angle. Computerized tomography, with or without intravenous contrast enhancement, plays the major role in differntial diagnosis. Briefly, some things to be considered are as follows. Meningiomas are usually dense even before intravenous contrast enhancement due to the presence of psamonian bodies and their intense vascularity. These lesions also show enhancment with intravenous contrast agents to confirm the diagnosis.

By their fatty nature, epidermoid tumors tend to be low in density, although isodensity epidermoids have been reported. These lesions usually show enhancement around their periphery and are very poorly circumscribed on CT scanning. If a tumor mass in the pontocerebellar angle has somewhat diffuse margins, is flattened against the posterior surface of the temporal bone, and has a low density center, it is almost certainly an epidermoid tumor.

Metastatic tumors and lobulated tumors of the pons may show staining surrounding areas of edema and mass effect on CT scanning. Their final diagnosis depends on complete neurological evaluation and a comparison of the CT findings with the patient's total clinical picture.

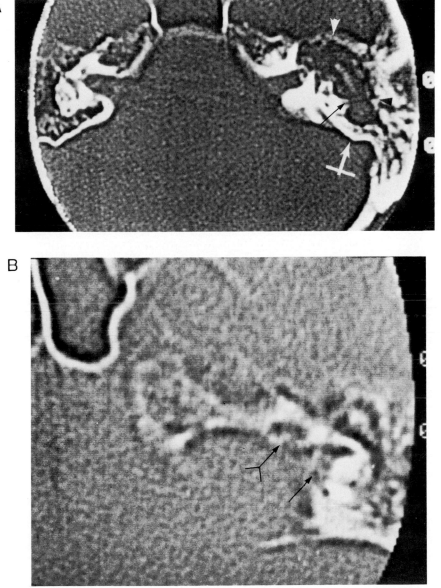

Figure 4.   (A) Large primary cholesteatoma (right) that has essentially destroyed the semicircular canal system and has passed medial to the otic capsule (arrowhead). The horizontal semicircular canal is eroded (→), and only a portion of the posterior limb remains. Despite such extensive erosion the sigmoid plate (↣) is intact. (B) Primary cholesteatoma of the right petrous apex that has eroded the internal auditory canal and has invaded the region of the vestibule (→) and modiolus of the cochlea (⤳). The more laterally placed middle ear cavities are all within normal limits.

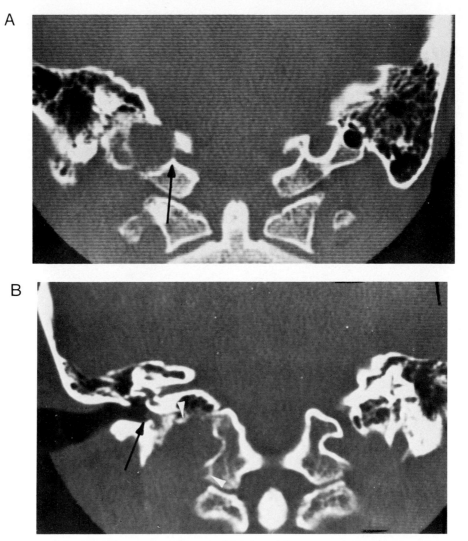

Figure 5.   Glomus jugulare as shown by coronal CT scans. (A) Extensive destruction about the region of the jugular foramen, with the erosion extending to the region of the hypoglossal canal (→). (B) More anteriorly placed scan showing that the tumor has eroded into the hypotympanum (→). The major destruction of the inferior surface of the temporal bone is well delineated (arrowhead).

REFERENCES

1. Davis, K. R., Parker, S. W., New, P. F. J., Roberson, G. H., Tareras, J. M., Ojemann, R. J., and Weiss, A. D., Computed tomography and acoustic neuroma. *Radiology,* 1977, **124:**81–86.
2. Dolan, K. D., Babin, R. W., and Jacoby, C. G., Asymmetry of the internal auditory canals without acoustic neuroma. *Ann. Otol., Rhinol., Laryngol.,* 1978, **87:**815–820.
3. Hanafee, W., Computerized tomography in hearing loss and disequilibrium states. *Otolaryngol. Head Neck Surg.,* 1981 (in press).
4. Hanafee, W. N., Gussen, R., and Rand, R. W., Laminography of the mastoid in the basal projection. *Am. J. Roentgenol., Radium Ther. Nucl. Med.,* 1970, **110:**111–118.
5. Hatam, A., Moller, A., and Olivecrona, H., Changes of internal auditory meatus. *Neuroradiology,* 1978, **16:**454–455.

6. Mancuso, A., and Hanafee, W. N., *Computed Tomography of the Head and Neck*. Williams & Wilkins, Baltimore, Maryland (in press).

7. Metzger, J., Sterkers, J. M., Dorland, P., Pertuiset, B., and Dufor, M., Les neurones de l'acoustique et leur diagnostic différentiel. In: *Traité de Radiodiagnostic: Temporal fosses nasales cavités accessoires* (J. Vignaud, ed.). Masson, Paris, 1974:304–341.

8. Valavanis, A., Schubiger, O., and Wellauer, J., Computed tomography of acoustic neuromas with emphasis on small tumor detectability. *Neuroradiology*, 1978, **16**:598–600.

9. Valvassori, G. E., The radiological diagnosis of acoustic neuromas. *Arch. Otolaryngol.*, 1966, **83**:92–97.

10. Ziedes des Plantes, B. E., Een byzondere Methode voor bet maken van roentgenfot's Van Schedelen. *Inverrelkeom. Med. Tidschr. Geneeskd.*, 1931, **75**:5219.

Approach to the Dizzy Patient

ROBERT W. BALOH

Department of Neurology
School of Medicine, University of California Los Angeles
Los Angeles, California

HISTORY

Although many technological advances have occurred in the field of neurotology (e.g., computed X-ray tomography, brainstem evoked responses, and quantitative rotatory testing), the history remains the most important part of the evaluation of a patient complaining of dizziness. A complete history should include a description of (a) the character of the dizziness, (b) the time course, (c) precipitating factors, (d) associated symptoms, and (e) predisposing factors

CHARACTER OF THE DIZZINESS

Often a patient will use the term "dizziness" to describe a sense of imbalance or dysequilibrium unrelated to an abnormal sensation within the head. This type of dizziness occurs when the patient is moving while standing or walking and disappears when he is still. It suggests bilateral symmetric vestibular loss, proprioceptive loss, or cerebellar dysfunction. An illusion of movement is specific for vestibular system disease. The most common illusion is that of rotation (vertigo), although occasionally a patient will complain of linear displacement or tilt. Damage to a semicircular canal or its afferent nerve decreases tonic activity from neurons innervating sensory cells all oriented in the same direction and produces a sensation similar to that experienced with physiological stimulation, i.e., a sensation of angular rotation in the plane of the damaged canal. A lesion involving all the canals of one labyrinth produces a sensation of rotation in a plane determined by the balance of afferent signals from the contralateral canals (usually near the horizontal since the vertical canals partially cancel each other). An illusion of linear movement is rare, probably because macular lesions decrease afferent activity from neurons innervating sensory cells oriented in multiple directions, producing a sensation unlike anything previously experienced by the patient.

Although an illusion of movement always indicates an imbalance in the vestibular

NYSTAGMUS AND VERTIGO: CLINICAL
APPROACHES TO THE PATIENT WITH DIZZINESS

system, its absence does not rule out a vestibular lesion. Other descriptions of the sensation associated with vestibular dysfunction include giddiness, swimming in the head, floating, and drunkenness.

The nonspecific sensation of light-headedness is most often associated with chronic anxiety and hyperventilation. The patient describes the feeling of an impending faint and often goes on to lose consciousness. Associated symptoms include frequent sighing, air hunger, perioral numbness, paresthesias of the extremities, lump in the throat, and tightness in the chest. Hyperventilation causes dizziness by lowering the carbon dioxide content of the blood, thus producing constriction of the cerebral vasculature. This type of dizziness must be recognized early to prevent needless diagnostic studies, which invariably increase the patient's chronic anxiety.

Many patients complain of dizziness when they first wear glasses; they experience a vague feeling of disorientation often accompanied by headache. Dizziness most frequently accompanies correction of astigmatism but also occurs after a change in magnification. A similar sensation is produced by imbalance in the extraocular muscles. After an acute muscle paralysis, looking in the direction of the paralyzed muscles causes dizziness (in addition to diplopia), but within a short time the nervous system adapts to the altered spatial information. Patients with symmetric bilateral vestibular loss complain of blurred vision and/or oscillopsia when they make rapid head movements or walk because of impaired vestibuloocular reflexes. Oscillopsia is also frequently associated with acquired primary position nystagmus of any type. Finally, autonomic symptoms such as nausea and vomiting nearly always accompany dizziness caused by vestibular lesions, and occasionally vegetative symptoms are the only manifestation of such lesions.

TIME COURSE OF THE DIZZINESS

The nervous system has a remarkable capacity to compensate for an imbalance within the vestibular system, and thus dizziness due to vestibular lesions usually occurs in bouts. Of the commonly encountered vestibular syndromes, brief episodes lasting only seconds are typical of so-called benign paroxysmal positional vertigo. Episodes lasting minutes are characteristic of vascular syndromes such as transient vertebrobasilar insufficiency and migraine. Vertigo during a typical bout of Ménière's syndrome lasts for 3 to 4 hours, although the patient often complains of a vague sense of dizziness for a day or so thereafter. Viral labyrinthitis and mononeuritis of the vestibular nerve are characterized by the acute onset of severe vertigo followed by a gradual decrease in intensity over several days. The rapidity of compensation depends on the patient's age and the functional status of the other body-orienting systems. A young, healthy patient suffering an acute peripheral vestibular insult is usually able to return to work in 2 to 4 weeks.

Continuous dizziness without fluctuation for a long period of time is not typical of vestibular disorders.

PRECIPITATING FACTORS

Dizziness caused by vestibular lesions is usually worsened by rapid head movements since the new stimulus is sensed differently by the intact and the abnormal labyrinth, and existing asymmetries are accentuated. Episodes may be precipitated by turning over in bed, sitting up from a lying position, extending the neck to look up, or bending over and straightening up. Patients with a perilymph fistula have brief episodes of vertigo precipitated by changes in middle ear pressure (coughing, sneezing). Occasionally, loud noises induce transient dizziness in patients with endolymphatic hydrops (Tulio phenomena).

ASSOCIATED SYMPTOMS

Unfortunately, a description of the dizziness associated with lesions of the vestibular system does not help one to differentiate the location of the lesion. One must rely on the associated symptoms (Table 1). Lesions of the labyrinth or eighth nerve usually produce auditory symptoms such as hearing loss, tinnitus, a sensation of pressure or fullness in the ear, and pain in the ear. As with dizziness, the time course of the hearing loss is important. Fluctuating hearing loss and tinnitus are characteristic of Ménière's syndrome. Patients with this disease usually notice a buildup of pressure in the ear just before the onset of hearing loss, tinnitus, and dizziness. Sudden, complete unilateral deafness and dizziness occur with viral or bacterial labyrinthitis and vascular occlusion to the inner ear. A slow, progressive unilateral hearing loss strongly suggests the existence of an acoustic neuroma in the internal auditory canal or the cerebellopontine angle. Lesions in the former location are often associated with ipsilateral facial weakness, whereas those in the latter location may cause ipsilateral facial numbness and weakness and ipsilateral extremity ataxia.

Since vestibular pathways run throughout the brainstem and cerebellum, it is not surprising that vestibular symptoms are common with lesions involving these structures. At the same time, because of the close approximation of other neuronal centers and fiber tracts in the brainstem and cerebellum, it is unusual to find lesions that produce isolated vestibular syndromes. Lesions of the brainstem are associated with other cranial nerve and long tract symptoms. For example, with transient vertebrobasilar insufficiency, vertigo is associated with other brainstem and occipital lobe symptoms such as diplopia, hemianoptic field defects, drop attacks, weakness, numbness, dysarthria, and ataxia. Lesions of the cerebellum (e.g., infarction or

TABLE 1
SYMPTOMS COMMONLY ASSOCIATED WITH VERTIGO CAUSED BY LESIONS AT DIFFERENT
NEUROANATOMICAL SITES

Labyrinth	Brainstem
Hearing loss	Diplopia
Tinnitus	Visual hallucinations (unformed)
Pressure	Dysarthria
Pain	Drop attacks
	Extremity weakness and numbness
Internal auditory canal	
Hearing loss	Cerebellum
Tinnitus	Imbalance
Facial weakness	Incoordination
Cerebellopontine angle	Temporal lobe
Hearing loss	Absence spells
Tinnitus	Visual hallucinations (formed)
Facial weakness and numbness	Visual illusions
Extremity incoordination	Olfactory or gustatory hallucinations

hemorrhage) may be relatively silent but are invariably associated with extremity and truncal ataxia in addition to vertigo. Hearing loss for pure tones is unusual with brainstem lesions, even in the late stages.

Vertigo can occur as part of an aura of temporal lobe seizures. The cortical projections of the vestibular system are activated by a focal discharge within the temporal lobe. Such vertigo is nearly always associated with other typical aura symptoms such as an abnormal taste or smell and distortion of the visual world (hallucinations and illusions). Occasionally, however, vertigo can be the only manifestation of an aura. In such cases the association with typical "absence" spells should lead one to the correct diagnosis.

PREDISPOSING FACTORS

The medical history of a patient complaining of dizziness should focus on the items listed in Table 2. Although uncommon in the era of antibiotics, chronic middle ear infections may lead to bacterial labyrinthitis or serous labyrinthitis, and patients with bacterial meningitis can develop bacterial labyrinthitis through the direct cerebrospinal fluid–perilymph connections. Patients with viral labyrinthitis and vestibular mononeuritis frequently report an upper respiratory tract illness either within 2 or 3 weeks before or at the time of onset of vertigo. Head injury often results in labyrinthine trauma, producing a single prolonged episode of dizziness or, more commonly, recurrent episodes of positional vertigo. Dizziness results from surgery in or about the ear, even when confined to the middle ear. For example, more than 50% of patients undergoing stapedectomy for otosclerosis complain of dizziness during the postoperative period.

The medical history should focus on chronic medical illnesses that might predispose the patient to vestibular system damage such as diabetes mellitus, atherosclerotic vascular disease, syphilis (congenital or acquired), and major allergies. Important disorders with genetic predisposition include Ménière's syndrome, otosclerosis, neurofibromatosis, and spinocerebellar degeneration. Congenital malformations of the inner ear are often associated with other congenital malformations. Ototoxic drugs, such as the aminoglycosides and salicylates, occasionally cause vertigo but more often produce imbalance from bilateral symmetric vestibular end organ damage.

EXAMINATION

The critical areas in the examination of a patient complaining of dizziness are summarized in Table 3. The examination should include a complete head and neck and neurological evaluation. Bedside examination of the vestibular system is usually

TABLE 2
PREDISPOSING FACTORS

Infectious disease
Head trauma
Surgery on the ear
Vascular disease
Metabolic disease
Neoplasia
Developmental disorders
Ototoxic drugs

TABLE 3
EMPHASIS IN EXAMINATION OF THE DIZZY PATIENT

General: heart and major vessels
    (hypertension, murmurs, bruits, etc.)
Head and neck: external auditory canal and tympanic membrane
    (trauma, infection, cholesteatoma, etc.)
Neurological: cranial nerves and coordination
    (nystagmus, hearing loss, facial weakness, imbalance, etc.)

limited to a search for imbalance within the vestibulospinal and vestibuloocular reflexes.

TESTS OF VESTIBULOSPINAL FUNCTION

As a general rule, bedside tests of vestibulospinal function lack specificity and sensitivity. It is difficult to distinguish vestibular signs from those resulting from lesions of the proprioceptive and cerebellar pathways. Furthermore, an acute vestibulospinal imbalance is rapidly compensated for so that a chronic lesion may be undetectable even when the tests are performed with the patient's eyes closed.

"Past pointing" refers to a reactive deviation of the extremities caused by an imbalance in the vestibular system. The test is performed by having the patient place his extended index finger on that of the examiner, close his eyes, raise the extended arm and index finger to a vertical position, and attempt to return his index finger to the examiner's. Consistent deviation to one side is termed "past pointing." As with all tests of vestibulospinal function, extralabyrinthine influences should be eliminated as much as possible by having the patient seated, with eyes closed and arms and index fingers extended throughout the test. The standard finger-to-nose test does not identify past pointing since joint and muscle proprioceptive signals permit accurate localization even when vestibular function is lost. Patients with acute peripheral vestibular damage past point toward the side of loss, but compensation rapidly corrects the past pointing and can even produce a drift to the other side.

For the Romberg test the patient stands with feet together, arms folded against the chest, and eyes closed. Patients with acute unilateral labyrinthine lesions sway and fall toward the damaged side. Like the past pointing test, however, the Romberg test is not a good indicator of chronic unilateral vestibular impairment, and sometimes the patient will fall toward the intact side. The sharpened Romberg test is often a more sensitive indicator of vestibular impairment. For this test the patient stands with feet aligned in the tandem heel-to-toe position with eyes closed and arms folded against the chest. Normal subjects can stand in this position for 30 sec, whereas patients with unilateral or bilateral vestibular impairment can rarely sustain the position.

When performed with the patient's eyes open, tandem walking or heel-to-toe walking is usually a test of cerebellar function since vision compensates for chronic vestibular and proprioceptive deficits. Acute vestibular lesions, however, may impair tandem walking with the patient's eyes open. Tandem walking with the patient's eyes closed provides a good test of vestibular function as long as cerebellar and proprioceptive function are intact. As with other tests of vestibulospinal function, however, the direction of falling in patients with chronic lesions is not a reliable indicator of the side of the lesion. So-called stepping or marching tests have the same limitations as the tandem walking test.

TESTS OF VESTIBULOOCULAR FUNCTION

Spontaneous Vestibular Nystagmus

Imbalance within the vestibuloocular reflex leads to nystagmus, a nonvoluntary rhythmic oscillation of the eyes. "Spontaneous nystagmus" refers to nystagmus that occurs with the patient seated, eyes in the primary position and without external stimulation such as movement of the head or surroundings. A decrease in the spontaneous flow of action potentials from a single semicircular canal results in vestibular nystagmus in the plane of that canal with a slow conjugate deviation toward the damaged side interrupted by a quick corrective movement in the opposite direction. Since a selective loss of tonic afferent signals from one canal is unusual, vestibular nystagmus is usually rotatory because of the combined effects of altered vertical and horizontal canal input. The horizontal component is most prominent, however, because the components from the two vertical canals partially cancel each other. Gazing in the direction of the fast component increases the frequency and amplitude, whereas gazing in the opposite direction has the reverse effect (Alexander's law). Vestibular nystagmus resulting from lesions of the labyrinth or eighth nerve (i.e., peripheral lesions) is strongly inhibited by fixation. Unless the patient is seen within a few days of the acute episode, spontaneous nystagmus will not be present when fixation is permitted (i.e., on routine examination). In this instance, Frenzel glasses (+20 lenses) are particularly useful for abolishing fixation and uncovering spontaneous vestibular nystagmus. Acquired spontaneous nystagmus that is not inhibited by fixation usually indicates a lesion in the brainstem and/or cerebellum. Other features that help to distinguish spontaneous nystagmus of peripheral and central origin are summarized in Table 4.

Positional Nystagmus

Nystagmus that is not present while the patient is in the sitting position but is present while the patient is in some other head and body position is called positional nystagmus. This definition excludes nystagmus present while the patient is in a sitting position that is modified by a change in position. Two general types of positional

TABLE 4
CHARACTERISTICS OF DIFFERENT VARIETIES OF NYSTAGMUS ASSOCIATED WITH VESTIBULAR LESIONS

Type	Characteristics
Spontaneous peripheral vestibular	Unidirectional; rotatory; inhibited with fixation except during acute stage of disease process
Spontaneous central vestibular	May change direction in different gaze positions; often purely horizontal or vertical; not inhibited by fixation
Peripheral static positional	Direction-fixed or direction-changing; rotatory; inhibited with fixation except during acute stage
Central static positional	Direction-fixed or direction-changing; often purely horizontal or vertical; not inhibited with fixation
Peripheral paroxysmal positional	In direction of posterior canal of down ear, i.e., torsional with large upbeat vertical component; brief duration (<30 sec); latency; fatigues with repeated positioning
Central paroxysmal positional	Multidirectional in different positions (often downbeat); no latency, does not fatigue

nystagmus can be identified on the basis of nystagmus regularity: static and paroxysmal. One induces static positional nystagmus by slowly placing the patient into the supine, right lateral, and left lateral positions. This type of positional nystagmus persists as long as the position is held. Paroxysmal positional nystagmus, on the other hand, is induced by a rapid change from erect sitting to supine head hanging left, center, or right position. It is initially high in frequency but rapidly dissipates within 30 sec to 1 min. The characteristics of each type of positional nystagmus are summarized in Table 4.

Static positional nystagmus is usually not associated with vertigo and is seldom seen without the aid of Frenzel glasses to inhibit fixation. It may be unidirectional in all positions or direction-changing in different positions. Both direction-changing and direction-fixed static positional nystagmus occur most commonly with peripheral vestibular disorders, but both also occur with central lesions. Their presence merely indicates a dysfunction in the vestibular system and is without localizing value; thus, they have the same significance as vestibular nystagmus. As with vestibular nystagmus, however, lack of suppression with fixation and signs of associated brainstem dysfunction suggest a central lesion.

The most common variety of *paroxysmal positional nystagmus* (so-called benign paroxysmal positional nystagmus) usually has a 3- to 10-sec latency before onset and rarely lasts longer than 15 sec. The nystagmus is always torsional, with fast phase directed upward, i.e., toward the forehead. It is prominent in only one head-hanging position, and a burst of nystagmus in the reverse direction usually occurs when the patient moves back to the sitting position. Another key feature is that the patient experiences severe vertigo with the initial positioning, but with repeated positioning the vertigo and nystagmus rapidly disappear.

Benign paroxysmal positional nystagmus is a sign of vestibular end organ disease. It can be the only finding in an otherwise healthy individual, or it may be associated with other signs of peripheral vestibular damage, such as vestibular nystagmus and unilateral caloric hypoexcitability. In those instances in which an abnormality is identified on caloric testing, the nystagmus will invariably occur when the patient is positioned with the damaged ear down. Benign paroxysmal positional nystagmus is a common sequella of head injury, viral labyrinthitis, and occlusion of the vasculature to the inner ear. In the majority of cases, however, it occurs as an isolated symptom of unknown cause.

Paroxysmal positional nystagmus can also result from brainstem and cerebellar lesions. This type does not decrease in amplitude or duration with repeated positioning, does not have a clear latency, and usually lasts longer than 30 sec. The direction is unpredictable and may be different in each position. It is most often purely vertical, with fast phase directed downward, i.e., toward the cheeks.

Induced Vestibular Nystagmus

Two methods are used for clinical evaluation of the vestibuloocular reflex: rotation and caloric stimulation. Neither of these methods is particularly effective at the bedside because the fixation pursuit system normally overrides vestibular induced eye movements. In an alert subject rotating the head back and forth in the horizontal plane (the so-called doll's eye test) induces compensatory eye movements (i.e., in the opposite direction of head movement) that are entirely dependent on the fixation pursuit system. The same eye movements are seen in a patient with complete loss of vestibular function. The doll's eye test is useful, however, in a comatose patient since fixation pursuit is absent. Slow conjugate compensatory movement in this setting indicates normally functioning vestibuloocular pathways.

The caloric test uses a nonphysiological stimulus to induce endolymphatic flow in the horizontal semicircular canal and thus horizontal nystagmus by creating a temperature gradient from one side of the canal to the other. Because of its availability, iced water (approximately 0°C) is usually used for bedside testing. A major advantage over rotatory testing is that caloric testing allows selective stimulation of one labyrinth at a time. It is usually performed with the patient in the supine position, head tilted 30 deg up, placing the horizontal canal in the vertical plane. To avoid inadequate stimulation, 10 cc of iced water should be used. After infusion of the water into the external canal, the endolymph circulates because of the difference in specific gravity on the two sides of the canal. This induces a brief burst of nystagmus (1 to 2 min in duration), with slow phase toward and fast phase away from the side of stimulation. In a comatose patient only a slow tonic deviation toward the side of stimulation is observed. In normal subjects the duration and speed of induced nystagmus varies greatly depending on the size of the external canal, the thickness of the temporal bone, the circulation to the temporal bone, and the subject's ability to use fixation to suppress the nystagmus. In any given subject, however, the responses tend to be symmetric. Greater than 20% asymmetry in nystagmus duration is usually abnormal.

SUGGESTED READING

Baloh, R. W., and Honrubia, V., *Clinical Neurophysiology of the Vestibular System*. Davis, Philadelphia, Pennsylvania, 1979.

Goodhill, V., *Ear Diseases, Deafness and Dizziness*. Harper & Row, Hagerstown, Maryland, 1979.

Schuknecht, H. F., *Pathology of the Ear*. Harvard Univ. Press, Cambridge, Massachusetts, 1974.

Evaluation of Rotatory Vestibular Tests in Peripheral Labyrinthine Lesions

VICENTE HONRUBIA,[1] HERMAN A. JENKINS,[2] ROBERT W. BALOH,[1] and
CLIFFORD G. Y. LAU[1]

[1]Division of Head and Neck Surgery (Otolaryngology)
School of Medicine
University of California Los Angeles
Los Angeles, California

[2]Department of Otorhinolaryngology and Communicative Sciences
Baylor College of Medicine
Houston, Texas

PHYSIOLOGICAL BASIS OF ROTATORY TESTS

The need for improvement in the diagnosis of peripheral labyrinthine disorders has led to the increased use of controlled rotatory stimulation and rigorous quantitative methods of data analysis in vestibular testings. The apparent anatomical simplicity of the elementary three-neuron vestibuloocular reflex (VOR) arc, consisting of a primary afferent neuron, vestibular nuclei, and oculomotor neurons (12), and recent advances in understanding the physiology of vestibular receptors have led to the development of theoretical studies for predicting VOR responses. It has been assumed that measurements of eye movements following rotatory stimulation provide information on the functional state of the labyrinthine organs when the remainder of the VOR arc is intact (1,8,9,11,18,22,24). In particular, measurements of the velocity of the eye during the slow-component phase of the resultant nystagmus have been accepted as indicators of the activity of the eighth nerve and vestibular receptor organs.

VESTIBULAR END ORGAN AND NERVE PHYSIOLOGY

Central to the design and selection of a vestibular rotatory test is an adequate understanding of the vestibular end organ and nerve physiology. The pendulum model of vestibular function (21,24) can be an aid in predicting the quantitative characteristics of nystagmus responses. The vestibular nerve responses in the squirrel monkey to sinusoidal rotational stimuli of frequencies between 0.0125 and 0.2 Hz

57

can be approximately described by the transfer function $H(j\omega)$ according to the following equation (6,16,20):

$$H(j\omega) = K/(1 + Tj\omega) \tag{1}$$

Given a general system with an input $u(t)$ and an output $y(t)$, the transfer function is defined as the ratio of the output function to the input function. In Laplace notation this is usually represented as $H(s) = Y(s)/U(s)$. The suffix (s) can be replaced by $j\omega$ if the stimulus is a sinusoidal function where the angular frequency in complex notation is $j\omega$ ($\omega = 2\pi f$). T is the time constant of the system response, approximately 6 sec, and K represents a sensitivity coefficient relating the change in the firing frequency of action potentials of neurons in the eighth nerve to the stimulus acceleration. The predictions of Eq. (1) are graphically represented in Figure 1 for sinusoidal accelera-

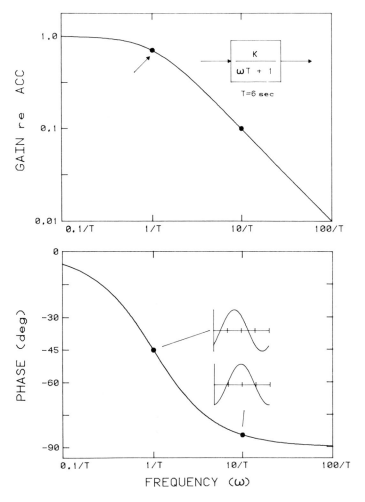

Figure 1.   Graphs showing the relationship between the gain and phase of the response predicted by the transfer function of the first-order system shown in the inset. The graph at the top shows the relationship between the logarithms of gain (ordinate) and of frequency (abscissa). Gain is defined as the ratio of the response magnitude to the stimulus magnitude (ACC, acceleration), and frequency as $1/T$, where $\omega = 2\pi f = 1/T$. The graph at the bottom shows the phase-angle difference (in degrees) between the response and the stimuli as a function of frequency ($1/T$).

tion of maximum amplitude α and angular frequency ω. These plots indicate the normalized gain (top) and phase (bottom) of the response as a function of the frequency of rotation. Gain is defined as the ratio of the peak (or maximum) response amplitude to the peak stimulus amplitude. For any stimulus of frequency ω, the response of the vestibular organ and nerve is under the control of two parameters, K and T. The sinusoidal response has an amplitude AR and phase θ,

$$AR = \alpha K([1 + (\omega T^2)]^{1/2} \tag{2}$$
$$\theta = -\arctan \omega T \tag{3}$$

where AR is given in units of (spikes/sec)/(deg/sec^2) and θ in degrees, both in relationship to the head acceleration stimulus (16).

Maximum response occurs at very low frequencies ($f << 0.02$ Hz) in which the denominator of Eq. (2) assumes a value close to 1 (since $\omega T \to 0$), and the response AR approaches αK; i.e., gain approaches the value of K. As the frequency of stimuli increases, gain decreases in such a way that, when $\omega = 1/T$, the gain is $K(2)^{1/2}$ 0.7 maximum, as indicated by the arrow in Figure 1 (top). In the squirrel monkey, where $T \sim 6$ sec, the gain is 70% of maximum when the frequency is 0.026 Hz. At higher frequencies (i.e., $f >> 0.1$ Hz), Eq. (2) reduces to

$$AR \approx \alpha K/T\omega \tag{4}$$

Hence, when $\omega = 10/T$, the gain is 1/10 of maximum. Also, since $\alpha = V\omega$, where V is the stimulus velocity, Eq. (4) can be further reduced to

$$AR \approx VK/T \tag{5}$$

The response magnitude for high frequencies is therefore proportional to the velocity of the stimulus rather than the acceleration α. That is, if the peak velocity is the same, the response magnitude is independent of the frequency of stimulation.

The system responses [Eq. (3)] show an increasing lag with the stimulus as the frequency increases. Characteristically, there is a 45-deg delay between the stimulus and the response when $\omega = 1/T$, and the phase lag reaches 90 deg, a quarter-cycle delay, at higher frequencies. Because of the coincidence of the response phase with that of the stimulus velocity [Eq. (3)] and the constant gain for higher frequencies [Eq. (5)], the vestibular organs are often referred to as angular velocity detectors, although the natural stimulus is the head angular acceleration.

An alternative method to the use of sinusoidal angular acceleration for the assessment of the eighth nerve function is the use of impulse acceleration. Because unit impulses with infinitesimal duration are unrealizable for clinical tests, in practice this is accomplished by suddenly starting or arresting a constant-velocity moving platform. Currently available mechanical devices allow changes in velocity as large as 200 deg/sec in a fraction of a second, a sufficiently short time to obtain adequate estimation of vestibular dynamics. The temporal course of the response of the system, with the transfer function given by Eq. (1), to an impulse of angular acceleration is illustrated in Figure 2. As impulses are generated by sudden changes in rotational velocity ΔV, the responses follow the equation

$$AR = K(\exp -t/T) \Delta V/T \tag{6}$$

where exp is the base of natural logarithms, t is in seconds, and ΔV, K, and T have been defined. The stimulus ΔV is measured in degrees per second. Immediately

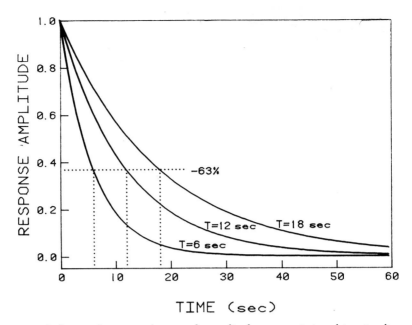

Figure 2.   Graph showing the temporal course of normalized responses to impulsive stimuli as predicted by Eqs. (1) and (6). Three different unit impulse responses are illustrated corresponding to those of systems with three different time constants: 6, 12, and 18 sec. The ordinate indicates the magnitude of response and the abscissa the time line after the stimuli.

after the impulse or when $t \approx 0$, the value of the exponential term is close to 1 and the response AR is

$$AR = \Delta V \, K/T \tag{7}$$

Thereafter, as illustrated in Figure 2, AR exponentially decays with a time constant T. The longer the time constant, the longer it takes for the response to decline to a given value, as shown by the three different curves corresponding to three different time constants. Of interest is the value of the response when $t = T$. The exponential term then is equal to 0.3678 and the response has decayed 63% of maximum. Measurements of the slope of the response decay have traditionally been used to obtain the value of T (11,22,24).

Since ΔV is known and AR and T can be measured, K can be computed. If the model is linear and time invariant, the value of T, obtained from measurements of the time decay of the impulse response, can be used to predict the phase of the response to sinusoidal stimulation at low frequency by using Eq. (4). The similarity between Eqs. (5) and (7) indicates that the response is the same during impulse stimulation and high-frequency sinusoidal rotation if $\Delta V = V(t)$.

CONTRIBUTION OF VESTIBULAR END ORGANS TO THE PRODUCTION OF VOR RESPONSES

Normally, during sinusoidal rotation in the plane of the horizontal semicircular canals, both labyrinths contribute equally to the production of VOR reflexes. The total VOR response represents the combined effect of the ampullopetal deviation of the cilia of hair cells in one crista (ARP) and the ampullofugal deviation of the cilia of hair cells in the crista of the opposite side (ARF) during each half-cycle of rotation. What changes do labyrinthine lesions produce in the VOR? Intuitively, one may anticipate that, after the complete destruction of a single labyrinth, two major changes in the VOR response would occur. The amplitude of the response should decrease as a result of the loss of input from one labyrinth. There should also be an asymmetry in the responses to clockwise (CW) and counterclockwise (CCW) rotations as a consequence of the inherent asymmetry in the ampullopetal versus ampullofugal eighth nerve responses (7). This asymmetry is usually referred to as Ewald's second law of labyrinthine function. Goldberg and Fernández (7) found that the sensitivity of the primary afferent vestibular neuron [the value of K in Eq. (2)] assumed the magnitudes of 2.44 and 1.6 (spikes/sec)/(deg/sec^2) during ampullopetal and ampullofugal stimulation, respectively. Likewise, the value of T was direction dependent, being 6.7 and 5.2 sec for ampullopetal and ampullofugal stimulation, respectively. The magnitude of the responses during ampullopetal and ampullofugal stimulations according to Eq. (3) should be frequency dependent; e.g., the ratio of the average afferent vestibular neuron responses ARP/ARF is 1.4 at 0.0125 Hz, 1.2 at 0.05 Hz, and 1.1 at 0.1 Hz. In summary, after unilateral labyrinthectomy if an algebraic addition of the two end organ outputs to the final VOR response is assumed, a 50% reduction in eye velocity measurements would occur. In addition, the amplitudes of the half-cycle responses should directly reflect the ampullopetal–ampullofugal asymmetry, leading to asymmetric eye velocity responses. Further theoretical analyses predict slight changes in phase-angle relationships in responses of patients with total unilateral labyrinthine paralysis compared to responses of normal subjects due to small differences in the value of T controlling the ampullopetal and ampullofugal responses.

In the study described in this chapter, the results of measurements of VOR responses in two groups of patients with partial and complete unilateral peripheral labyrinthine paralysis indicate that the mechanisms controlling the production of the VOR are more complex than anticipated with the use of engineering circuits based on the simple pendulum model and the elementary three-neuron reflex arc. The use of rotatory tests is not consistently effective in separating vestibular patients from normal subjects because of the large variance associated with the test results in normal subjects. These variabilities are also reflected in the computation of model parameters, which limits their clinical usefulness. In addition, it appears that the nervous system reacts to lesions of the labyrinthine organs by changing the characteristic of the output responses in a progressive manner after injury. This creates additional limitations for the use of such measurements as indicators of the functional state of the labyrinthine organs. A model based on known anatomical and physiological properties of the VOR is proposed to help explain some of the changes observed in the present data that were not predicted by earlier models.

PATIENTS

The data for this study were obtained from 12 normal subjects and 27 patients with significant unilateral labyrinthine damage as determined by caloric examination. Thirteen patients had significant unilateral decreased responses, with the maximum slow-component eye velocity of the caloric nystagmus being at least 27% smaller than that of the other ear. We used 44° and 30°C water temperatures. A 20% difference is the 95% confidence limit of our normal subject population. The computation of the paralysis was made according to the standard formula

$$\frac{[\text{Right ear (cold + hot responses)}] - [\text{left ear (hot + cold responses)}]}{[\text{Right ear (cold + hot responses)}] + [\text{left ear (hot + hot responses)}]}$$

These patients are referred to as the "partial group."

Fourteen patients had complete lack of caloric response from one ear. These patients are referred to as the "unilateral total paralysis group." Eight of the latter had previously undergone eighth nerve sectioning for acoustic neuromas or Ménière's disease. All of the patients had chronic vestibular lesions, except for three who had surgery 1 week before testing.

TEST METHODOLOGY

The test subjects underwent a series of sinusoidal rotations in the dark at a peak velocity of 60 deg/sec and frequencies of 0.0125, 0.05, and 0.2 Hz, using an Inland Control Rate Table. In addition, 9 of the normal subjects and 10 of the patients were tested with pulses of accelerations generated by sudden changes in velocity of 60 deg/sec in the CW and CCW directions.

Analysis of eye movement data was conducted with the aid of a LSI-11 minicomputer system. Details of the stimulating, recording, and on-line analysis systems have been previously published (3).

The digitized eye position data were differentiated to obtain the instantaneous eye velocity. Data associated with the nystagmus fast-component motion were automatically removed and a Fourier analysis performed on the remaining slow-component eye velocity measurement. Figure 3 shows examples of computer outputs from two programs used to evaluate the nystagmus data. One illustration corresponds to the response of a normal subject (top) and the other, to that of a patient (bottom) with an asymmetric response of the type often found in unilateral labyrinthine patients.

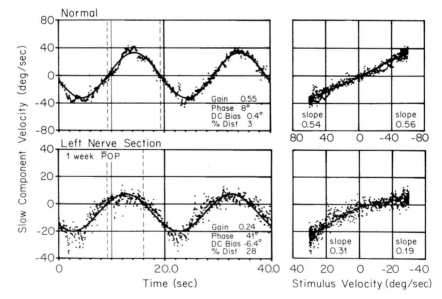

Figure 3. Graphs illustrating the methods used to evaluate the nystagmus responses of a normal subject (top) and a patient (bottom). Details are given in the text.

Several aspects of the computer-generated data are important for proper use of the measurements.

One computer program performs a Fourier analysis of the slow-component eye velocity, and the output (plots on left) provides the magnitude of the dc term, the gain (estimated as the ratio of the amplitude of the fundamental to that of the stimulus), the phase of the fundamental component, and the percentage of distortion (estimated as the ratio of the power of the first harmonic to that of the fundamental).

In normal subjects with symmetric and linear responses, the phase value derived from Fourier analysis and that which could be obtained directly from the graph by measuring the delay of the zero crossing of the fitted curve to the stimulus are identical for each half-cycle of response. In patients, because of the possibility of significant biases and large distortions in the responses, special precautions had to be taken in evaluating the results. For example, in the patient illustrated in Figure 3 (bottom) with a bias of 6.4 deg/sec and 28% distortion, the computer-determined phase lead was 41 deg. However, from direct measurements on the plot, at the time when the response has a zero value illustrated by the dashed vertical line, we can see that the CW response leads by 10 deg but that the CCW response lead is approximately 45 deg.

Gain measurements can be obtained from either one of two computer outputs: from the value of the fundamental components of the Fourier analysis, as provided by the program used to generate the outputs on the left side, or from a least-square regression analysis of the eye velocity versus stimulus velocity, as shown on the right side. With the latter method a plot is made comparing the eye velocity to the stimulus velocity after the two signals are aligned. For this, their phase-angle differences are corrected by the amount indicated from the Fourier analysis performed with the first method. When this approach is taken, the gain is obtained after computation of the slope of the least-square regression line fitted to the corresponding eye and stimulus velocity values.

If the response is linear and symmetric, as in the case of normal subjects, the difference of gain obtained by the two methods is less than 1%. If the response is linear (i.e., distortion is less than 5%) but there is a bias, the gain is also estimated by using the magnitude of the fundamental obtained from the Fourier analysis as in the first method. However, the maximum eye velocity in this situation is equal to the peak value corrected by the magnitude of the bias. If the bias is negative (CCW direction), the maximum velocity during CCW eye movement is the sum of the bias and the peak eye velocity of the fundamental. The maximum eye velocity during CW rotation is equal to the peak velocity of the fundamental minus the bias.

A point of concern is the fact that patients' responses often have a large distortion together with asymmetries, as in the case of the patient data illustrated in the bottom plots of Figure 3. In our sample data it was observed that the magnitude of the asymmetry correlated with the magnitude of the distortion, as shown in Figure 4. In this illustration, which includes data from normal subjects and patients, a comparison is made between the magnitude of the asymmetry (estimated as the percentage ratio of maximum eye velocity measurements × 100) and the magnitude of the distortion as obtained from Fourier analysis of the data from normal subjects and patients. Because of the significant distortion in patients, a reasonable way to estimate the value of the gain is by using the least-square linear regression analysis methods (as in Figure 3, right-side plots) to obtain the coefficient of the slope of the line as the

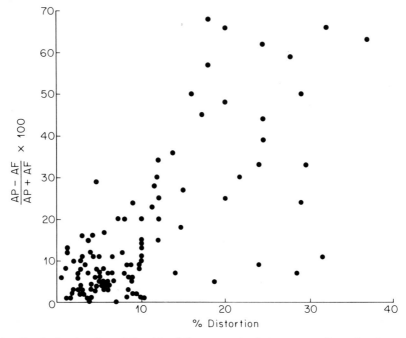

Figure 4. Graph showing the relationship of the asymmetry between ampullopetal and ampullofugal responses to the magnitude of distortion. The ordinate indicates the asymmetry expressed as 100 times the ratio of the difference to the sum of the ampullopetal and ampullofugal responses; the abscissa the distortion expressed as the percentage of the power in the first harmonic to the power on the fundamental.

estimation of gain. In the patient data illustrated in the bottom left scatter plot of Figure 3, there is a bias (the intercept of the lines is not at the origin of the cartesian coordinates), and the slopes of the lines for each half-cycle have different values (0.31 during CW rotation and 0.19 during CCW rotation).

Clinical reports often overlook the complexities associated with the evaluation of the VOR responses. Frequently, the necessary equipment is not available to perform a detailed analysis of the eye velocity data, and the reports are based on estimated gain using the maximum eye velocity from direct visual observation obtained with analog devices and displayed on the polygraph charts. In our experience this simple method of obtaining gain, which ignores, for example, the presence of bias, results in an enhancement of the asymmetries. Since the method gives erroneous estimates of gain, it enhances the differences among patients' records and those of normal subjects. We use the maximum eye velocity value for computation of different parameters to facilitate comparison with previous studies, as in Figures 8, 9, and 11. For more accurate descriptions, we use more rigorous treatment of the amplitude data, as in Figures 10 and 13. For the purpose of uniformity in the description of data, the results are described in terms of the direction of motion of the cupula in the remaining or healthier horizontal semicircular canal. If the disease process was located in the left ear, the responses induced by CW head rotation are referred to as the ampullopetal responses (of the right labyrinth), and those following CCW rotation as ampullofugal.

ROTATORY TEST RESULTS

A representative example of the nystagmus reactions following rotatory stimulation of a patient with total unilateral labyrinth paralysis is shown in Figure 5. The patient was a 50-year-old woman with a 5-year history of Ménière's disease who had undergone a left vestibular nerve sectioning 1 week before this test battery was performed. Her preoperative rotatory responses were within the normal range, and caloric testing showed only a significant directional preponderance. During the postoperative rotatory test, a marked asymmetry developed, as demonstrated in the nystagmus records on the left side of the figure. During CW, or ampullopetal, stimulation of the right horizontal semicircular canal, the nystagmus was most prominent. Coun-

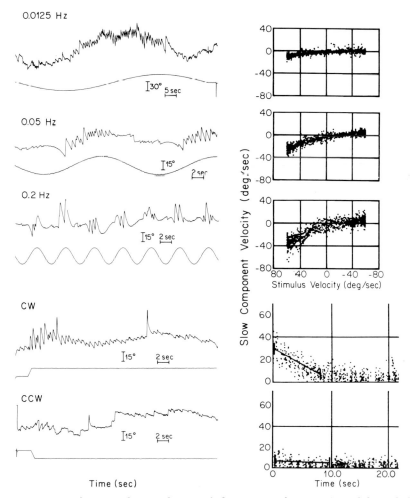

Figure 5.   Responses of a patient (history of Ménière's disease, 1 week postoperative, left vestibular nerve section) to different vestibular rotatory stimulations. At the left, reproduction of the nystagmus records and the trajectory of the stimulus velocity. The top three plots on the right show the computerized measurements of the slow-component eye velocity versus the stimulus velocity. The bottom two right graphs show the temporal course of the slow-component eye velocity following impulsive stimuli.

terclockwise, or ampullofugal, stimulation induced only a small amount of nystagmus during the 0.0125- and 0.05-Hz tests or merely the slow compensatory eye movements, as with 0.2 Hz. The computer-derived plots of the slow-component velocity versus the stimulus velocity after the phase shift had been removed, as shown on the right of the figure, further illustrate the asymmetry in responses. For example, during the 0.05-Hz test, the maximum slow-component velocity was 26 deg/sec during the CW, or ampullopetal, and 6 deg/sec during the CCW, or ampullofugal, rotations. The patient had a spontaneous nystagmus in the dark for only 4 deg/sec.

Another pattern of response found in the patient group is illustrated in Figure 6. This patient also had a history of Ménière's disease and had undergone right vestibular nerve sectioning 1 year before being subjected to this series of tests. In contrast to

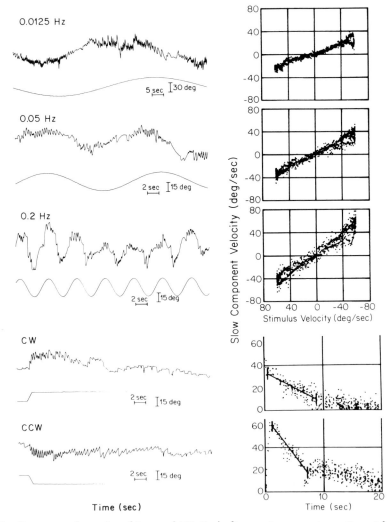

Figure 6. Responses of a patient (history of Ménière's disease, 1 year postoperative, right vestibular nerve section) to different vestibular rotatory stimulations. See legend to Figure 5.

the patient in Figure 5, this patient did not demonstrate marked asymmetry on the nystagmus reaction. The plots of the slow-component velocity on the right show approximate symmetric responses. The maximum velocity during CCW ampullopetal rotation was only slightly greater than the CW responses for all tests.

Measurements of phase and gain were obtained in each of the normal subjects and patients tested. Figure 7 summarizes the results of phase measurements with respect to velocity as a function of frequency of rotation. Phase measures the difference between the eye velocity response and the head velocity stimulus. An additional 180-deg phase difference has been removed to emphasize the compensatory nature of the response during high-frequency rotation; i.e., zero phase indicates that the eye velocity response is compensatory (180-deg differential) for the head movement. The eye velocity responses are in phase or lead the stimulus velocity at all frequencies.

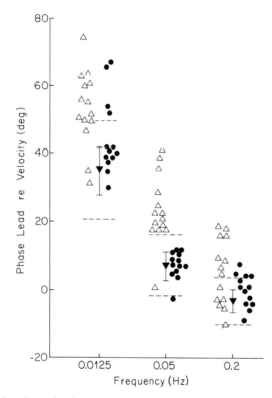

Figure 7. Phase-angle relationship between the slow-component eye velocity and the head velocity for three different stimulation frequencies in normal subjects and patients. Phase-angle relationships are expressed as the differences in degrees between the head (or stimulus) velocity and the Fourier analysis-obtained curve describing the fundamental component of the eye velocity data. A constant value of 180 deg was added to the responses in order to indicate that when phase angle is zero the eye velocity response is compensatory for the motion of the head as it occurs with high-frequency (0.2–Hz) stimuli. Positive phase leads, as shown for the lowest frequency (0.0125 Hz), indicate that the eye velocity leads the head velocity by the amount indicated in the ordinate. The results of measurements in normal subjects are shown by the solid triangles and bars, each representing the mean ±1 standard deviation (SD). The dashed horizontal lines above and below the bars indicate twice the SD value. Open triangles represent the phase measurements for the total unilateral labyrinthine paralysis patients and filled circles, the measurements in partial unilateral labyrinthine paralysis patients.

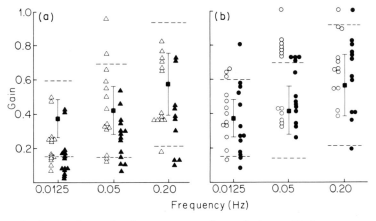

Figure 8.   Graphs showing the results of measurements of eye velocity amplitude responses as a function of the frequency of stimulation in the normal subjects and in the "total" patients (a) and "partial" patients (b). The results are expressed in terms of gain determined as the ratio of the peak or maximum eye velocity response to the peak of maximum velocity of the stimuli. The results from normal subjects are indicated by the solid squares and bars, each representing the mean ±1 SD. The horizontal lines above and below the bars indicate the range corresponding to 2 SD. Data obtained during ampullopetal stimulation of the remaining or healthy labyrinth are indicated by the open symbols, and data obtained during ampullofugal stimulation are indicated by the solid symbols.

The magnitude of the lead is dependent on the frequency of stimulation, being minimal at 0.2 Hz and maximal at 0.0125 Hz. Separation of the patients with total and partial paralysis occurred most effectively during the 0.05-Hz test, with only one "total" falling within the 2-SD interval, and one "partial" falling below the normal range of phase lead. The data show more scatter at other frequencies, with values falling on both sides of the dashed lines. A statistical evaluation comparing the two groups of patients with the normal population showed the confidence level of significance to be higher for the "totals" at the 0.0125-Hz and the 0.05-Hz test ($p < .002$). The other groups ("totals" at 0.2 Hz and "partials" at 0.05 and 0.2 Hz) failed to show a significant difference from the normals.

The results of the gain measurements are shown in Figure 8. In this figure, the "totals" (triangles) and "partials" (circles) have been separated, as have the ampullopetal and ampullofugal responses, to provide further insight into the measurements. There is a great deal of overlap of individual values in both groups of patients with the data of the normal group as well as the data between the ampullopetal and ampullofugal responses. Table 1 summarizes the result of gain for the

TABLE 1
AVERAGE GAIN MEASUREMENTS FOR NORMAL SUBJECTS AND PATIENTS

| Frequency (Hz) | Normal | Total | | Partial | |
		Ampullopetal	Ampullofugal	Ampullopetal	Ampullofugal
0.0125	0.37 ± 0.12	0.22 ± 0.12	0.15 ± 0.12	0.41 ± 0.16	0.36 ± 0.21
0.05	0.45 ± 0.16	0.44 ± 0.24	0.26 ± 0.14	0.62 ± 0.23	0.52 ± 0.16
0.2	0.59 ± 0.19	0.58 ± 0.21	0.37 ± 0.23	0.68 ± 0.20	0.60 ± 0.28

groups of normal subjects and patients. In the "total" paralysis group, the mean of the gain responses for ampullopetal stimulation was greater than that for the ampullofugal stimulation for frequencies of 0.0125 and 0.2 Hz ($p < .01$) but failed to show a statistically significant difference at 0.05 Hz. The "partial" group showed a significant difference at all three frequencies ($p < .002$ for 0.0125 and 0.05 Hz, and $p < .01$ for 0.2 Hz).

No differences were found between the responses of normal subjects and the responses of patients in the "partial" group. The totals showed significant differences at 0.0125 Hz for both directions ($p < .01$) and for the ampullofugal responses at 0.05 and 0.2 Hz ($p < .02$ and .01, respectively).

A further comparison of the differences in ampullopetal and ampullofugal responses is shown in Figure 9. The ordinate represents the difference ratio, computed as the difference in the maximal eye velocity during ampullopetal and ampullofugal stimulations, divided by the sum of the two responses. With few exceptions, all of the difference ratios were positive (i.e., ampullopetal responses were greater than ampullofugal), but less than 25% of the difference ratios were greater than 2 SD from the normal population mean for difference in CW and CCW stimulation (dashed lines).

Additional information on the characteristics of the data is shown in Figure 10. The bias magnitude (degrees per second) as obtained from the Fourier analysis is plotted for both normal subjects and patients. Biases in the ampullopetal direction are shown

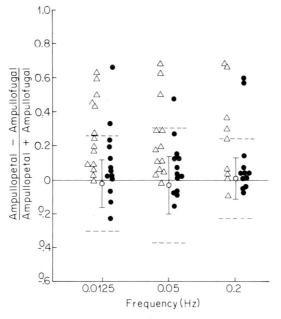

Figure 9. Graph showing the relationship between the frequency of stimuli and the magnitude of the asymmetry between ampullopetal and ampullofugal responses. In the normal subjects the results indicated by the open circles and cross bars (mean ±SD) represent the difference between clockwise and counterclockwise rotations. The results from patients indicate the difference between the ampullopetal and ampullofugal stimulus responses of the remaining or healthier labyrinth. Data from total unilateral labyrinthine paralysis patients are indicated by open triangles and data from partial unilateral labyrinthine paralysis patients, by circles. The dashed lines above and below the bars for normal subjects indicate the width of the 2-SD values.

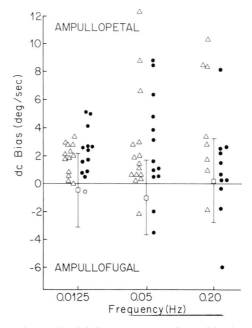

Figure 10.   Graph showing the results of dc bias component obtained by the Fourier analysis of the eye velocity measurements on normal subjects (●) and patients (△). Mean dc bias on normal subjects is less than 1 deg/sec.

as positive values and in the ampullofugal direction, as negative values. Most of the patients' biases are similar to those of normal subjects ($< \pm 4$ deg/sec). However, the direction of the patients' biases is usually in the expected ampullopetal direction, with a few exceptions. The discriminating power of the bias for differentiating patients from normal subjects is smaller than that of gain or percent difference (Figures 8 and 9, respectively).

Comparisons were made between the results of impulse testing and sinusoidal testing to evaluate the theoretical predictions. It has been pointed out that sinusoidal rotations at high frequency and impulse stimuli should have the same gain [Eqs. (5) and (7)] and that the phase obtained during sinusoidal testing could be predicted using Eq. (3) (and the value of T obtained from impulse data).

A comparison of the gain measurement between the two tests is shown in Figure 11. The lines in the plot represent the locus of equal values. Both normal subjects and patients had data distributed around the bisecting line of the plot. The mean gain of normal subjects was 0.58 ± 0.19 for 0.2 Hz and 0.62 ± 0.19 for the impulse test. For the patients' ampullopetal responses, mean gains were 0.63 ± 0.20 and 0.72 ± 0.17 for the sinusoidal and impulse tests, respectively. For ampullofugal responses, mean gains were 0.48 ± 0.25 and 0.59 ± 0.27. The number of patients that had data for both sets of stimuli is relatively small, but both tests produced similar information about the gain of the VOR.

Once the value of T is obtained from impulse tests, Eq. (4) can be used to compute the phase of the response to any frequency of stimulation (ω). A comparison of the phase measured at 0.0125 Hz and that predicted by Eq. (4) is shown in Figure 12. The lines in the plot indicate again the locus of equal values. Most of the data fall

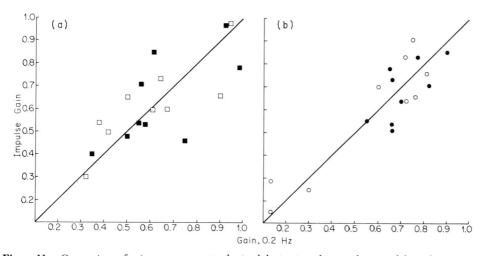

Figure 11. Comparison of gain measurements obtained during impulsive and sinusoidal accelerations at 0.2-Hz frequencies in normal subjects (a) and patients (b). In normal subjects the data are separate to indicate clockwise (□) and counterclockwise (■) directed stimuli. In patients, however, the data are separate to indicate ampullofugal (○) and ampullopetal (●) directed stimuli of the remaining or healthier horizontal semicircular canal as in other figures.

below the bisecting line, indicating that the phase predicted from impulse measurements is less than that obtained from sinusoidal stimulation. In other words, the value of T from impulse is smaller than the one controlling the response during sinusoidal tests. A least-square regression line fitted to the data points showed a slope in the normal subjects of 0.77 with a correlation coefficient of 0.94. The patient data showed a slope of 0.79 with a correlation coefficient of 0.88. In both cases there is a consistent underestimation of the phase from impulse data. However, as indicated by

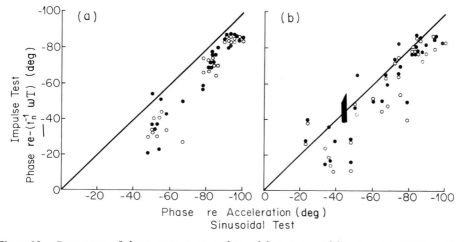

Figure 12. Comparison of phase measurements obtained during sinusoidal testing at 0.0125 Hz with the phase predicted using Eq. (3) and the value of T obtained from impulse responses. The data for normal subjects (a) indicate whether the predicted phase was obtained using clockwise (○) or counterclockwise (●) directed impulses. The data for the patients (b) indicate whether the value T was obtained during ampullofugal (○) or ampullopetal (●) directed impulses. The phase of the sinusoidal stimuli (0.0125 Hz) was obtained from Fourier analysis of the eye velocity measurements.

the significant correlation coefficient, the intrinsic mechanism controlling the phase shift has not changed in the patient population, and the predicted value of the test is similar in the two groups.

Discussion

Previous reports from this laboratory on patients with only one functional labyrinthine organ have provided a conditional confirmation of Ewald's second law of vestibular function (2,4,10). Ampullopetal stimulation of the remaining horizontal semicircular canal consistently resulted in greater responses than did ampullofugal stimulation, when the sinusoidal rotatory stimuli (0.05 Hz and impulse accelerations) were of large magnitude (i.e., peak velocities greater than 100 deg/sec). It was postulated that this asymmetry was due mainly to the existence of an amplitude nonlinearity in response to large ampullofugal stimuli. Because of this nonlinearity, a complete inhibition of the spontaneous neural activity was reached during ampullofugal stimulation, whereas the spontaneous activity continued to increase during ampullopetal stimulation. Using even lower frequencies and moderate stimulus amplitudes, Mathog and Wolfe *et al.* reported differences in ampullopetal and ampullofugal responses (15,23). The question was raised as to whether on the basis of available physiological information such results could be expected. A theoretical study undertaken in this laboratory suggested that, indeed, differences between ampullopetal and ampullofugal responses should be more significant at lower than at higher frequencies, as the above authors claimed. However, changes in phase-angle relationships failed to be predicted by this theoretical study, although they were significant in our data and in those of other investigators (23).

In view of our present results, several observations can be made regarding the usefulness of rotatory tests for diagnostic purposes, and some suggestions may help explain the findings. The responses from the group of unilateral total labyrinthine paretic subjects changed according to prediction based on physiological data (Table 1). These patients as a group had weaker responses than the group of normal subjects. The ratio of the mean ampullopetal to ampullofugal responses was approximately the same at all three frequencies: 1.5 at 0.0125 and 0.2 Hz, and 1.6 at 0.5 Hz. Although these ratios are greater than predicted, they nevertheless corroborate Ewald's second law. However, the clinically significant question is whether the response from an individual patient can be statistically identified as different from that of the group of normal subjects. In our experience, measurements based on response amplitude rarely meet this criterion in patients regardless of the parameter used for evaluation. Few of the individual results were outside the 2-SD range of values. The observation that the results of these patients as a group conform to the prediction of Ewald's second law of labyrinthine function is of theoretical value but of limited practical value.

The theoretically unanticipated change in phase-angle relationship between stimulus and response is a more consistent discriminator of patients than gain measurements of the rotatory test, at least for the patient group with unilateral total paralysis. Results of phase measurement in the majority of patients with partial loss of semicircular canal function, however, were not significantly different from those in normal subjects.

The results of the comparison of rotatory and caloric test data are somewhat disappointing. Patients with significant asymmetries in caloric test results often had rotatory responses within the normal range. Even patients with unilateral absence of response to caloric tests had rotatory responses that were many times within the range of normal values (see Table 1). One reason for the lack of sensitivity of the rotatory tests is the large variance associated with response amplitude of rotatory tests in normal subjects. During rotatory testing both labyrinths are simultaneously activated, whereas during the caloric test each ear is stimulated independently. Demonstrating differences in function, such as in cases of complete unilateral paralysis, is easier with the caloric test.

Another reason for the lack of sensitivity of the rotatory test is indicated by the data in Figure 13. This illustration (top) shows the frequency dependence of gain in our group of normal subjects and selected patients. The data correspond to those ob-

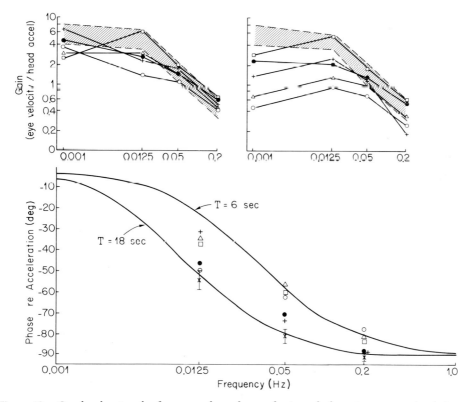

Figure 13. Graphs showing the frequency dependence of gain and phase to rotatory stimulations in normal subjects and in five patients with complete unilateral labyrinthine paralysis. The shaded areas of the graphs on the top show the range of gain of normal subjects covering ±1 SD around the mean value for each stimulus. Responses from individual patients are indicated by different symbols and joined by continuous lines. Two patients were tested 1 year (●, □), two patients within 1 week (○, △), and one patient within 2 weeks (+) after surgical section of the vestibular nerve. Gain measurements from patients indicate responses during ampullopetal (left) or ampullofugal (right) directed stimuli from the remaining labyrinth. The low-frequency (≈0.01-Hz) response is predicted by Eq. (7) using impulsive stimuli data (gain K and time constant T). The bottom graph shows the phase obtained in normal subjects (mean ±SD), indicated by the cross and the vertical bar, and the results of individual phase measurements in the same group of patients. The lines are theoretical predictions of phase using Eq. (3) and a time constant T of 18 and 6 sec, as indicated. Phase represents the lag in degrees of the eye velocity response to the head acceleration and shows increased lag with increased frequency.

tained with three different stimuli: 0.2, 0.05, and 0.0125 Hz. Also included is the predicted gain for a very low frequency or constant accelerations derived using Eq. (5). The gain for these stimuli corresponds to the value of K obtained by dividing the response amplitude following the impulse test by the time constant T of the response decline. Data corresponding to ampullopetal or ampullofugal stimuli are shown on the left and right graphs, respectively. The summarized data from 12 normal subjects are plotted as a shaded area. The width of this area covers the range of ± 1 SD around the mean values. The data from the patients are individually shown. As indicated, these patients had operations at different times before the tests were made.

Ampullopetal responses in the group of patients are closer to normal values than are ampullofugal responses. Patients tested within 2 weeks of surgery had ampullofugal gains that were lower than those of patients tested 1 year after surgery.* Thus, the difference between ampullopetal and ampullofugal measurements observed here is smaller than that which would have been obtained if the effect of bias due to a spontaneous nystagmus had been considered. It appears that the process of compensation leads to a continuing improvement of the VOR response, particularly the ampullofugal response. The recovery process appears to be progressive, and the responses return to normal after less than 1 year of surgery. In view of these data it is reasonable to assume that the compensation process interacts with the pathological process to minimize the disease-induced changes in VOR function. Only after acute, total, or virtually complete loss of function is the effect of peripheral lesions significant. For smaller changes in function or in chronic situations, the differences between ampullopetal and ampullofugal responses are smaller.

The changes in the phase measurements are another interesting aspect of the data, as illustrated at the bottom of Figure 13. The phase data from normal subjects indicated by bars (mean $\pm$ SD) coincide with the predictions of Eq. (3) using a time constant of 18 sec, as shown by the lower curve. In patients the changes are consistently toward a decrease in phase lag whereby the phase of the VOR response resembles more the phase of the vestibular nerve response. For comparison, the predicted phase of the nerve responses with a time constant of 6 sec is shown by the upper curve.

The characteristics of the VOR response are quantitatively different from those predicted from the model describing the behavior of vestibular afferent neurons. However, qualitatively, the response has many features in common with the pendulum model of vestibular function. The similarity of responses shown in Figure 13 and those predicted by Figure 1 is remarkable. The model provides a way of describing the data in the framework of mathematical expression rather than in qualitative terms; however, one should exercise caution in using the data to derive model parameters. As an example, in normal subjects, the low time constant T obtained from impulse responses has a mean value of 12 sec, but the value of T predicted from measurements of phase is closer to 18 sec (Figure 13). It is likely that differences between values of T obtained from two methods—sinusoidal and impulsive—are due to the effect of adaptation during the postrotatory nystagmus in the impulse test. A theoretical analysis of the use of the more complex adaptation pendulum model of vestibular function showed that the duration of postrotatory nystagmus following

---

*Gain for the data in the plot in Figure 13 was measured as the slope of the least-square line obtained during a linear regression analysis of the eye velocity versus stimulus velocity, as in Figure 3 (right-side plots.)

impulse stimuli reaches a maximum of 30 to 35 sec due to the effect of adaptation (19,24). Because of this limited duration, the postrotatory reaction responses to stimuli larger than 100 deg/sec declines at rates greater than those of responses to smaller stimuli. Likewise, gains predicted using Eq. (7) for constant acceleration or for very low frequency overestimate their true value since adaptation that has a time constant of 80 sec (19) would become important at these frequencies.

Besides the information obtained about the usefulness of rotatory testing in peripheral labyrinthine disease, what do the present data suggest about the function of the VOR? A comparison of response phase measurements that would be obtained from a "typical" right eighth nerve and a neuron in the right vestibular nucleus with the average measurements of slow-component eye velocity in human subjects at the three different frequencies is shown in Figure 14. At the top is the temporal course of the stimulus in terms of sinusoidal angular acceleration. A typical primary afferent neuron with a time constant of 6 sec shows an increase in phase lag with an increase in frequency, e.g., 25 deg at 0.0125 Hz (equivalent to a delay of 5.5 sec), 61 deg at 0.05 Hz (3.4 sec), and reaches 82 deg at 0.2 Hz (0.1 sec). This phase lag is due mainly to the canal dynamics. At the vestibular nuclei, as shown by Buettner *et al.* (5), there is another significant shift. The phase response of these neurons in relation to the head acceleration is 43 deg at 0.0125 Hz (9.4 sec). The delay between the response of the

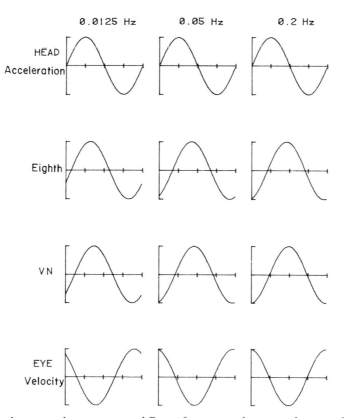

Figure 14. Graph generated to compare at different frequencies the temporal course of the stimulus (head acceleration) and the response (change in firing rate) of a vestibular afferent neuron (eighth), a second-order vestibular neuron (VN), and the eye velocity of the vestibuloocular reflex response.

eighth nerve and the vestibular nucleus is greater than could be anticipated from the delay due to synaptic transmission in one neuron. This increased delay amounts to 5 sec at 0.0125 Hz, to 0.7 sec at 0.05 Hz, and to 0.05 sec at 0.2 Hz.

In normal subjects, average eye velocity measurements, represented at the bottom of Figure 14, show further increase in phase lag. It is 54 deg at 0.0125 Hz (12 sec) and (<0.1 sec) at 0.05 Hz 79 deg. Because of the cross-connection between the right vestibular system and the left abducens motor neurons, the eye velocity trajectory is inverted. The immediate benefit of this connection is that, at high frequencies, the eye velocity is opposite to that of head; thus, the VOR response compensates for the velocity of head motion.

The phase of eye velocity measurement in complete unilateral labyrinthine paretic patients resembles the characteristics of the eighth nerve more than the measurement of normal subjects. How does this occur? Why there is an increased delay in the responses from the vestibular nuclei to the eye movement, and why the time constant of the VOR response of the patient changes, are important questions without firm answers. A heuristic model of the VOR that simulates the delay at the vestibular nuclei has been postulated (5). The model presumes the existence of positive feedback in vestibular nuclei neurons through an interneuron. Anatomical evidence for the existence and the role of internuncial neurons in the VOR was presented about 50 years ago by Lorente de Nó (13,14). He described two basic loops of interneurons in open and closed circuits. We have incorporated these ideas into another model that simulates many of our observations (Figure 15). The interneurons are represented as two systems. The ipsilateral system combines the open or cascade chains of neurons in closed-loop connection, shown at the top. The second feedback loop originates with an axon collateral from the vestibular nuclei from the opposite VOR. The first interneuronal synapse, we postulate, is located in the contralateral brainstem and represents one of the secondary vestibular inhibitory neurons described by Precht and Shimazu (17). Axons from this interneuron connect with another open-loop system of neurons in the ipsilateral side. Because of the similarities between the input from the two vestibular organs and the change in sign of the signal at the inhibitory interneuron, the final effect of the second loop of interneuron is equivalent to a second positive feedback loop acting on the ipsilateral vestibular nucleus. A diagram of these circuits is illustrated in the lower half of Figure 15. At the top is a positive feedback loop similar to that proposed earlier by Buettner *et al.* (5), and at the bottom is a second loop, whose input originates in the contralateral ear. Although increasing the number of synapses leads to increased delay, it can be shown that it is the combination of the two systems, the closed and opened loops, that produces the greatest delay. Preliminary computations of this circuit show remarkable similarities between the results of unilateral labyrinthine patients and the changes resulting from interruption of the input from the contralateral labyrinth. The interruption of the contralaterally originated feedback loop leads to a decrease in gain, as intuitively anticipated, but also to a decrease in phase lag or delay because of the loss of inputs from the reverberating circuits activated from the contralateral side.

Making improvements in diagnostic tests is not as easy as one would hope. Through these efforts, however, a better understanding of the problem is evolving, which in the final analysis should be our main objective if we are to help patients with vestibular disorders.

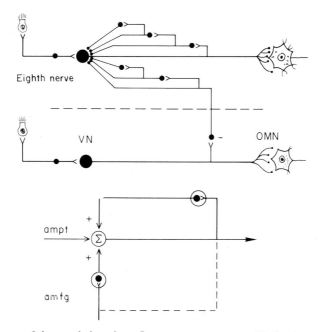

Figure 15. Diagram of the vestibuloocular reflex connections responsible for the increased phase lag between the afferent vestibular nerve responses and the second-order vestibular nuclei neuron (VN) response. Reverberating circuits of internuncial neurons provide positive feedback to the vestibular nuclei neuron. For each vestibular nucleus there are two feedback loops of interneurons. As shown for the vestibular nuclei, the top of the loop receives input from the ipsilateral vestibular nuclei neuron (shown above); the second loop, from the contralateral vestibular neuron (shown below). While the contralateral neuron response during physiological stimulation is of opposite phase than that of the ipsilateral vestibular nuclei neuron, the input signal is changed by the first synaptic step in the inhibitory interneuron. The change in the input signal to the lower loop of interneuron leads to the creation of a second positive feedback loop to the ipsilateral vestibular nuclei neuron. Bottom diagram shows the equivalent engineering circuit corresponding to the diagrams at the top.

ACKNOWLEDGMENTS

We wish to thank Leonard Jones for help with the preparation of illustrations, Susan Sakala, who helped in the collection of data, Melody Horner for editorial aid, and Virginia Herrera for secretarial services. Financial support was obtained from USPHS NS 09823, USPHS NS 08335, and Herman Jenkins' Teacher Investigator Award.

REFERENCES

1. Baloh, R. W., and Honrubia, V., *Clinical Neurophysiology of the Vestibular System.* David, Philadelphia, Pennsylvania, 1979.
2. Baloh, R. W., Honrubia, V., and Konrad, H. R., Ewald's second law re-evaluated. *Acta Oto-Laryngol.*, 1977, **83:**475–479.
3. Baloh, R. W., Langhofer, L., Honrubia, V., and Yee, R. D., On-line analysis of eye movements using a digital computer. *Aviat. Space Environ. Med.*, 1980, **51**(6):563–567.
4. Baloh, R. W., Sills, A. W., and Honrubia, V., Impulsive and sinusoidal rotatory testings: A comparison with results of caloric testing. *Laryngoscope*, 1979, **89:**646–654.
5. Buettner, U. W., Buttner, U., and Henn, V., Transfer characteristics of neurons in vestibular nuclei of the alert monkey. *J. Neurophysiol.*, 1978, **41:**1614–1628.

NEW TRENDS IN CLINICAL TESTING OF THE VESTIBULOOCULAR REFLEX

Technical Problems in Stimulation, Recording, and Analysis of Eye Movements

R. SCHMID

Istituto di Informatica e Sistemistica
Università di Pavia
Pavia, Italy

INTRODUCTION

In each test of ocular motility we can distinguish three different issues: stimulation, recording, and analysis of eye movement. The first two take place simultaneously, whereas the analysis of eye movement can be made either (a) immediately, by means of on-line computer programs or special instrumentation or (b) off-line, by simple eye inspection of the records, by hand measurement of the response parameters, or by the use of automatic systems.

For each test of ocular motility we have to answer the following questions: What is the "best" stimulation? What is the "best" way of recording eye movement? What are the "best" parameters that can be computed from the response? Obviously, no answer can be given unless we have clarified what "best" means. Since the tests of ocular motility are performed for diagnostic purposes, the best solution is that which satisfies the following two conditions. First, it must be feasible. Second, it must provide the highest clinical information. Feasibility should be examined by taking into account the state of the patient, the available technology, and the cost of the instrumentation. For what constitutes the clinical information of a test, useful suggestions can be obtained from physiological considerations and from what we know of the clinical history of the patient.

Because of the variety of tests of ocular motility, very little general information can be given about stimulation, recording, and analysis of eye movements. In a short communication, it is almost impossible to discuss each test separately and to suggest a solution for the many technical problems related to its execution. Thus, only a few conceptual problems will be considered here, using an approach that is typical of system theory and biomedical engineering.

81

NYSTAGMUS AND VERTIGO: CLINICAL
APPROACHES TO THE PATIENT WITH DIZZINESS

STIMULATION OF EYE MOVEMENT

Among the classical tests of ocular motility, those that give rise to major problems from the standpoint of stimulation are the vestibular tests evoking nystagmic eye movements.

The first dilemma is choosing between caloric and rotatory tests. The main arguments for performing caloric tests relate to the cost of the instrumentation and the ability to produce unilateral vestibular stimulations. A water or air irrigation system with a reliable control of temperature and flow is usually less expensive than the most economical apparatus for rotatory stimulations, e.g., a mechanical pendular chair for torsion swing tests.

During unilateral caloric tests only one ear is stimulated. Therefore, it was concluded that the right and left vestibuloocular pathways connected to each labyrinth could be explored separately by these tests. This conclusion would be entirely valid if the two pathways did not interact at many levels—first of all at the level of the vestibular nuclei through contralateral inhibitory projections. The survival of a bidirectional rotatory nystagmus in hemilabyrinthectomized animals after the disappearance of spontaneous nystagmus indicates that under normal conditions as well the vestibuloocular response is the result of two synergistic actions: an excitation of the ipsilateral vestibuloocular pathway and an inhibition of the contralateral one. Thus, during unilateral caloric tests, although only one labyrinth is stimulated, both vestibuloocular pathways participate in the generation of nystagmus. The push–pull organization of vestibularly induced eye movements that originates at the level of the semicircular canals during rotatory stimulations is, in the case of unilateral caloric stimulation, simply postponed to take place at the level of the vestibular nuclei.

Caloric stimulations produce a convection motion of endolymph in the horizontal canals when these canals are placed in the vertical plane by an appropriate head tilt. This motion of the endolymph has been considered perfectly equivalent to that produced by head rotations about the vertical axis. Attempts have been made to establish a scale of equivalence between caloric and rotatory stimulations.

Let us suppose that we are able to compute the bilateral caloric stimulation producing the same endolymph flow in the two horizontal canals as a given angular acceleration, and let us produce these two stimulations. Will eye movement be the same in the two cases? Probably not. Recent findings by Taglietti and Nishimura (personal communication) on isolated semicircular canals of the frog indicate that the discharge characteristics of the ampullary receptors vary with the temperature of the endolymph. In particular, the resting discharge increases with the temperature. Thus, even in the absence of endolymph flow, a different temperature of the endolymph in a pair of semicircular canals would create an imbalance between the right and left vestibular pathways. Then, during caloric stimulations, a bias component would be superposed on the eye movement induced by the convection motion of the endolymph in the canals. It has been shown by Bock and colleagues (2) that there is no adaptation in the vestibular nystagmus induced by a prolonged constant irrigation of one ear. Once steady-state conditions have been reached in the irrigated ear, the nystagmus remaining could be a proof of the existence of a bias component due to a static imbalance of the peripheral vestibular system.

It is likely, although not yet proved, that the dynamic characteristics of the

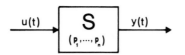

Figure 1.   Dynamic system (S) characterized by n parameters $p_1, \ldots, p_n$. $u(t)$, system input; $y(t)$, system output.

mechanoneural transduction in the vestibular receptors also depend on the temperature of the endolymph.

Clinical tests are performed to investigate whether a particular function is preserved. Test conditions should conform as closely as possible to those occurring in everyday life. Unnatural patterns of stimulation could produce central reactions masking the normal behavior of the investigated organ.

From this viewpoint, the unnatural condition of unilateral caloric stimulations cannot be disregarded. In everyday life, vestibular stimulations are always bilateral. When the discharge frequency of primary vestibular neurons increases on one side, it decreases in parallel on the other side. How do the central neural mechanisms responsible for on line control of the vestibulooocular reflex react when this general rule is violated? It is reasonable to suspect that the control exerted by the central nervous system on the vestibuloocular reflex in unnatural situations created by caloric stimulations is not the same as that produced during rotatory stimulations.

Finally, the stimulus produced during a caloric test cannot be easily quantified. This represents a serious handicap when vestibular nystagmus is used to identify some parameters of the vestibuloocular reflex through a comparison between recorded responses and responses predicted by some model of the vestibuloocular reflex.

This discussion does not prove that caloric tests are useless. Such a conclusion would be contradicted by clinical experience. This simply suggests that caloric and rotatory tests could be substantially different, and the results obtained from the two types of test cannot easily be compared.

Nonetheless, let us assume that, for some reason, we have decided that rotatory stimulations are better than caloric stimulations. Then, we shall be rather embarrassed by the number of rotatory tests that have been proposed: postrotational and perrotational tests, pendular tests, torsion swing tests, pseudorandom acceleration tests, and so on. Each of them has been proposed with different parameters.

Is there any criterion for an a priori judgment of the significance of a test? Systems theory can give us some useful suggestions. We shall state the problem in the following way. Let S be a dynamic system characterized by a number of parameters, say, $p_1, \ldots, p_n$ (Figure 1). Let Ω be the set of all the possible input functions $u(t)$. Each input produces an output $y(t)$ that can be used to estimate the system parameters. Which one is the input $u(t)$ belonging to Ω that produces the best output from the viewpoint of system parameter estimation? Obviously, the greater the output sensitivity to the variation of one parameter, the higher is the accuracy in estimation of that parameter. In other words, a parameter can be accurately estimated if, for a given input, small variations of it produce large variations of the output. Then, for each parameter p_i and for each input function we can define a sensitivity coefficient σ_{p_i} as the ratio between output variation and parameter variation (13), that is,

$$\sigma_{p_i}(t) = \frac{\partial y(t)}{\partial p_i}$$

or, better, as the ratio between output variation and relative parameter variation, that is,

$$\sigma_{p_i}(t) = \frac{1}{p_i}\frac{\partial y(t)}{\partial p_i} = \frac{\partial y(t)}{\partial \ln p_i}$$

Provided that all the inputs give the same noise-to-signal ratio at the output, we can reasonably assume that the best input from the viewpoint of system parameter estimation is that producing the highest sensitivity coefficients.

The same input can produce large sensitivity coefficients for some parameters and small sensitivity coefficients for other parameters. It is therefore important to specify which parameters we want, to see whether they are changed with respect to normal values. In order to establish the test to be used for a clinical investigation, we should first use the available a priori clinical information to define the suspected pathology. Knowledge of physiology will then indicate those parameters of the system that are likely to be varied. Only then can the more appropriate test be selected. For each type of pathology there will be one test that is better than the others, that is, the test giving the largest sensitivity coefficients for the parameters likely to be varied in that pathology.

Sensitivity analysis can do even more. If we consider the time course of the sensitivity coefficients, we can establish which periods of the response are more strictly related to the different system parameters. Actually, if one sensitivity coefficient maintains high values during a given period of the response, whereas the remaining coefficients are small, we can assume that that period is the best one for the estimation of the parameter corresponding to that sensitivity coefficient.

Sensitivity analysis is based on the assumption of small parameter variations. A large variation of just one parameter may drive the system to a working point far from normal. Then, the conclusions of a sensitivity analysis made with reference to normal conditions might not be valid. On the other hand, if large parameter variations produce large variations of the output, then the choice of the input (test) is much less critical.

In our case, the system S is the vestibuloocular reflex (VOR), the main parameters of which are the gain K, the long time constant T_1 of the semicircular canals, the time constant T_2 of the mechanoneural transduction, and the time constant T_3 of the central leaky integrator (Figure 2). The input is head angular velocity $\dot{\Theta}_H$. The possible input functions are the various velocity profiles used in rotatory tests: a step input in the case of postrotational tests, a trapezoid input in perrotational tests, a sinusoidal input in pendular tests, a damped sinusoidal input in torsion swing tests,

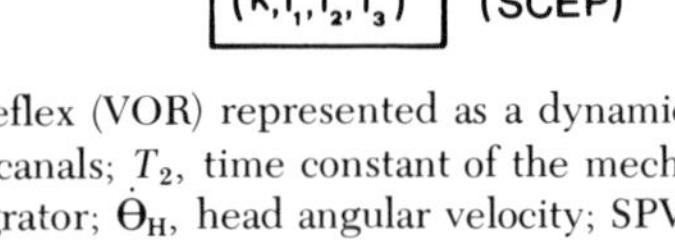

Figure 2. The vestibuloocular reflex (VOR) represented as a dynamic system. K, VOR gain; T_1, long time constant of the semicircular canals; T_2, time constant of the mechanoneural transduction; T_3, time constant of the central leaky integrator; Θ_H, head angular velocity; SPV, nystagmus slow-phase velocity; SCEP, nystagmus slow cumulative eye position.

and a pseudorandom input in pseudorandom acceleration tests. The output can be either the slow-phase velocity (SPV) or the slow cumulative eye position (SCEP) of nystagmus.

Zambarbieri and I have examined the sensitivity of SCEP to VOR parameter variations in postrotational and torsion swing tests (16). The following transfer function between SCEP and head angular velocity $\dot{\Theta}_H$ has been used to describe VOR:

$$\frac{SCEP(s)}{\dot{\Theta}_H(s)} = \frac{KT_2T_3s^2}{(1 + sT_1)(1 + sT_2)(1 + sT_3)} \tag{1}$$

The time course of SCEP sensitivity coefficients in a postrotational test is shown in Figure 3. The values assumed as normal values for the parameters K, T_1, T_2, and T_3 are given in the upper right-hand corner. It should be noted that the parameter here denoted by K is not the VOR gain as usually defined. The latter corresponds to the ratio K/T_1.

Those familiar with the time course of SCEP in postrotational tests can easily recognize that the time course of the sensitivity coefficient σ_K repeats that of SCEP. The peak of σ_K occurs at the end of the primary phase, whereas the declining part of the diagram of σ_K corresponds to the secondary phase of postrotational nystagmus.

From the analysis of the time course of the remaining sensitivity coefficients, the following conclusions can be derived. The primary phase of postrotational nystagmus is dominated by the long time constant T_1 of the semicircular canals; it is little influenced by the dynamics of the mechanoneural transduction and even less by that of the central integrator. In contrast, the secondary phase is very sensitive to the dynamics of the mechanoneural transduction. The dynamics of the leaky integrator influence only the last part of the secondary phase, which is usually less reliable. Thus, the error in the estimation of T_3 is normally large.

The time course of the sensitivity coefficients σ_K, σ_{T_1}, and σ_{T_2} in a torsion swing test performed with an initial deviation of the chair of 180 deg and a period of oscillation of 20 sec is shown in Figure 4. The time course of the sensitivity coefficient σ_{T_3} has not been represented since the values assumed by this coefficient were too small. By inspection of Figure 4 it can be concluded that only the parameters K and T_1 can be estimated with some accuracy from the nystagmus recorded in torsion swing tests.

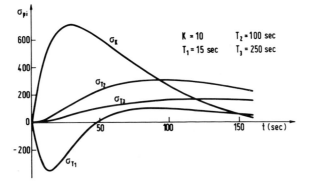

Figure 3. Time course of SCEP sensitivity coefficients in a postrotational test ($A = 120$ deg/sec). Subscripts of σ indicate the parameter of VOR to which the SCEP sensitivity coefficient is referred.

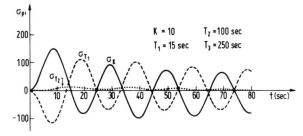

Figure 4. Time course of SCEP sensitivity coefficients in a torsion swing test (θ_{e1} = 180 deg). Notation as in Figure 3.

Let us now discuss the potential significance of the pendular tests normally performed in the clinical environment. It is well known from systems theory that a complex dynamic system cannot be identified by using a sinusoidal input at only one frequency. If a low frequency is chosen, only those parts of the system that present slow dynamics (long time constants) will reasonably be identified. The converse will be true if a high frequency is used. On the other hand, if an intermediate frequency is considered, all the system time constants will probably be incorrectly estimated.

Pendular tests are usually performed at a frequency of 0.05 Hz. What part of VOR can reasonably be investigated by using this frequency? Owing to the normal values of VOR time constants, the frequency of 0.05 Hz falls near the corner frequency corresponding to the long time constant of the cupula–endolymph system. Since the gain and the phase shift sensitivity to variations of a time constant are maximal when the adopted frequency in radians per second is close to the inverse of the time constant (corner frequency), it can be concluded that pendular tests performed at 0.05 Hz are likely to provide reliable information only about the dynamics of the semicircular canals. The same conclusion could have been reached by the analysis of the sensitivity coefficients shown in Figure 4 and referred to a torsion swing test performed at the same frequency of 0.05 Hz.

In order to identify VOR completely, the gain and phase diagrams of VOR frequency response should be constructed. This implies that pendular tests should be repeated at different frequencies. Alternatively, a single pseudorandom acceleration test can be performed. By using the pseudorandom binary sequence of rotational accelerations suggested by O'Leary and Honrubia (8), we can produce a vestibular stimulus containing all the components of the frequency spectrum ranging between 0.01 and 2 Hz. Under the assumption that VOR behaves like a linear system, which could be rather arbitrary in pathological situations, the SPV of the corresponding nystagmus will contain all the harmonics of the input signal amplified and phase-shifted according to VOR frequency response. A spectral analysis of nystagmus SPV will then provide all the information about the gain and dynamic characteristics of the vestibuloocular reflex of the examined subject.

Unfortunately, pseudorandom acceleration tests present two serious disadvantages. First, they require complex instrumentation for the control of chair movement. Second, the responses obtained in these tests cannot be examined by eye inspection of the records or by hand. Classical parameters such as the number of beats, their frequency or amplitude, the duration of some phases of nystagmus are completely meaningless in the case of responses obtained in the pseudorandom acceleration tests. Also, the time course of nystagmus SPV or SCEP cannot be interpreted in functional terms. Information can be made available only through a comparison of the input (acceleration) and output (SPV or SCEP) power spectra. A computer analysis is therefore absolutely necessary.

RECORDING OF EYE MOVEMENT

Several techniques have been proposed for recording eye movements (15). Cost considerations reduce the choice in clinical applications to traditional electrooculography or infrared electrooculography. The former is simpler to use and cheaper but significantly less precise than the latter. The artifacts due to variations of the basic corneoretinal potential or to changes in skin or electrode impedance can obviously be avoided in infrared electrooculography. Nevertheless, if this technique is used in rotatory vestibular tests (particularly in postrotational tests) and the light emitters and receivers are mounted on a pair of glasses or on a helmet, there can be some difficulty in avoiding a relative motion between the subject's head and light emitters and receivers. If such a relative motion occurs after the calibration of eye movement, a later quantitative analysis of nystagmus will be seriously compromised. Finally, infrared electrooculography is not particularly appropriate for recording vertical eye movements.

The real problem is: What is the precision needed in recording eye movements for clinical purposes? The highest precision is required to record saccades. Nevertheless, the variations of saccade parameters in pathological situations where the saccadic mechanism is impaired are normally much greater than the difference in precision between traditional and infrared electrooculography. We thus conclude that traditional electrooculography can be conveniently used for recording any type of eye movement in clinical tests of ocular motility. Only when the pathology affects small or microsaccades should traditional electrooculography be replaced by more precise techniques.

The second classical problem in recording eye movement regards the filtering of electrooculographic signals. What level of filtering can be tolerated without loss of clinical information? Smooth eye movements, whether pursuit movements or slow phases of vestibular or optokinetic nystagmus, present a frequency spectrum with significant components not exceeding 20 Hz. Thus, they can be conveniently filtered below 50 Hz (60 Hz) in order to eliminate the power supply noise.

The real filtering problem occurs in recording saccadic movements. We have investigated this problem by examining saccades evoked by step displacements of a visual target and recorded by infrared electrooculography. Recorded signals were low-pass-filtered with three different cutoff frequencies (200, 100, and 50 Hz) and converted from analog to digital at a sampling frequency of 500 Hz. By the use of an interactive computer program (4), the amplitude, duration, and peak velocity of each saccade were measured for each frequency of filtering.

The regression lines of the experimental data concerning the amplitude–duration and the amplitude–peak velocity characteristics are shown in Figure 5. When the filter cutoff frequency was decreased from 200 to 100 Hz, no significant difference was found in the values of saccade duration. Saccade peak velocity was not significantly altered by this change in the filter parameters, except for larger saccades. On the contrary, a remarkable change in the amplitude–duration and amplitude–peak velocity characteristics was observed when the filter cutoff frequency was decreased

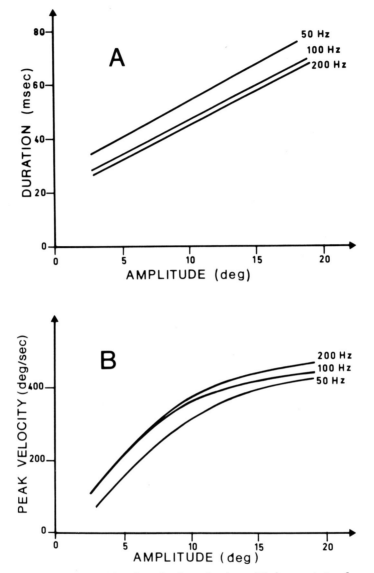

Figure 5. Amplitude–duration (A) and amplitude–peak velocity (B) characteristics of saccades low-pass-filtered at 50, 100, and 200 Hz.

to 50 Hz. The computed saccade duration increased, and the peak velocity decreased.

The conclusion of this analysis is that saccades can be recorded by using low-pass filters to reject high-frequency noise, but the filter cutoff frequency should not be less than 100 Hz.

ANALYSIS OF EYE MOVEMENT

The analysis of eye movement may be completely different depending on whether computer programs or other automatic systems are available for on-line or off-line data processing. Let us focus our attention on the analysis of vestibular nystagmus.

A simple inspection of the records by eye can reveal only modifications in the morphology of the response. Rhythm deviations and nystagmus irregularities, such as pauses, arhythmias, dismetrias, salvos, intermittent fast phases, crochetages, or other types of group formations, can be appreciated without the need for any measurement. In many cases, this very crude analysis of nystagmus can provide enough information for discriminating between normal and pathological situations. In other cases, a more quantitative analysis of the response is needed.

The number of nystagmus beats and their mean frequency in given periods of the response are two parameters that can easily be computed by hand. In response to sinusoidal stimulations, a different number of beats during rotations in the clockwise (CW) and counterclockwise (CCW) direction indicates an asymmetry between the left and the right vestibuloocular pathway. Nevertheless, if the SPV or the SCEP is not computed, it will be difficult to establish whether this asymmetry is due to a different gain of VOR during rotations to the right and to the left, or to a different threshold of the saccadic mechanism in triggering the fast phases of nystagmus. In the former case, the asymmetry would be more likely, although not exclusively, indicative of a peripheral pathology. In the latter case, the asymmetry would be indicative of a central disorder.

Nystagmus SPV and SCEP are the two parameters of a nystagmic response that are more representative of the behavior of the vestibuloocular reflex. Since their computation by hand is time-consuming and subject to trivial errors, many computer programs have been made available for on-line or off-line measurement of nystagmus SPV and SCEP (1,3,6,9,11,12). One of these programs has been developed in our institute, and it is now implemented on a microprocessor-based system for automatic vestibular analysis (VAMP 1 system) (5).

A block diagram of the system is shown in Figure 6. The system consists of a rotating chair driven by a servo dc motor; a light panel for the calibration of eye movements; a recording chain composed of a preamplification unit, a device for offset compensation, an amplifier with adjustable gain, and an A/D converter; a recording

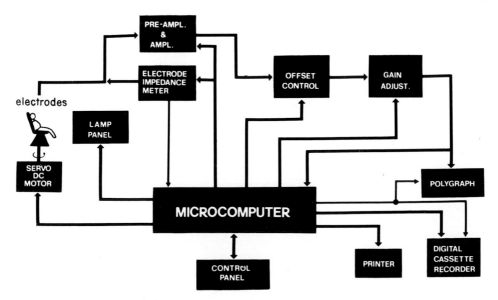

Figure 6.   Block diagram of VAMP 1 system for automatic vestibular analysis.

unit equiped with a polygraph and a digital cassette recorder; a microprocessor Z80 with a 6 Kbyte memory; a control panel; and a printer.

The analysis of nystagmus is made on line. The beginning and the end of each slow and fast phase of nystagmus are automatically recognized, and the corresponding coordinates are stored in a scratch memory. At the end of the response, the number, the mean frequency, and the mean amplitude of nystagmus beats in each period of nystagmus in one direction are printed. The diagrams of SPV and SCEP can be either plotted on paper or presented on a graphic display.

What kind of analysis can then be made off line in order to quantify the vestibuloocular response? In postrotational responses, the peak values of SPV and SCEP and the time-to-SCEP peak (or time-to-SPV zero crossing) can easily be computed (Figure 7). The first parameter is related strictly to the gain of the vestibuloocular reflex. The second one depends on both the gain and the dynamic characteristics of VOR. The third parameter depends almost exclusively on the dynamics of the semicircular canals.

In response to sinusoidal stimulations, the predominance of nystagmus in one direction can be appreciated as continuous drift of the SCEP diagram in the direction opposite to the predominant side (Figure 8). The asymmetry of the response can be quantified by the ratio of the average peak-to-peak amplitude of SCEP in the two directions. For each direction the same parameter gives a measure of VOR gain for rotations in the opposite direction. VOR dynamics can roughly be appreciated by computing the phase shift between the SCEP diagram and that of chair position or, alternatively, between the SPV diagram and that of chair velocity. In the case of asymmetric responses, the phase shifts during rotations to the right and to the left can be computed separately.

If a spontaneous nystagmus (SN) due to a static imbalance between the right and left vestibuloocular pathway is present, its contribution should be eliminated from the diagrams of SCEP or SPV in order to estimate correctly the parameters of the response evoked by the vestibular stimulation. To a first approximation, the contribution of SN to the SCEP diagram is a ramp with a slope corresponding to the average slow-phase velocity of SN. In some cases, if the effect of SN is not taken into account, both a gain and a dynamic asymmetry will appear in the original diagrams of SPV and SCEP unless an asymmetry actually exists in the evoked response.

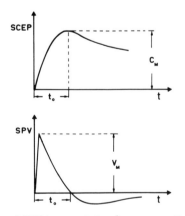

Figure 7.   Parameters of SCEP and SPV in postrotational responses. C_M, peak value of SCEP; V_M, peak value of SPV; t_0, time-to-SCEP peak or time-to-SPV zero crossing.

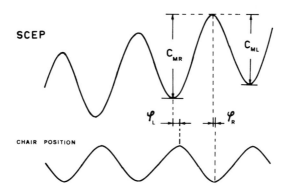

Figure 8.   Parameters of SCEP in a response to a sinusoidal stimulation. A predominance of nystagmus to the left was assumed. C_{MR} and C_{ML}, peak-to-peak displacement to the right and to the left, respectively; ϕ_R and ϕ_L, phase shift between SCEP and chair position during rotations to the left and to the right, respectively.

Rhythm deviations and nystagmus irregularities, which are often signs of central vestibular disorders, cannot be easily quantified by an automatic computer analysis. In a previous paper we suggested using the histogram of the ratio between the durations of each pair of successive intersaccadic intervals (DRH) and that of the ratio between the amplitudes of each pair of successive fast components (ARH) (3). Actually, it was reasonable to expect that in the case of rhythmic and regular nystagmus both these histograms would present a sharp distribution with mean value of unity and a small standard deviation. In contrast, changes in nystagmus rhythm and regularity would flatten these distributions with a significant increase in the standard deviation.

This expectation was confirmed by the results obtained from many normal and pathological responses. The upper part of Figure 9 shows the nystagmus recorded from a normal subject during a postrotational test of 120 deg/sec. The amplitude and duration of nystagmus beats varied progressively according to the time course of nystagmus SPV. Nevertheless, no abrupt changes of these parameters in successive beats could systematically be observed. The response can be classified as rhythmic and regular. This conclusion, derived by eye inspection of the response, is quantita-

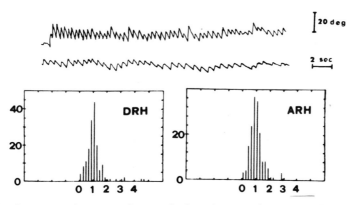

Figure 9.   Top: Postrotational response of a normal subject (A = 120 deg/sec; CCW). DRH, histogram of the ratio between the durations of each pair of successive intersaccadic intervals; ARH, histogram of the ratio between the amplitudes of each pair of successive fast components.

tively confirmed by the DRH and ARH histograms shown in the lower part of the figure. They both present a symmetric sharp distribution around a mean value close to 1 (1.05 with an SD of 0.51 for DRH, and 1.06 with an SD of 0.49 for ARH).

The postrotational response of a patient with a brainstem lesion is recorded in the upper part of Figure 10. Eye inspection of the record shows that the major deviations are concerned with nystagmus regularity. Mainly in the second part of the record, the response is characterized by sequences of small beats interrupted by fast phases of larger amplitude. The variations in successive intersaccadic intervals are less significant. The response can be classified as rhythmic but irregular. The DRH and ARH histograms shown in the lower part of the figure confirm this conclusion. DRH presents a mean value of 1.11 and an SD of 0.66. It is therefore perfectly comparable with the corresponding histogram in Figure 9. In contrast, ARH is flattened and presents a mean value of 1.14 and an SD of 0.87.

If appropriate computer programs for system parameter identification are available, an additional effort can be made to define the state of the vestibuloocular reflex quantitatively. All the parameters so far considered have been parameters of the response and not of the system that produced the response, i.e., VOR. Therefore, the values assumed by those parameters in a vestibuloocular response depend not only on the state of the examined subject, but also on the type and the modalities of the vestibular stimulation adopted in the test. Then, if two tests are not performed in exactly the same way, the values assumed by those parameters in the corresponding responses cannot be compared. Only a strict standardization of the vestibular tests and of the way of computing the response parameters can make the results obtained by different groups of investigators comparable. This standardization is far from being established. On the other hand, if ever established, it will not be easily accepted. Then, each group will have its own statistics for discriminating between normal and pathological situations.

The situation would be completely different if the nystagmic response were used not to compute some parameters of the response, but to estimate the parameters of some model of VOR. The general scheme for this analysis of nystagmus is shown in Figure 11. The VOR model is simulated on a digital computer, and normal values are initially assigned to its parameters. The predicted output to an input reproducing the

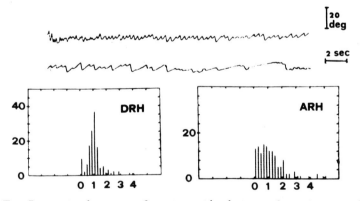

Figure 10.   Top: Postrotational response of a patient with a brainstem lesion (A = 150 deg/sec; CW). DRH, histogram of the ratio between the durations of each pair of successive intersaccadic intervals; ARH, histogram of the ratio between the amplitude of each pair of successive fast components.

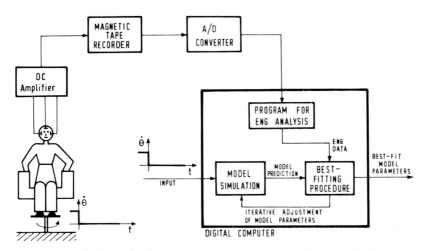

Figure 11.   General scheme for the estimation of VOR parameters from recorded nystagmus.

vestibular stimulation adopted in the test is computed. Model prediction and experimental data obtained from the nystagmus recorded during the test are then compared, and the values of model parameters are automatically adjusted through a best-fitting procedure until the best matching between predicted and experimental data is obtained. Under the assumption of linearity, the values so determined for the model parameters will depend only on the state of the examined subject and not on the vestibular stimulation used in the test.

This approach has been used by Schmid and colleagues for the identification of VOR from postrotational responses (7,10) and by Wall and colleagues (14) from responses recorded during pseudorandom acceleration tests. The identification of VOR from postrotational responses was made in the time domain by comparing the SCEP predicted by the transfer function [Eq. (1)] with $\dot{\Theta}_H(s) = A/s$ (Laplace transform of a step input with amplitude A) with the SCEP reconstructed from the postrotational nystagmus.

The identification of VOR from responses to pseudorandom accelerations was made in the frequency domain. Gain and phase estimates were first determined by calculating the ratio between the cross-power spectrum of nystagmus SPV and the power spectrum of the input signal. Then, the experimentally determined gain and phase values were used to estimate the parameters of a transfer function of the form

$$H(s) = \frac{K\Pi_i(1 + A_i s)s^k}{\Pi_j(1 + sT_j)}$$

through a least-squares fit procedure. Here, K, A_i, and T_j are the parameters in question, and s is the Laplace operator.

The major criticism that can be made against the use of this approach in clinical applications regards the assumption of linearity. Suppose that VOR behaves like a linear system in normal conditions, is it correct to assume linearity in pathological conditions as well? If the nystagmic response is clearly asymmetric for rotations in the two directions, linear system analysis based on VOR frequency response cannot be further applied. Owing to the unidirectionality of the stimulus produced in postrotational tests, a time domain analysis of the CW and CCW postrotational response should be preferred. Nevertheless, what kind of VOR transfer function should be used to fit the experimental data? If structural modifications occurred in the system due to the pathology, the fitting of the experimental data by an inappropriate transfer function might also indicate variations of parameters referring to parts of the system that are actually perfectly normal. On the other hand, if we let both the VOR transfer function and its parameters be identified from the experimental data of the examined patient, which is theoretically possible, how can the results then be interpreted from a clinical viewpoint? All these questions should be answered adequately in order to avoid unjustified mistrust or disappointment due to premature use of models for clinical diagnosis.

ACKNOWLEDGMENT

The work described in this chapter was supported by the Italian National Research Council (CNR), Rome, Italy.

REFERENCES

1. Anzaldi, E., and Mira, E., An interactive program for the analysis of ENG tracings. *Acta Oto-Laryngol.*, 1975, **80**:120–127.
2. Bock, O., Koschitzky, H. V., and Zangemeister, W. H., Vestibular adaptation to long-term stimuli. *Biol. Cybernet.*, 1979, **33**:77–79.
3. Buizza, A., Schmid, R., Zanibelli, A., Mira, E., and Semplici, P., Quantification of vestibular nystagmus by an interactive computer program. *ORL*, 1978, **40**:147–159.
4. Cabiati, C., and Pastormerlo, M., *Un Sistema per l'Analisi Automatica dei Movimenti Saccadici degli Occhi*. D. Thesis, University of Pavia, 1979.
5. Dotti, D., Lombardi, R., and Schmid, R., VAMP 1: A microprocessor-based system for vestibular analysis. *Proceeding of the Second Mediterranean Conference on Medical and Biological Engineering, Marseille, 1980:*135–136.
6. Michaels, D. L., and Tole, J. R., A microprocessor-based instrumentation for nystagmus analysis. *Proc. IEEE*, 1977, **65**:730–735.
7. Mira, E., Schmid, R., and Stefanelli, M., Application clinique d'un modèle mathématique du système vestibulo-oculomoteur. *Acta Oto-Rhino-Laryngol Belg.*, 1975, **29**:29–55.
8. O'Leary, D. P., and Honrubia, V., On-line identification of sensory systems using pseudo-random binary noise perturbations. *Biophys. J.*, 1975, **15**:505–532.
9. Oman, C. M., Allum, H. J., Tole, J. R., and Young, L. R., Automated nystagmus analysis. *AGARD Conf. Proc.*, 1973, **AGARD-CP-128**(A22):1–9.
10. Schmid, R., Buizza, A., and Zambarbieri, D., Modelling of the vestibulo-ocular reflex and its use in clinical vestibular analysis. In: *Applied Physiological Mechanics* (D. N. Ghista, ed.). Harwood Academic Publ., Chur, Switzerland, 1979:1:779–893.
11. Sills, A. W., Honrubia, V., and Kunley, W., Algorithm for multi-parameter analysis of nystagmus using a digital computer. *Aviat. Space Environ. Med.*, 1975, **46**:934–942.
12. Tole, J. R., and Young, L. R., MITNYS: A hybrid program for on-line analysis of nystagmus. *Aerosp. Med.*, 1971, **42**:508–511.
13. Tomovic, R., *Sensitivity Analysis of Dynamic Systems*. McGraw-Hill, New York, 1963.
14. Wall, C., III, O'Leary, D. P., and Black, F. O., Systems analysis of vestibulo-ocular system response using white noise rotational stimuli. In: *Vestibular Mechanisms in Health and Disease* (J. D. Hood, ed.). Academic Press, New York, 1978:157–164.
15. Young, L., and Sheena, D., Survey of eye movement recording methods. *Behavior Res. Methods Instrum.*, 1975, **7**:397–429.
16. Zambarbieri, D., and Schmid, R., Sensitivity analysis of vestibular nystagmus induced in post-rotational and torsion swing tests. *Proc. Int. Conf. Med. Biol. Eng.*, *12th, 1979*, Part II, Paper 47.3.

Low-Frequency Harmonic Acceleration in the Evaluation of Patients with Peripheral Labyrinthine Disorders

JAMES W. WOLFE,[1] *EDWARD J. ENGELKEN,*[1] *and JAMES E. OLSON*[2]

[1]*USAF School of Aerospace Medicine, Brooks Air Force Base, San Antonio, Texas*
[2]*Wilford Hall USAF Medical Center, Lackland Air Force Base, San Antonio, Texas*

INTRODUCTION

The study described in this chapter was designed to evaluate vestibular responses to low-frequency harmonic acceleration in patients with peripheral or end organ pathology and to determine whether this form of testing would provide information not available from standard bithermal caloric tests.

In its basic form, the semicircular canal system consists of a mechanical transducer (canals in the plane of rotation), central neural pathways, and effectors (extraocular muscles). In caloric stimulation of the labyrinth, a single semicircular canal is stimulated by heating or cooling the endolymphatic fluid within the canal, leading to a displacement of the cupula in a utriculopetal or utriculofugal direction and thereby simulating an angular acceleration or deceleration of the canal. One major problem with caloric stimulation has been the inability to determine or control the intensity of the stimulus, since it is impossible to specify the amount of energy actually transmitted to the end organ.

Recent clinical studies of vestibulooculomotor reflex (VOR) function in man (2, 13, 14) have attempted to develop more repeatable tests of vestibular function through the use of rotational stimuli. The development of precision dc torque motors has made it possible to control and specify stimulus input accurately, and computer technology has allowed investigators to analyze more precisely the vestibulooculomotor response. The adequate stimulus for the vestibular system is angular or linear acceleration. In the semicircular canals, changes in head velocity lead to compensatory eye movements and, in order to have a stabilized retinal image, the eye must move at the same velocity as the head but in the opposite direction. A number of studies (5, 8) have shown that the dynamic characteristics of the VOR are such that at frequencies from approximately 0.1 to 5 Hz, the system operates as an

NYSTAGMUS AND VERTIGO: CLINICAL
APPROACHES TO THE PATIENT WITH DIZZINESS

integrating accelerometer so that eye velocity is exactly 180 deg out of phase with head velocity. As pointed out by Cramer (5, p. 401), "At higher frequencies the eye tends simply to oscillate harmonically to compensate for rapid low amplitude movements of the head." On the basis of these facts, it is apparent that, if the input velocity to the head can be accurately controlled and the eye movement output reliably measured, it should be possible to determine the gain, phase, and left–right symmetry of the VOR in response to angular acceleration. Normally, the VOR functions in conjunction with vision, and either saccadic or slow pursuit eye movements can be used to acquire and track a target. However, visual oculomotor control is limited to tracking fairly low velocity targets (40 to 50 deg/sec) (6). Even with predictable sinusoidal targets, the upper limit is approximately 1 Hz in normal subjects. Therefore, a loss of visual input at frequencies below 1 Hz (which occurs during rotational testing in the dark) results in a decrement in the gain and phase of the oculomotor reflex. Although the gain of the VOR is highly sensitive to the state of arousal of the individual and his frame of reference (3), the phase relationships between the input head velocity and output eye velocity are very repeatable in normal subjects.

We have shown in previous studies with infrahuman primates (16) that the loss of one labyrinth leads to a permanent deficit in the phase relationships of the animal's eye movements in response to low-frequency harmonic acceleration. On the basis of these data, patients with peripheral deficits in labyrinthine function were selected from a large patient population referred to the Otolaryngology Service at Wilford Hall U.S. Air Force Medical Center and the Clinical Sciences Division of the U.S. Air Force School of Aerospace Medicine. Patients were evaluated periodically for up to 3 years.

METHODS AND MATERIALS

Each patient received a complete vestibulooculomotor evaluation, including tests of saccadic eye movements, sinusoidal pursuit tracking, optokinetic tracking, spontaneous and positional nystagmus, bithermal calorics, and harmonic acceleration.

Sinusoidal acceleration was generated by a dc torque motor (Contraves-Goerz, Pittsburgh, Pennsylvania, model DP-300) in a turntable system fabricated locally. This system consists of an encapsulated lightproof drum; communication is maintained through an intercom system. Each subject's head was positioned so that the horizontal canals were in the plane of rotation. All trials were conducted in the dark with the subject's eyes open. Conversation, including various questions, was used in an effort to maintain alertness. There was an initial 10-min period of dark adaptation and a 5-min interval between trials.

The torque motor was driven by a PDP-11/34 digital computer at five separate frequencies one octave apart, ranging from 0.01 to 0.16 Hz. Peak velocity was 60 deg/sec at all frequencies and acceleration varied from 3.8 deg/sec^2 at 0.01 Hz to 60 deg/sec^2 at 0.16 Hz. Eye movements were measured using standard electrooculography recording techniques and amplified by a locally assembled system consisting of an Analog Devices AD 283J isolation amplifier followed by a precision 3-sec time constant high-pass filter and then an Analog Devices 610J instrumentation amplifier.

The summated horizontal eye movement data were passed through a 15-Hz LP 4-pole Butterworth filter and sampled at 61.44 Hz. Digital filters were used to process the sampled electronystagmography (ENG) recording and to compute eye velocity and acceleration as well as correct for the effect of the high-pass filter used in the ENG recording system. The fast phases were removed from the velocity data by comparing the eye velocity and acceleration data to threshold values consistent with the amplitude and duration of fast-phase activity. Once identified, the fast phases were removed by linear interpolation between adjacent slow-phase velocity segments. Therefore, the resulting velocity record consisted only of slow-phase eye velocity. Frequency domain analysis techniques were then used to compare the stimulus signal (turntable acceleration) to the resulting slow-phase eye velocity signal. This analysis provided gain and phase estimates at the five stimulus frequencies as well as an assessment of the even and odd harmonic distortion components and system noise. As a result, the eye movement response was factored into a linear component described by the gain and phase at the five stimulus frequencies, a stationary nonlinear component indicated by the labyrinthine preponderance and harmonic distortion products, and a noise component represented by nonharmonically related components. Table 1 is a typical computer printout after completion of the five rotation trials. Since the terms in this table will be used in discussing patient responses in this study, an attempt will be made to delineate clearly the meaning of each term. Spectral purity (SP) is the percentage of the stimulus and/or response power which is at the input frequency. For example, at 0.01 Hz, the input stimulus frequency had an SP approaching 100%. The nystagmic response had a spectral purity of 77% at 0.01 Hz. The remainder of the response was made up of odd and even harmonic distortion (HD), which was minimal, and 19% noise. Spectral purity is

TABLE 1
HARMONIC ACCELERATION DATA ANALYSIS OUTPUT

	Spectral purity	HD odd	HD even	Noise
Frequency 0.01 Hz				
Stimulus	1.0000	0.00000	0.00000	0.00000
Response	0.77657	0.02454	0.00458	0.19431
Gain 0.14	Phase[a] 42.60		LP 8.45%L	
Frequency 0.02 Hz				
Stimulus	1.00000	0.00000	0.00000	0.00000
Response	0.93259	0.00785	0.00146	0.05810
Gain 0.22	Phase[a] 24.95		LP 2.32%R	
Frequency 0.04 Hz				
Stimulus	1.00000	0.00000	0.00000	0.00000
Response	0.93051	0.01146	0.00455	0.05348
Gain 0.35	Phase[a] 17.42		LP 2.30%R	
Frequency 0.08 Hz				
Stimulus	0.99999	0.00000	0.00000	0.00000
Response	0.88578	0.02701	0.02479	0.06241
Gain 0.42	Phase[a] 10.25		LP 0.04%L	
Frequency 0.16 Hz				
Stimulus	0.99999	0.00000	0.00000	0.00000
Response	0.89062	0.00613	0.01539	0.08786
Gain 0.47	Phase[a] 3.38		LP 10.24%R	

[a] Phase in degrees with reference to velocity (compensatory eye movements = ϕ degrees phase).

basically the percentage of the slow-phase output power which is at the stimulus frequency. Gain is determined by taking the ratio of the cross-power spectral density function (of the stimulus and response) and the autopower spectral density function (of the stimulus). The magnitude of this ratio at the stimulus frequency is taken as the system gain. Phase is given by the arctangent of the ratio of the imaginary and real components of the cross-spectral density function at the stimulus frequency. Labyrinthine preponderance (LP) was determined by separately integrating the total slow-phase velocity to the left and to the right and taking the following ratio:

$$\frac{\text{Slow-phase velocity left} - \text{slow-phase velocity right}}{\text{Slow-phase velocity left} + \text{slow-phase velocity right}}$$

Unlike the preponderance of caloric nystagmus, which is based on the direction of the fast phase, our analysis of asymmetry is based on slow-phase eye deviation when accelerated to the left or right. This should not be confused with caloric directional preponderance. For example, a patient with total loss of function on the right (in the uncompensated state) would have a labyrinthine preponderance of 50 to 60% to the left.

As shown in Table 1, these measures are computed at each frequency. If the spectral purity is fairly high (greater than 75%), one can be confident that the gain and phase measures are accurate descriptors of the response. Figure 1 is a summary of the method of analysis.

A total of 215 patients were included in the study as follows: 20 patients with surgically documented acoustic neuromas, 7 patients who underwent vestibular nerve section, 95 patients with a diagnosis of Ménière's disease, and 93 patients with hearing loss but no history or evidence of vestibular system pathology. The neuroma patients ranged in age from 23 to 63 years with a mean age of 39 and a standard deviation of 10 years. The patients with Ménière's disease ranged in age from 14 to 68 years with a mean of 40 and a standard deviation of 13. The patients with hearing loss were from 25 to 56 years of age with a mean of 37 and a standard deviation of 10. Data

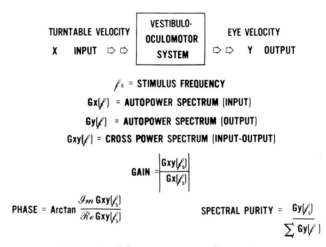

Figure 1.   Schematic summary data analysis.

from the 215 patients were compared with responses from 50 normal subjects accumulated in a previous study (15).

RESULTS

Figure 2A shows grouped data for phase and labyrinthine preponderance measures from 20 patients with surgically confirmed acoustic neuromas. These patients were selected from a larger group ($N = 32$) of tumor patients on the basis of having no central signs either before or after surgery. The tumors ranged in diameter from 1.5 to 2.5 cm. As a group, these patients showed a significant deficit ($p < .01$), one-way analysis of variance) in their phase relationships at frequencies of 0.01, 0.02, and 0.04 Hz and a significant asymmetry at 0.01 and 0.02 Hz when compared with our normal subjects (Figure 2A). Seventeen of the patients received both caloric and harmonic acceleration tests, and responses were within normal limits [based on 2 standard deviations (SD)] in 4 of the patients. Six had abnormal responses to caloric and harmonic stimulation. However, 6 patients had abnormal caloric responses with the harmonic responses within normal limits. Only 1 of the patients had an abnormal harmonic test and a normal caloric test.

After sectioning of the vestibular nerve, *each of seven patients* had a significant deficit in phase reference velocity at 0.01, 0.02, and 0.04 Hz and preponderance at all frequencies, which ranged from 25 to 95% toward the intact side.

The seven patients selected for vestibular nerve section showed similar phase deficits pre- and postoperatively, as did the neuroma patients (Figure 2B). However, as a group, they did not show any significant labyrinthine preponderance preoperatively. After surgery, they also showed a significant labyrinthine preponderance toward the intact ear.

In those patients with a diagnosis of Ménière's diesease, 80 of 95 completed all of the caloric and harmonic acceleration test sequence. Both tests were within normal limits in 39% of the patients. Twenty-eight percent had deficits in their responses (again based on an arbitrary limit of 2 SD) to both caloric and harmonic acceleration; 11% had only an abnormal caloric; and 21% had only an abnormal harmonic. Therefore, the caloric test identified 39% as abnormal, whereas the harmonic test identified 49%; the combination of the two tests identified 61% as abnormal.

A group comparison of the 95 patients with a diagnosis of Ménière's disease with our 50 normal subjects showed a significant deficit ($p < .01$, ANOVA) in phase at 0.01 and 0.02 Hz and a significant ($p < .01$) labyrinthine preponderance at the same frequencies. However, when their phase shifts were regrouped on the basis of a decrement at the lowest frequency (0.01 Hz), as shown in Figure 2C, approximately 55% were within 2 SD of the normal mean. Twenty-eight percent of the total (27 patients) were over 2 SD from normal at 0.01 and 0.02 Hz. There was also a corresponding increase in the percentage of patients with a significant unilateral weakness as a function of the decrement at 0.01 Hz.

The 93 patients with hearing loss and no history of vestibular problems did not differ significantly from the normal subjects at any frequency in response to rotational testing (Figure 2D). In fact, this group showed less asymmetry in response to harmonic acceleration, which is probably a reflection of their younger age as compared to our original normal group.

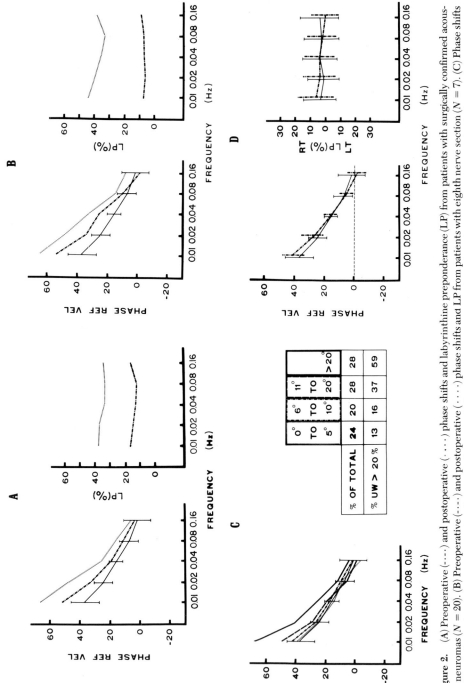

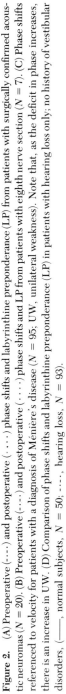

Figure 2. (A) Preoperative (····) and postoperative (-·-·) phase shifts and labyrinthine preponderance (LP) from patients with surgically confirmed acoustic neuromas ($N = 20$). (B) Preoperative (····) phase shifts and LP from patients with eighth nerve section ($N = 7$). (C) Phase shifts referenced to velocity for patients with a diagnosis of Ménière's disease ($N = 95$; UW, unilateral weakness). Note that, as the deficit in phase increases, there is an increase in UW. (D) Comparison of phase shifts and labyrinthine preponderance (LP) in patients with hearing loss only; no history of vestibular disorders. (——, normal subjects, $N = 50$; -·-·, hearing loss, $N = 93$).

Discussion

The commonly accepted belief that the central nervous system (CNS) can totally compensate for the loss of one labyrinth (or even its impairment) is not true. The extreme of this hypothesis is found in the following statement: "A fairly common example of the brain repairing itself is the recovery from a sudden peripheral vestibular lesion. Spontaneous nystagmus and dizziness result. These symptoms diminish over the next two to three weeks and, in a few months, not a trace of the disorder remains" (11, p. 413). Robinson further states that the cerebellum acts like a "motor repair shop for the gain of the vestibulo-ocular reflex" (11, p. 415). We would agree that the loss of a labyrinth leads to changes in gain and symmetry of the vestibuloocular reflex and, in time, this aspect of the response becomes more orthometric. However, this is only one measure of the system's performance (and also the most variable one). We believe that it is important to distinguish between repair and compensation. Repair implies that the impaired system returns to its previous unimpaired state and functions normally in all respects. Compensation implies that the system's "design goals" are achieved but via a different (compensatory) mechanism. In the case of unilateral labyrinthectomy, we have observed significant low-frequency phase deficits years after surgery; clearly, no repair has taken place. Figure 3 shows data from a patient who had a 2.5-cm right neuroma removed via a translabyrinthine approach. This patient had a 30% unilateral weakness before surgery and harmonic responses well within the normal range. The tumor was an encapsulated mass and did not appear to involve the brainstem or cerebellum.

Since this patient works in our facility, it was possible to test him with rotational stimulation on a periodic basis. Following transection of the eighth nerve (coincident with removal of the tumor), he showed a marked deficit in his phase measures at all frequencies tested below 0.16 Hz and a 30 to 50% preponderance to the left. As can be seen from Figure 3, even after 3 years there was no improvement in his low-frequency responses based on the phase relationships of his VOR to acceleration. After 2 years, he had become perfectly symmetric based on his LP. However, his 3-year follow-up test reflected a further deficit in his phase relationships at 0.08 and 0.16 Hz and an increase in his asymmetry. Unfortunately, 1 month before this test, he had suffered a severe retinal detachment of the right eye that had not fully resolved at the time of testing. It would appear that normal binocular visual input plays an important role in compensating for vestibular asymmetry. In over 40 patients that we have tested before and after labyrinthectomy, the same pattern has emerged and *all* have had permanent deficits in the phase relationships of their VOR to the input acceleration at 0.01, 0.02, and 0.04 Hz. Figure 4 shows data from a 23-year-old patient before and after removal of a 2.5-cm tumor; within 3 months his asymmetry had decreased almost to his preoperative level. We have noted (as have many clinicians) that the younger the patient the more rapidly compensation takes place. However, symptoms remit and symmetry improves as a result of compensation, not repair. If compensation is assumed to be a "conditioned response" following a learning period, then we would expect it to work well in a situation in which a disease state (or surgical procedure) resulted in a permanent, stationary impairment. Compensation would be much less effective in the case of Ménière's disease, in which the pathological process is characterized by fluctuant behavior.

Most models of the vestibulooculomotor system (4, 10, 12) ignore the fact that the

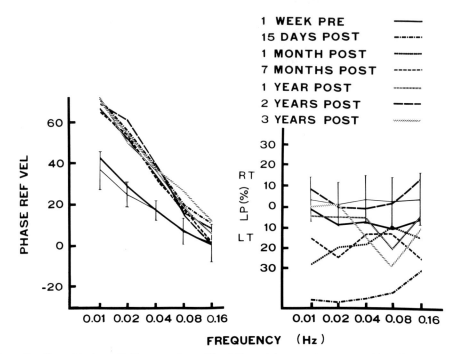

Figure 3. Repeat test results from a patient with a 2.5-cm right acoustic neuroma. Note that asymmetry 15 days postoperative is greatest at the lowest frequencies.

semicircular canals are synergistic accelerometers and represent canal dynamics by a single formula. If a model does include two canals, their output is represented as a differential input into a common summing junction, which then combines this information into a single input to the CNS. More recently, Furman (7) has proposed that the phase of the VOR is a function of the summation of the phase properties of

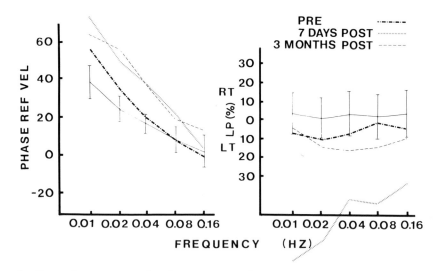

Figure 4. Pre- and postoperative data from a patient with a 2.5-cm right acoustic neuroma. Note that asymmetry is greater at the lowest frequencies.

individual fibers involving both the direct and indirect pathways. The phase characteristics of these connections are integrated in such a manner that a change in the relative weighting of the indirect pathways results in a low-frequency phase deficit. Although, as pointed out by Precht (9), a strict dichotomy probably does not exist between these pathways, it appears from our data that information from a single horizontal canal can be processed to maintain the correct phase relationships within the dynamic range above 0.1 Hz. This apparently involves the more direct pathways. However, destruction of Scarpa's ganglion or sectioning of the eighth nerve leads to a permanent deficit in phase relationships at lower frequencies (in our case, below 0.04 Hz) and appears to involve the indirect pathways; it also interferes with commissural interaction due to a loss of cell bodies within the ipsilateral Scarpa's ganglion and/or vestibular nuclei.

Recent studies (1, 2) have also implied that utriculopetal and utriculofugal stimulation lead to asymmetric output only at very high accelerations. This may be true in the compensated state, but it does not appear to be valid within the first few months after damage to an end organ or the eighth nerve. In fact, data from our studies clearly show that the response (based on total slow-phase output) shows the greatest asymmetry at the lower frequencies and accelerations. Furthermore, the asymmetry is usually compensated for within 1 month to 2 years, depending on the age of the patient. However, the phase shifts at frequencies below 0.04 Hz reflect a permanent deficit in function.

It is also apparent that the choice of stimulus input parameters and eye movement output measures are critical factors. The use of a single stimulus frequency or a single output measure (such as maximum slow-phase velocity) clearly is an incomplete test and results in an incomplete description of the VOR. Our data indicate that a single semicircular canal can provide adequate information to the CNS within the dynamic range of the system; however, below this range, both horizontal canals are necessary for optimal function.

Subjectively, the patient is unaware of any deficit in phase relationships at these very low frequencies since, in his everyday environment, vision is primary in controlling compensatory eye movements within this range. It is interesting that patients who are a few years post-eighth nerve section report no significant problem with orientation unless they suddenly lose vision (such as when the light is turned out in a room or upon entering a darkened theater), at which time they note a brief feeling of disorientation. However, certain patients (such as those with Ménière's disease) who show marked asymmetries are typically dizzy and disoriented, even when they have visual input. This is probably due to the nonstationarity of the disease process. Essentially, then, decrements in phase shifts at the very low frequencies correlate with the degree of peripheral impairment, and the labyrinthine preponderance correlates with subjective dizziness.

The question of whether rotational testing, regardless of the test design, is better than caloric testing misses the point. Our data support doing both types of testing. In the case of acoustic neuromas, it is obvious that the caloric test is more sensitive in detecting a unilateral weakness. Only 1 of 17 patients who received both caloric and rotational tests had an abnormal harmonic and a normal caloric, whereas in those patients with Ménière's diesease a combination of the two tests markedly increased the percentage of patients identified as abnormal (see results). Harmonic acceleration tests do have some advantages over caloric tests:

TABLE 2

MEAN VALUES FOR DATA FROM TWENTY-FIVE NORMAL SUBJECTS:
CROSS-POWER SPECTRAL DENSITY ANALYSIS[a]

Frequency (Hz)	Spectral purity	HD odd	HD even	Noise		Phase[b]	Gain	LP (%)
0.01	0.92	0.01	0.01	0.06	$\bar{\chi}$	42	0.47	4 L
					SD	7	0.12	15
0.02	0.93	0.01	0.01	0.05	$\bar{\chi}$	25	0.54	2 L
					SD	5	0.15	12
0.04	0.91	0.02	0.01	0.06	$\bar{\chi}$	15	0.57	5 L
					SD	7	0.18	15
0.08	0.91	0.01	0.01	0.07	$\bar{\chi}$	9	0.66	6 L
					SD	5	0.16	12
0.16	0.91	0.01	0.01	0.07	$\bar{\chi}$	3	0.66	8 L
					SD	3	0.16	14

[a] Standard deviations (SD) are not shown for values that are not normally distributed.
[b] Phase in degrees with reference to velocity.

1. The input stimulus can be controlled and clearly specified.

2. Very young children can be tested with practically no trauma. We have evaluated children as young as 2 years of age with excellent results and have been able to provide the clinician with information he would otherwise have lacked.

3. As has been shown in numerous studies, the phase measures are very repeatable and show relatively low variability within subjects. Therefore, a patient can be evaluated periodically to determine whether his pathology is progressing or is stable.

4. Patients can be tested very soon after middle and inner ear surgery, which is not practical or desirable with either water or air calorics.

5. It is possible to evaluate objectively the course of central compensation in a patient and correlate these findings with his subjective feelings.

Currently, the major disadvantage of rotational testing is the high cost of the equipment. Our method of using discrete frequencies is also time-consuming (45 min). However, this is the only method in which asymmetry can be assessed as a function of frequency. Other methods, such as pseudorandom noise, have been shown to give essentially the same phase measures in human beings, but only a single measure of asymmetry is obtained (13). Another advantage of single sinusoids is that all of the stimulus power is at the desired frequency; this results in a very good response with high spectral purity. Table 2 lists the results from 25 normal subjects. Note that the lowest spectral purity is 91%; with this high spectral purity, one can be confident that the phase and gain are reliable measures of the system's performance. We are now in the process of implementing two tests: one that uses a sum of sinusoidal stimulus and frequency analysis and one that employs varying acceleration at a single frequency. These two tests take only 15 min to accomplish, but they assess phase, gain, and labyrinthine preponderance.

SUMMARY

Vestibulooculomotor responses from patients with peripheral labyrinthine pathology were evaluated by on-line computer techniques in response to sinusoidal accelerations. Data from sinusoidal acceleration revealed that peripheral deficits can be reliably documented on the basis of phase measures at very low frequencies (0.01 and 0.02 Hz). Phase abnormalities appear to be a function of the extent of peripheral end organ damage. Results clearly show that low-frequency harmonic acceleration provides information to the clinician that can be useful in diagnosis and in the evaluation of subsequent therapy.

ACKNOWLEDGMENTS

The authors wish to acknowledge the editorial assistance and cooperation of H. H. Hanna, M.D., Chief, Otolaryngology Branch, Brooks Air Force Base (AFB), Texas. The authors thank John W. Docken, Daniel E. Dreher, Lloyd J. Loup, and LaVerne A. Spriggs for their technical assistance.

The research reported in this paper was conducted by personnel of the Clinical Sciences and Data Sciences Divisions, USAF School of Aerospace Medicine, Aerospace Medical Division, AFSC, Brooks AFB, San Antonio, Texas; the Otolaryngology Service, Wilford Hall USAF Medical Center, Aerospace Medical Division, AFSC, Lackland AFB, San Antonio, Texas. The voluntary informed consent of the subjects used in this research was obtained in accordance with AFR 80-33.

REFERENCES

1. Baloh, R. W., Honrubia, V., and Konrad, H. R., Ewald's second law re-evaluated. *Acta Oto-Laryngol*, 1977, **83**:475–479.
2. Baloh, R. W., Sills, A. W., and Honrubia, V., Impulsive and sinusoidal rotatory testing: A comparison with results of caloric testing. *Laryngoscope*, 1979, **89**:646–654.
3. Barr, C. C., Schultheis, L. W., and Robinson, D. A., Voluntary, non-visual control of the human vestibulo-ocular reflex. *Acta Oto Laryngol.*, 1976, **81**:365 375.
4. Chun, K. S., and Robinson, D. A., A model of quick phase generation in the vestibulo-ocular reflex. *Biol Cybernet.*, 1978, **28**:209–221.
5. Cramer, R. L., The dynamic characteristics of the vestibulo-ocular reflex are after prolonged stimulation. *Biomed. Sci. Instrum.*, 1963, **1**:401–406.
6. Engelken, E. J., and Wolfe, J. W., A modeling approach to the assessment of smooth pursuit eye movement. *Aviat. Space Environ Med.*, 1979, **50**:1102–1107.
7. Furman, J. M., *Linear Systems Analysis of the Horizontal Vestibulo-Ocular Reflex of the Alert Rhesus Monkey*. Ph.D. Thesis, University of Pennsylvania, Philadelphia, 1979.
8. Jones, G. M., and Milsum, J. H., Spatial and dynamic aspects of visual fixation. *IEEE Trans. Biomed. Eng.*, 1965, **BME-12**:54–62.
9. Precht, W., The functional synaptology of brainstem oculomotor pathways. In: *Control of Gaze by Brain Stem Neurons* (R. Baker and A. Berthoz, eds.). Elsevier North-Holland Biomedical Press, Amsterdam, 1977:131–141.
10. Robinson, D. A., Models of oculomotor neural organization. In: *The Control of Eye Movements* (P. Bach-y-rita, C. C. Collins, and J. E. Hyde, eds.). Academic Press, New York, 1971:519–539.
11. Robinson, D.A., How the oculomotor system repairs itself. *Invest. Ophthalmol. Visual Sci.*, 1975, **14**:413–415.
12. Robinson, D. A., Vestibular and optokinetic symbiosis: an example of explaining by modeling. In: *Control of Gaze by Brain Stem Neurons* (R. Baker and A. Berthoz, eds.). Elsevier/North-Holland Biomedical Press, Amsterdam, 1977:49–58.
13. Wall, C., Black, F. O., and O'Leary, D. P., Clinical use of pseudorandom binary sequence white noise in assessment of the human vestibulo-ocular system. *Ann Otol., Rhinol., Laryngol.*, 1978, **87**:845–852.
14. Wolfe, J. W., Engelken, E. J., Olson, J. E., and Kos, C. M., Vestibular responses to bithermal caloric and harmonic acceleration. *Ann. Otol., Rhinol., Laryngol.*, 1978, **87**:861–868.
15. Wolfe, J. W., Engelken, E. J., Olson, J. E., and Kos, C. M., Low-frequency harmonic acceleration as a test of labyrinthine function: Basic methods and illustrative cases. *Trans. Am. Acad. Ophthal. Otolaryngol.*, 1978, **86**:130–142.
16. Wolfe, J. W., and Kos, C. M., Nystagmic responses of the rhesus monkey to rotational stimulation following unilateral labyrinthectomy: Final Report. *Trans. Am. Acad. Ophthalmol. Otolaryngol.*, 1977, **84**:38–45.

Use of Pseudorandom Angular Accelerations in the Evaluation of Vestibuloocular Function

DENNIS P. O'LEARY,[1] JOSEPH M. FURMAN,[2] and JAMES W. WOLFE[3]

[1]Division of Vestibular Disorders, Eye and Ear Hospital, Department of Otolaryngology, University of Pittsburgh School of Medicine, Pittsburgh, Pennsylvania
[2]Department of Neurology, Center for the Health Sciences, University of California Los Angeles, Los Angeles, California
[3]USAF School of Aerospace Medicine, Brooks Air Force Base, San Antonio, Texas

INTRODUCTION

The use of rotational stimulation for analysis of the vestibuloocular reflex (VOR) was reexamined during the 1970's (1, 5, 9, 10). Sinusoidal oscillations or unidirectional accelerations have been used, often with the aid of small computers both to control the stimulus and to analyze the eye movement responses. An alternative stimulus profile is obtained by the use of a pseudorandom rotational acceleration as adapted from control engineering for the analysis of control system parameters. Pseudorandom testing was first applied to the vestibular system at UCLA in studies of eighth nerve responses in guitarfish (7). The efficiency and success of these studies suggested that they would also be valuable for analysis of the vestibuloocular system. The purpose of this chapter is to delineate the practical aspects of pseudorandom protocols that are useful for vestibuloocular testing and to describe current applications using combinations of these stimuli.

METHODS

Single periods of a pseudorandom binary sequence (PRBS) of rotational acceleration and velocity are shown in Figures 1D and 1C, respectively, in comparison with single periods of a sinusoidal stimulus profile, shown in Figures 1A and 1B. In practice, either stimulus form would be repeated periodically and used to control the motion of a rotating chair or turntable (5). An intuitive difference between the two

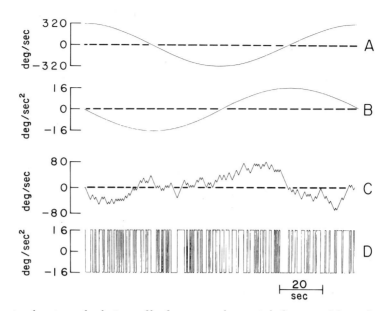

Figure 1.   Acceleration and velocity profiles for one complete period of a sinusoidal stimulus and a PRBS stimulus. (A) Sinusoidal velocity profile of frequency 0.0078 Hz and amplitude ±318 deg/sec. (B) Sinusoidal acceleration profile corresponding to A. (C) PRBS velocity profile generated by a length 255 sequence with state duration of 500 msec and an amplitude of ±16 deg/sec². (D) Acceleration profile corresponding to C; the bandwidth of this waveform is 0.0078 to 0.66 Hz. From Furman *et al.* (5) by permission.

stimuli is the inherent randomness, or "unpredictability," of the PRBS, in contrast to the smoothly varying, or "pendular," profile of the sinusoid. The unpredictability derives from the fact that a PRBS is a "white noise" signal equivalent to mixing 255 different stimulus frequencies, spaced equally across a two-decade frequency range. Therefore, in addition to its unpredictability, a PRBS stimulus is efficient in the sense of testing the VOR across a broad frequency range simultaneously, and under the same state of arousal, instead of testing with a series of individual sinusoidal frequencies. The PRBS can be generated by a low-cost computer hardware circuit formed by a shift register with digital feedback (3). Alternatively, we generated the PRBS with a PDP-11 computer program and a relay to control the timing and acceleration direction to produce the stimulus profiles shown in Figures 1C and D (5).

The resulting eye movements were recorded by electrooculography, digitized at 100 samples per second, and then analyzed by a computer program that performed four operations: (a) Fast phases of nystagmus were identified and removed by linear interpolation from adjacent slow phases. This resulted in a reconstructed slow-phase eye position (SEP) profile, as shown in Figure 2. (b) The SEP profile was differentiated. (c) Cross-correlation analysis was used to obtain a linear system impulse response, and cross-spectral analysis was applied to produce gain and phase characteristics. (d) The gain and phase values were fitted by a nonlinear regression program that yielded transfer function parameters (8). These operations produced three types of response characteristics. First, the system impulse response is a characteristic "signature" in the time domain depicting how the system responds to a sharp impulse of acceleration. It is obtained indirectly through cross-correlation of the PRBS with the eye movement response but is somewhat analogous to a "cupulometry" response

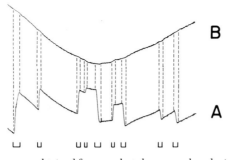

Figure 2. Eye position responses obtained from an alert rhesus monkey during PRBS rotational acceleration. (A) Eye position showing typical vestibular nystagmus with fast phases interrupting slow-phase
movements. A computer algorithm searched for fast phases by means of minimum velocity and minimum
time duration criteria. The brackets mark the position of the detected fast phases. Eye position during each
fast-phase epoch was then reconstructed using information about the previous slow-phase eye movement.
(B) Slow-phase eye position following application of reconstruction algorithm, which substituted a linear
extrapolation of the previous slow-phase movement for each detected fast phase. The next slow-phase data
were then concatenated with the termination of the extrapolation. From Furman et al. (5) by permission.

obtained by suddenly stopping a subject rotating at constant velocity. Second, the
gain and phase characteristics are frequency-dependent descriptors that can be compared directly with similar values obtained from discrete sinusoidal frequency testing
used previously (1, 5, 10). Finally, the fitted transfer function parameters describe the
system in the form of an equivalent linear system model, and, for the VOR, the
number of parameters is small for an acceptable approximation (5, 9).

RESULTS

We tested these methods by applying them to computer simulations of models of
the VOR with known system characteristics and determining that the analysis produced accurate estimates of the known characteristics (5). In addition, our studies
with rhesus monkeys showed similar gain and phase results from both PRBS and
sinusoidal testing (Figure 3), implying that the "predictable" nature of sinusoids did
not systematically bias the VOR responses, at least for the short-time stimulus protocols employed. However, it is still possible that stimulus-dependent differences
based on prediction could result from the use of either longer stimulus protocols at
each period or particular stimulus combinations.

The state of arousal is known to affect VOR responses during rotational testing,
often through supression of eye movements (5). Pharmacological agents such as
amphetamines have been used to maintain alertness in animals, but their use could
also affect central vestibular processing. We compared the VOR effects of amphetamines with those resulting from the use of a behavioral task based on a classical
conditioning fruit-juice-reward paradigm. An audible click, generated randomly by
the computer program, signaled the monkey to lick a nipple within 2 sec in order to
obtain a fruit juice reward. This paradigm alerted the animal throughout the protocol,
resulting in VOR responses that were uniform and comparable to those obtained in
other experiments using the same animals kept alert by amphetamines. Moreover,
the similar results obtained from both the behavioral task and the pharmacological
alertness paradigms were significantly different from those obtained without any
arousal methods (6). These quantitative results confirmed earlier qualitative observa-

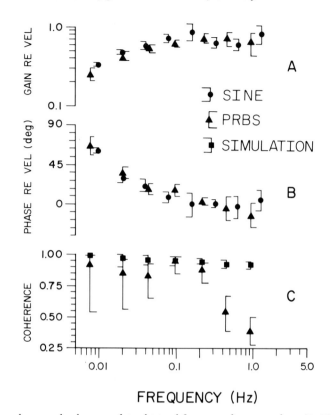

Figure 3.   Gain, phase, and coherence data obtained from one rhesus monkey. (A, B) Gain and phase data obtained from PRBS and sinusoidal stimulation. Pseudorandom testing used 5 cycles of a length 255 sequence with state durations of 100 and 500 msec. Single-frequency stimulation consisted of approximately 10 cycles at each frequency. Error bars represent 90% confidence intervals for PRBS and 1 standard deviation for sinusoids. (C) Coherence values calculated from pseudorandom testing. For comparison, the coherence for both the simulations and the physiological testing is shown. From Furman *et al.*, (5) by permission.

tions concerning the importance of alertness in obtaining accurate and uniform VOR response characteristics.

Although a PRBS stimulus is composed of a broad range of frequencies delivered simultaneously, the stimulus amplitude in units of rotational acceleration is the same at each frequency. Furman (4) tested whether the VOR system responded linearly in amplitude by using the same PRBS, but with stepwise increases in amplitude, in separate experimental protocols. If the VOR system responded linearly, a doubling of the PRBS stimulus amplitude would result in a doubling of the VOR response amplitude. A linear result was found to be valid in monkeys over an amplitude range from 2 to at least 256 deg/sec² and similar protocols with discrete sinusoidal frequencies showed equivalent results. Therefore, a nonlinear rolloff in VOR amplitude must occur at higher stimulus amplitudes as determined approximately by other techniques (D. A. Robinson, personal communication). But a major advantage of PRBS protocols is their use at *low* stimulus amplitudes, either as a minimally disturbing stimulus for clinical use, or in combination with other ongoing motions as a small-signal test perturbation. In these applications, resolution of the resulting system parameters is enhanced by averaging responses to 5 to 10 successive stimulus periods and then cross-correlating the average with the PRBS input in order to minimize the effects of VOR responses that are unrelated to the stimulus.

Eye movement responses from the optokinetic system are conducive to experimental and modeling analyses that are similar to those used successfully in the VOR system (8). In addition to their use as a rotational stimulus only, we have explored the use of two-input PRBS stimuli with oculomotor responses in preliminary experiments that employ statistically independent PRBS's as commanding signals to both optokinetic and rotational stimulators. A servo-controller is used to control an optokinetic projector, positioned above the animal, which displays a pattern of moving vertical stripes on a surrounding cylindrical screen. The resulting eye movements are composite responses to both the optokinetic and the rotational inputs. How can they be separated into the response components of each separate input? From engineering applications of two-input PRBS analyses of industrial control processes, it is known that a cross-correlation of the composite output response with each of the separate PRBS inputs will yield a response component due to each input separately (2).

Figure 4 shows resulting eye movements from a rhesus monkey stimulated by simultaneously delivered vestibular and optokinetic inputs commanded by independent PRBS's and also the responses to each input delivered separately. A technical simplification resulted from the mathematical property that shifting a PRBS to another state in its period produces a stimulus that is statistically independent from the unshifted PRBS (2, 3). We therefore used the same PRBS to control each stimulus, but with a relative shift of half the PRBS period, to result in statistically independent rotational and optokinetic inputs. The result of cross-correlating the composite response with the PRBS is shown in Figure 5. An interesting result is a double impulse response (Figure 5f), with the early component due to the optokinetic response and the later component due to the vestibular (rotational) response. The optokinetic response component is inverted relative to the vestibular component because the eye movements were in opposite directions. Simulation studies with known linear system parameters have verified the validity of this operation (D. O'Leary, unpublished observations).

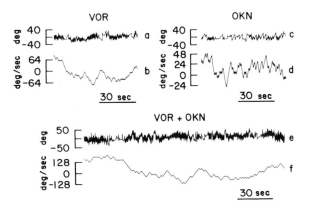

Figure 4. Eye movements evoked by PRBS stimuli commanding, respectively, (b) rotational acceleration (VOR); (d) optokinetic acceleration (OKN); (f) a superposition of *independent* PRBS's commanding VOR and OKN stimuli. Only the VOR stimulus is shown in f. The electro-oculographic responses are shown above each stimulus record as (a) vestibular, (c) optokinetic, and (e) combined stimulus.

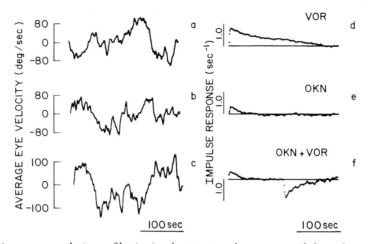

Figure 5.   Average eye velocity profiles (a–c) and system impulse responses (d–f) are shown corresponding to VOR, OKN, and OKN + VOR pseudorandom stimuli, respectively. Each system impulse response shown in the right column was obtained by cross-correlation of the pseudorandom angular acceleration stimulus with the adjacent eye velocity profile shown in the left column. The stimuli had 255 directional states of duration 1 second, and acceleration magnitudes of 16 and 32 deg/sec^2 for VOR and OKN stimuli, respectively. The number of stimulus periods used was 4, 6, and 5 for the responses shown in a–c, respectively. The impulse response profiles include certain distortions resulting from the stimulus transducers, which require frequency domain correction factors before determining gain, phase, and transfer functions.

A preliminary comparison of the impulse responses determined from each input delivered separately, and shown in Figures 5d and e, with those obtained from each component of the composite eye movement response in Figure 5f shows a strong similarity in the respective shapes of the response profiles. This implies that the optokinetic and vestibular responses resulted in a linear superposition, to a good approximation. However, a more detailed analysis and comparison of frequency domain transfer function parameters obtained from single versus double stimuli are necessary to determine quantitatively the range of similarity (6).

DISCUSSION

The use of pseudorandom rotational stimuli for analysis of the oculomotor system is based in control systems engineering and requires computerized signal processing for optimal results. Immediate advantages are the efficiency of the test and the accuracy of the resulting response parameters, as tested over a broad stimulus bandwidth simultaneously. The ability to use both relatively short-duration protocols and low-amplitude accelerations as compared with other VOR test protocols minimizes discomfort for clinical testing of vestibular patients who are prone to motion sickness. Finally, computerized eye movement analysis has the major advantage of rapid reporting of results for use in diagnostic evaluation.

In addition to their use for individual tests, pseudorandom stimuli can be used for multi-input testing, as shown by our preliminary results of combined VOR and OKN stimulation. Moreover, stimulus combinations that do not occur naturally can be achieved uniquely by this approach because of the statistical independence of the PRBS combination described in Figures 4 and 5. For example, motion of the head without visual fixation is usually accompanied by correlated apparent movement of the visual field in the opposite direction. But the responses of Figure 4e resulted from uncorrelated head and visual field movements that would not occur naturally. The "white noise" properties of these stimuli resulted in our ability to separate the respective components of each system.

Preliminary clinical trials of VOR responses using single input pseudorandom rotation have been described (9), and the sensitivity of the approach is presently being evaluated with patients having particular vestibular disorders (11).

In summary, we have described practical aspects of pseudorandom testing that we regard as advantageous to rotational testing as currently practiced, and we have shown preliminary results that point toward future uses with combinations of stimuli for more effective evaluation of vestibular function.

ACKNOWLEDGMENTS

The authors are grateful for the computer analysis of Agapi Svolou, technical assistance of Joseph Willy, and secretarial help of Catherine Seipe.

REFERENCES

1. Baloh, R. W., and Honrubia, V., *Clinical Neurophysiology of the Vestibular System.* Davis, Philadelphia, Pennsylvania, 1979.
2. Briggs, P. A. N., and Godfrey, K. R., Pseudorandom signals for the dynamic analysis of multivariable systems. *Proc. Inst. Electr. Eng.*, 1966, **113**:1259–1267.
3. Davies, W. D. T., *System Identification for Self-Adaptive Control.* Wiley, New York, 1970.
4. Furman, J. M. *Linear System Analysis of the Horizontal Vestibulo-Ocular Reflex of the Alert Rhesus Monkey.* Doctoral Thesis, University of Pennsylvania, Philadelphia, 1979.
5. Furman, J. M., O'Leary, D. P., and Wolfe, J. W., Application of linear system analysis to the horizontal vestibulo-ocular reflex of the alert rhesus monkey using pseudorandom binary sequence and single frequency sinusoidal stimulation. *Biol. Cybernet.*, 1979, **33**:159–165.
6. Furman, J. M., O'Leary, D. P., and Wolfe, J. W., Changes in the horizontal vestibulo-ocular reflex of the rhesus monkey with behavioral and pharmacological alerting, *Brain Res.*, 1981, **206**:490–494.
7. O'Leary, D. P., Dunn, R. F., and Honrubia, V., Analysis of afferent responses from isolated semicircular canal of the guitarfish using rotational acceleration white-noise inputs. *J. Neurophysiol.*, 1976, **39**:631–659.
8. Robinson, D. A., Vestibular and optokinetic symbiosis: An example of explaining by modeling. In: *Control of Gaze by Brain Stem Neurons, Developments in Neuroscience* (R. Baker and A. Berthoz, eds.). Am. Elsevier, New York, 1977:49–58.
9. Wall, C., O'Leary, D. P., and Black, F. O., System analysis of vestibulo-ocular system response using white noise rotational stimuli. In: *Vestibular Mechanisms in Health and Disease* (J. D. Hood, ed.). Academic Press, New York, 1978:157–166.
10. Wolfe, J. W., Engelken, E. J., and Olson, J. E., Use of rotatory test in the evaluation of patients with peripheral labyrinthine disorders. (*This volume.*)
11. Wall, C. W., Black, F. O., and O'Leary, D. P., Clinical use Pseudorandom Binary sequence white noise in assessment of the human vestibulo-ocular system. *Ann. Otol. Rhino. Laryngol.*, 1978, **87**(6):845–852.

The Correlation between Motion Sensation, Nystagmus, and Activity in the Vestibular Nerve and Nuclei

V. HENN

Department of Neurology
University of Zürich
Zürich, Switzerland

INTRODUCTION

Research in recent years has concentrated on the functional linkage of the neurons that constitute the vestibulooocular reflex (VOR). This has been complemented by detailed investigations of vestibular nystagmus in different planes of acceleration and its interaction with the visual system. Out of this work have evolved new concepts which have led to the formulation of functional models [for general review, see Henn *et al.* (16)]. The clinician, however, is still faced with the same problem: The patient complains of dizziness. Clinical tests of the vestibular system usually rely on the detection of pathological forms of nystagmus. These clinical signs are then used to localize the pathology. Therefore, it is necessary to know what the correspondence is between activity in the neuronal elements of the VOR, the direction and strength of nystagmus, sensation of motion, and its possible relation to motion sickness or dizziness. It will be shown that under normal physiological conditions these parameters can be widely dissociated.

METHODS

In human beings, eye position was measured with dc oculography, and subjective position or velocity was determined by rotating a handle fixed to the shaft of a potentiometer. Each full turn of the potentiometer corresponds to 360 deg subjective rotation. Animals and human beings were tested on servo-controlled turntables completely enclosed by an optokinetic drum that could be driven separately.

Techniques for single-unit recordings from the brainstem of alert monkeys are now standard and are basically similar in many laboratories [for details, see Waespe and Henn (27)]. Most data discussed below were obtained from chronically prepared alert

NYSTAGMUS AND VERTIGO: CLINICAL
APPROACHES TO THE PATIENT WITH DIZZINESS

rhesus monkeys. Horizontal and vertical eye positions were measured with dc electrodes implanted around the bony orbit, and single units were recorded with stereotaxically advanced tungsten microelectrodes.

ANGULAR ACCELERATION IN DARKNESS

If a monkey is exposed to a step of angular acceleration, the behavior of first-order vestibular units in the nerve as well as units in the vestibular nuclei can be recorded together with the nystagmus. An example of a vestibular nerve unit is given in Figure 1. The monkey is in total darkness and is accelerated by 40 deg/sec^2 to a constant angular velocity of 160 deg/sec. After 60 sec the monkey is decelerated. Unit activity initially builds up and reaches a peak near the end of the acceleration. Then, during the constant-velocity period, activity falls with a time constant of 5 to 6 sec. The time constant can be measured by setting the peak activity at the end of the acceleration at 100%. The amount of time it takes until activity has fallen to 37% is a measure of the time constant. It was found that *all* vestibular nerve fibers have very similar time constants of about 6 sec, although nystagmus always has a longer time constant; i.e., its decay is slower and its overall duration longer (4). This is also true of recordings from the nerve in the anesthetized squirrel monkey, in which more detailed studies have been done (11–13). Specifically, no difference was found in the time constants of neurons innervating the horizontal and vertical canals.

Recordings in central vestibular neurons show a very different picture. Time constants of vestibular nucleus neurons in alert animals are always longer than those of the nerve, and they normally correspond closely to the time constant of nystagmus. Figure 2 gives an example. The monkey was accelerated to a constant velocity of 40 deg/sec. Maximum activation or inhibition occurs at the end of acceleration, which is similar to the situation shown in Figure 1 for the peripheral neuron. However, in contrast to the behavior of the nerve, activity in this and all other central neurons returns to baseline level over a longer period of time parallel to the decline of nystagmus. Therefore, one decisive part of information processing between the first-order neuron in the nerve and second-order neurons in the nuclei is that time constants are prolonged (6). This is lost during anesthesia and was therefore not observed in experiments described in the older literature.

In human subjects two parameters can be measured during steps of angular veloc-

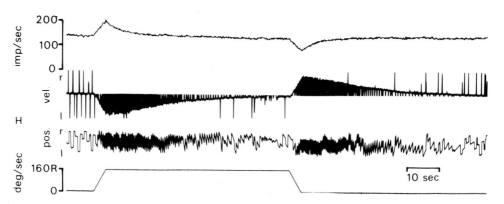

Figure 1. Vestibular nerve activity and nystagmus during angular acceleration of a monkey (4). From top: activity of single nerve fiber, horizontal eye velocity, horizontal eye position, and turntable velocity.

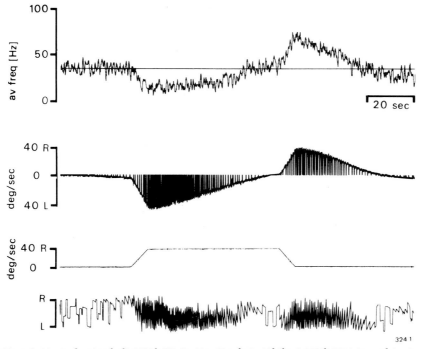

Figure 2. Activity of a vestibular nucleus neuron together with horizontal nystagmus during angular acceleration in the dark. From top: running average (over 250 msec) of unit activity, horizontal eye velocity, turntable velocity, and horizontal eye position. Occasionally, the modulation into the inhibitory direction is less than that into the excitatory direction, as in this neuron.

ity: nystagmus and subjective motion sensation. Figure 3 gives an example. After a step of angular velocity, nystagmus buildup and decline are the same in monkeys as in human subjects. Subjective motion sensation indicated by the human subject is also similar to nystagmus, although its time constant is usually slightly shorter.

Since the introduction of rotation tests for the evaluation of the vestibular system it has been noted that the duration of nystagmus can differ widely among normal subjects (22). This has been ascribed to habituation: Repeated exposure to the same vestibular stimulus can lead to a shortening of the duration of nystagmus and subjective motion sensation [recent reviews (8, 19)]. If one uses stimuli whose velocity changes with a sinusoidal profile, only frequencies below 0.1 Hz, i.e., periods longer than 10 sec, are effective (2, 18). Therefore, there exists no *single* normal value for the nystagmus time constant or, likewise, for the frequently used clinical measure of nystagmus duration. Instead, there is a wide range of normal values. The time constant of the peripheral nerve, which is 5 to 6 sec in the monkey and probably about 2 sec longer in human beings, is likely to constitute a lower limit below which the vestibular nystagmus time constant cannot fall. The largest time constants that we have measured in experimentally naive monkeys are 50 to 90 sec. Values outside this range have not been found in a series of 65 monkeys. If, during repeated testing of patients, time constants change, it must therefore be determined whether this might be an effect of habituation or the effect of a developing pathology.

In conclusion, during angular rotation about a vertical axis in total darkness, there is a close correlation between central vestibular unit activity, nystagmus, and motion

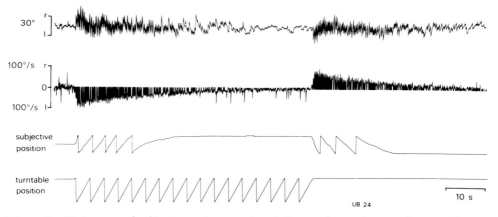

Figure 3. Nystagmus and subjective motion sensation during angular acceleration of a normal human subject in darkness. From top: horizontal eye position, horizontal eye velocity, subjective position, and turntable position. Turntable and subjective positions are measured with potentiometers that are reset at every full turn.

sensation, although motion sensation usually has a somewhat shorter duration. During such a stimulation, the canals—for practical purposes usually the horizontal canals—are exclusively stimulated. In normal subjects the wide range of time constants that can be observed depends on central factors and cannot be attributed to mechanical factors of the cupula or to different pressure gradients across it. Therefore, the earlier interpretations given within the framework of cupulometry should be reevaluated (15, 24).

OPTOKINETIC NYSTAGMUS

Optokinetic stimulation leads to nystagmus, which in the monkey can reach velocities of more than 160 deg/sec (7). In human beings the gain is usually below unity even at a stimulus velocity of 60 deg/sec. With stimulus velocities of up to 200 deg/sec, nystagmus velocity still increases, but gain progressively falls. Recordings in the vestibular nerve of monkeys never revealed any influence of a visual stimulus on unit activity (4, 21). Central vestibular units, however, do show a direction-specific modulation (9, 17). Unit activity increases in parallel with stimulus velocity, and therefore nystagmus velocity, up to 60 deg/sec on average (27). At higher stimulus velocities neuronal activation saturates, whereas nystagmus velocity still rises. Measurements in human beings show that nystagmus velocity and circular vection (the sensation of visually induced self-motion) can also rise to much higher values. This is an example of dissociation of unit activity in the vestibular nuclei and nystagmus velocity. It also shows that structures other than the vestibular nuclei are necessary to generate the high-velocity optokinetic response. The current hypothesis is that this is mediated by the flocculi (26).

By concentrating on a fixation point during full-field optokinetic stimulation, human beings can readily suppress all nystagmus but still have the full sensation of circular vection (3). Monkeys can be trained to suppress nystagmus. If unit activity is recorded in the vestibular nuclei during suppression of optokinetic nystagmus, it rises to a level that is not as high as that during nystagmus. This is an example of a visual stimulus influencing activity in the vestibular nuclei but simultaneously having no effect on vestibular nerve activity or nystagmus (5).

Visual-Vestibular Stimulation

Rotation of the animal or human subject inside the stationary illuminated optokinetic drum most closely mimics the natural condition, except that in our experiments all movements are passive rather than active. In the monkey, during acceleration, visual and vestibular inputs then combine to generate activity in the vestibular nuclei which is proportional to actual velocity independent of the value or duration of acceleration (29). Similarly, nystagmus velocity is unity (30). In human beings, nystagmus as well as subjective velocity sensation also reflects actual rotational velocity.

Vestibular Stimulation with Visual Fixation

Under natural conditions, during a goal-directed combined eye–head movement, vestibular stimulation occurs, but the VOR has to be suppressed. In the laboratory, a monkey can be trained to fixate continuously on a spot of light while being accelerated. That is, the monkey experiences a vestibular stimulus but suppresses the accompanying eye movements if a fixation light rotates with him in an otherwise dark environment. During the acceleration period, central vestibular unit activity is unchanged when compared to stimulation without fixation, but during the constant-velocity rotation the time constant of unit activity is shortened (5). Subjectively, during the acceleration period, the sensation of motion remains about equal to that during vestibular stimulation in total darkness.

Conflicting Visual-Vestibular Stimulation

For this paradigm the turntable and surrounding optokinetic drum are mechanically fixed together. During acceleration in the light, for the human subject, a literally nauseating conflict results: The vestibular end-organ measures and centrally transmits an acceleration signal, whereas the visual system cannot detect any visual displacement. Depending on the duration of such a stimulus, both human beings and monkeys suppress their nystagmus with accelerations up to 100 deg/sec (25). Vestibular nucleus activity shows changes in two respects: The decay time constant of unit activity falls to a value of about 6 sec, i.e., to a value that is similar to that of the peripheral nerve, and neuronal activation is attenuated, especially at low accelerations (28).

For human beings, motion sensation is attenuated in a similar fashion. At low accelerations, the vestibular signal might be totally canceled by the visual input, whereas at higher accelerations the attenuation is only small (25). These effects become more complicated if nystagmus cannot be completely suppressed. A vestibularly induced eye movement within a fixed visual field environment is often perceived as jitter or instability of the visual frame, which might then be interpreted as self-motion.

In conclusion, at accelerations below 5 deg/sec^2 central vestibular activity can be suppressed to such an extent that neither nystagmus nor motion sensation occurs, although there is appropriate activation in the vestibular nerve.

Vestibular Stimulation in Monkeys with Gaze Palsy

In some of the above-described experiments it was shown how suppression of nystagmus affects activity in the vestibular nuclei. The question therefore arises regarding the extent to which the occurrence of nystagmus itself feeds back and determines vestibular nucleus activity. To test this paradigm, unit activity and eye

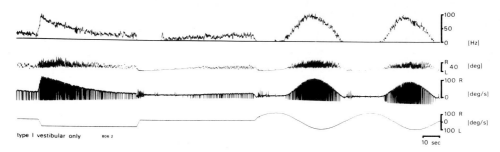

Figure 4. Single-unit recording from the vestibular nuclei in a monkey with a gaze palsy to the right. From top: running average of unit activity, horizontal eye position, horizontal eye velocity, and turntable velocity. The monkey is in the dark and exhibits spontaneous nystagmus to the left (far left in the figure). During acceleration and constant-velocity rotation to the left, there is activation of the unit and nystagmus as expected. During deceleration, unit activity is inhibited. The time it takes until the level of spontaneous activity is reached is similar both for the inhibitory and for the excitatory direction. The same applies to nystagmus. During sinusoidal rotation, there is symmetric unit activation and inhibition, but nystagmus occurs in only one direction.

movements were measured in monkeys with a unilateral gaze palsy. The gaze palsy was induced by an electrolytic or chemical lesion in the paramedian pontine retincular formation on one side (20). These monkeys then exhibited a total gaze palsy toward the ipsilateral side. Vestibular nucleus activity recorded on both sides of the brainstem remained symmetric with large time constants similar to those in normal monkeys (Figure 4). This shows that the occurrence of nystagmus itself is not the parameter that interacts with activity in the vestibular nuclei. Rather it is the combination of visual-vestibular stimuli that leads on the one hand to changes in vestibular nucleus activation and at the same time to partial or total suppression of nystagmus.

This also makes it plausible that one can estimate central vestibular time constants by using the parameter of motion sensation if eye movements cannot be measured in patients with gaze palsy or other peripheral oculomotor disorders.

ROTATION WITH ROTATING GRAVITY VECTORS

Vestibular tests are usually done in such a way as to test selectively one subsystem only, e.g., horizontal canals on the Bárány chair, the otoliths in positional maneuvers, or one labyrinth as in caloric tests. However, these tests cannot predict the performance of the system with more complex stimuli. One such stimulus is rotation about an off-vertical axis. If the rotation axis is tilted away from the vertical to 90 deg, i.e., into a horizontal orientation, this is also commonly described as "barbeque spit" rotation. With a velocity step, the initial nystagmus induced by the canals does not decline but continues as long as the rotation lasts. During deceleration, nystagmus declines with little or no postrotatory nystagmus. These effects already come into play with the rotation axis tilted by only 5 to 10 deg and reach a maximum with a tilt angle of 30 deg (1, 23, 31). Such persisting nystagmus can be observed whenever a rotating gravity vector is present, i.e., a continuous reorientation of the human subject or the animal toward gravity. Therefore, these phenomena can be observed whenever the rotation axis is not purely vertical, which besides "barbeque spit" rotation includes tumbling or somersaulting (Figure 5).

The mechanism that is responsible for the continuing nystagmus was recently clarified with recordings from semicircular canal and otolith afferents during off-

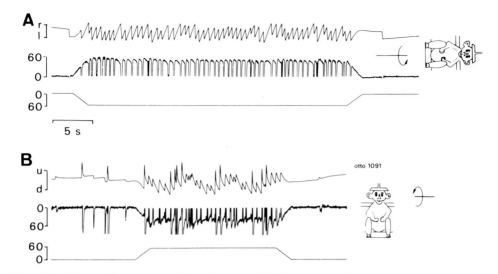

Figure 5. Off-vertical axis rotation of a monkey in total darkness. (A) "Barbeque spit" rotation; (B) somersaulting. From top: horizontal (A) or vertical (B) eye position, eye velocity, and turntable velocity. Note that nystagmus velocity represents actual head velocity during the whole period of rotation, which was done in complete darkness. During deceleration, nystagmus velocity declines to zero without any afternystagmus.

vertical axis rotation (14). Otolith afferents exhibited a sinusoidal modulation with each revolution. From this signal a head velocity signal had to be reconstructed centrally, since semicircular canal afferents showed no specific modulation.

CONCLUSION

The vestibular system seems to be the only sensory system whose dysfunction is routinely tested simply by observing a reflex motor response, i.e., nystagmus. Vestibular research has concentrated for a long time on the three-neuron reflex arc. In clinical practice, this reflex arc, in its pure form, is actually tested only if passive head movements or calorics are performed in a comatose patient. In all other cases, when nystagmus occurs, many more than just the three neurons, and many more pathways than the medial longitudinal fasciculus, are involved.

Only in the vestibular laboratory are the labyrinths exposed either to unilateral stimulation, as in caloric testing, or to selective stimulation of one pair of peripheral receptors. As pointed out above, the activities from the different sensory systems do not simply summate. Rather, peripheral inputs combine and are used to reconstruct a head velocity signal. The neuronal mechanism of this process has not been worked out. Therefore, the pathology connected with it cannot be predicted by testing single receptor systems.

We have discussed two basic paradigms of the way in which the vestibular system uses information, other than that from the semicircular canals, to reconstruct a head velocity signal. One is the use of visually mediated motion information. The other is the use of input from the otoliths, by which the vestibular system itself reconstructs a head velocity signal, if the rotation axis is not exactly vertical.

A situation can exist in which activity in the vestibular nerve is present, but there is no activity in central vestibular structures, no nystagmus, and no subjective motion sensation. This can occur during conflicting visual-vestibular stimulation. Suppression of optokinetic nystagmus leads to central activation without nystagmus. Finally, there can be high-velocity optokinetic nystagmus without sufficient activity in the vestibular nuclei to drive the eyes at such high velocity. These examples were chosen to demonstrate that, even under normal physiological conditions, activity in the nerve and central vestibular structures, nystagmus, and subjective motion sensation can differ widely. Therefore, the vestibular nuclei constitute only part of the central vestibular system, which must include the flocculi (see Zee, this volume) and probably other structures in the brainstem as well.

The vestibular system plays a complex role: It is the first central relay station of a sensory organ that indicates linear and angular acceleration or velocity. It also triggers motor reflex responses. For convenience of testing, nystagmus has generally been measured, but eye movements are also elicited and controlled by the visual system. This input is powerful enough that it can usually override vestibular input. Especially during goal-directed movements, when eyes and head together are turned toward a target, the VOR has to be suppressed. If patients cannot suppress such vestibularly induced nystagmus, they might complain of dizziness. Therefore, for clinical pupposes, it seems to be just as important to test not only whether nystagmus can be normally elicited, but also the extent to which it can be suppressed (10, 32). It is important that we sense active or passive head movements independent of eye movements or vestibulospinal reflexes that can be triggered with them. This way of thinking makes it easier to understand why a vestibular signal should still be relayed centrally even when all eye movements are suppressed.

All the animal experiments and measurements in human beings described above were carried out in normal subjects under physiological conditions with the exception of the animals with a gaze palsy. Whenever stimuli became more complex and involved more than the exclusive stimulation of the horizontal canals, complex relationships between activity in the vestibular nerve and nuclei, nystagmus, and subjective motion sensation evolved. These factors should be kept in mind if a patient complains about pathological forms of motion sensation or dizziness, yet no pathological nystagmus can be detected with standard testing methods.

SUMMARY

Single-unit recordings and nystagmus measurements were carried out in chronically prepared alert rhesus monkeys. In human beings nystagmus and subjective motion sensation were measured. Only during rotation about a vertical axis in darkness could a close correlation between single-unit activity, nystagmus, and motion sensation be established. Some dissociation became evident in most other paradigms: optokinetic nystagmus, visually suppressed vestibular nystagmus, and rotation about off-vertical axes.

REFERENCES

1. Benson, A. J., Modification of the response to angular accelerations by linear accelerations. In: *Handbook of Sensory Physiology* (H. H. Kornhuber, ed.). Springer-Verlag, Berlin and New York, 1974:6(2):281–320.
2. Blair, S., and Gavin, M., Response of the vestibulo-ocular reflex to differing programs of acceleration. *Invest. Ophthalmol.*, 1979, **18**:1086–1090.

3. Brandt, T., Dichgans, J., and Koenig, E., Differential effects of central versus peripheral vision on egocentric and exocentric motion perception. *Exp. Brain Res.*, 1973, **16**:476–491.
4. Büttner, U., and Waespe, W., Vestibular nerve activity in the alert monkey during vestibular and optokinetic nystagmus. *Exp. Brain Res.*, 1981, **41**:310–315.
5. Buettner, U. W., and Büttner, U., Vestibular nuclei activity in the alert monkey during suppression of vestibular and optokinetic nystagmus. *Exp. Brain Res.*, 1979, **37**:581–593.
6. Buettner, U. W., Büttner, U., and Henn, V., Transfer characteristics of neurons in vestibular nuclei of the alert monkey. *J. Neurophysiol.*, 1978, **41**:1614–1628.
7. Cohen, B., Matsuo, V., and Raphan, T., Quantitative analysis of the velocity characteristics of optokinetic nystagmus and optokinetic after-nystagmus. *J. Physiol. (London)*, 1977, **270**:321–344.
8. Collins, W. E., Habituation of vestibular responses with and without visual stimulation. In: *Handbook of Sensory Physiology* (H. H. Kornhuber, ed.), Springer-Verlag, Berlin and New York, 1974:6(2):369–388.
9. Dichgans, J., Schmidt, C. L., and Graf, W., Visual input improves the speedometer of the vestibular nuclei in the goldfish. *Exp. Brain Res.*, 1973, **18**:319–322.
10. Dichgans, J., von Reutern, G. M., and Rommelt, U., Impaired suppression of vestibular nystagmus by fixation in cerebellar and non-cerebellar patients. *Arch. Psychiatr. Nervenkr.*, 1978, **266**:183–199.
11. Fernández, C., and Goldberg, J. M., Physiology of peripheral neurons innervating semicircular canals of the squirrel monkey. II. Response to sinusoidal stimulation and dynamics of peripheral vestibular system. *J. Neurophysiol.*, 1971, **34**:661–675.
12. Goldberg, J. M., and Fernández, C., Physiology of peripheral neurons innervating semicircular canals of the squirrel monkey. I. Resting discharge and response to constant angular accelerations. *J. Neurophysiol.*, 1971, **34**:635–660
13. Goldberg, J. M., and Fernández, C., Physiology of peripheral neurons innervating semicircular canals of the squirrel monkey. III. Variations among units in their discharge properties. *J. Neurophysiol.*, 1971, **34**:676–684.
14. Goldberg, J. M., and Fernández, C., Responses to constant rotations about earth-horizontal axes in the squirrel monkey. *Ann. N.Y. Acad. Sci.*, 1981, **374**:40–43.
15. Groen, J. J., Cupulometry. *Laryngoscope*, 1957, **67**:894–905.
16. Henn, V., Cohen, B., and Young, L. R., Visual-vestibular interaction in motion perception and the generation of nystagmus. *Neurosci. Res. Program Bull.*, 1980, **18**:457–651.
17. Henn, V., Young, L. R., and Finley, C., Vestibular nucleus units in alert monkeys are also influenced by moving visual fields. *Brain Res.*, 1974, **71**:144–149.
18. Jaeger, J., and Henn, V., Habituation of the vestibulo-ocular reflex (VOR) in the monkey during sinusoidal rotation in the dark. *Exp. Brain Res.*, 1981, **41**:108–114.
19. Jaeger, J., and Henn, V., Vestibular habituation in man and monkey during sinusoidal rotation. *Ann. N.Y. Acad. Sci.*, 1981, **374**:330–339.
20. Jaeger, J., Henn, V., Lang, W., Miles, T. S., and Waespe, W., Vestibular unit activity in monkeys with horizontal gaze palsy. In: *Progress in Oculomotor Research* (A. Fuchs and W. Becker, eds.). Elsevier/North Holland, Amsterdam, 1981, 89–95.
21. Keller, E. L., Behavior of horizontal semicircular canal afferents in alert monkey during vestibular and optokinetic stimulation. *Exp. Brain Res.*, 1976, **24**:459–471.
22. Mowrer, O. H., The modification of vestibular nystagmus by means of repeated elicitation. *Comp. Psychol. Monogr.*, 1934, **9**:1–48.
23. Raphan, T., Cohen, B., and Henn, V., Effects of gravity on rotatory nystagmus in monkeys. *Ann. N.Y. Acad. Sci.*, 1981, **374**:44–55.
24. van Egmond, A. A. J., Groen, J. J., and Jongkees, L. B. W., The mechanics of the semicircular canals. *J. Physiol. (London)*, 1949, **110**:1–17.
25. Waespe, B., Waespe, W., and Henn, V., Subjective velocity estimation during conflicting visual-vestibular stimulation. *Arch. Psychiatr. Nervenkr.*, 1980, **228**:109–116.
26. Waespe, W., Büttner, U., and Henn, V., Input-output activity of the primate flocculus during visual-vestibular interaction. *Ann. N.Y. Acad. Sci.*, 1981, **374**:491–503.
27. Waespe, W., and Henn, V., Neuronal activity in the vestibular nuclei of the alert monkey during vestibular and optokinetic stimulation. *Exp. Brain Res.*, 1977, **27**:523–538.
28. Waespe, W., and Henn, V., Conflicting visual-vestibular stimulation and vestibular nucleus activity in alert monkeys. *Exp. Brain Res.*, 1978, **33**:203–211.

29. Waespe, W., and Henn, V., The velocity response of vestibular nucleus neurons during vestibular, visual, and combined angular acceleration. *Exp. Brain Res.*, 1979, **37**:337–347.

30. Waespe, W., Henn, V., and Isoviita, V., Nystagmus slow-phase velocity during vestibular, optokinetic, and combined stimulation in the monkey. *Arch. Psychiatr. Nervenkr.*, 1980, **228**:275–286.

31. Young, L. R., and Henn, V., Nystagmus produced by pitch and yaw rotation of monkeys about non-vertical axes. *Fortschr. Zool.*, 1975, **23**:235–246.

32. Zee, D. S., Suppression of vestibular nystagmus. *Ann. Neurol.*, 1977, **1**:207.

ROUTINE CLINICAL EVALUATION OF PATIENTS WITH PERIPHERAL LABYRINTHINE DISORDERS

A Report from Japan on the Routine Clinical Evaluation of Patients with Vestibular Disorders

JUN-ICHI SUZUKI

Department of Otolaryngology
Teikyo University School of Medicine
Itabashi-ku, Tokyo 173, Japan

Introduction

In 1957, the Japan Society for Vestibular Research was founded in Kyoto. The introduction of electronystagmography (ENG) into clinical use then followed. This technique has greatly facilitated both basic and clinical research in Japan, just as it has in the Americas and in Europe.

In 1965, an international symposium on oculomotor and vestibular systems was organized by Professor Kirikae in Tokyo (6). In 1975, the fifth extraordinary meeting of the Bárány Society was held in Kyoto and was chaired by Professor Morimoto (8). These international meetings have given us direct contact with colleagues from other countries and have encouraged our research activities.

In 1968, the Japan Society for Vestibular Research expanded to become the Japan Society for Equilibrium Research. This change reflected the shift from emphasis on the labyrinthine end organs to wider neurotological and oculomotor aspects. The new society developed standards of qualification for the nomination and acceptance of "active members," of whom there were 83 in 1979. The active members are expected to contribute to the elevation of academic and professional standards of the society and to promote research in this field.

The present report concerns our approach to vestibular examinations in Japan with emphasis on the aspects that may be especially characteristic of our country. The report is limited to the clinical tests that have originated or been further developed in Japan and at the same time have found wide acceptance and proved useful for diagnostic purposes.

NYSTAGMUS AND VERTIGO: CLINICAL
APPROACHES TO THE PATIENT WITH DIZZINESS

OBSERVATION AND EVALUATION OF SPONTANEOUS NYSTAGMUS WITH AND WITHOUT FRENZEL GLASSES

The clinical significance of the identification of spontaneous nystagmus need not be reemphasized. To observe vestibular nystagmus in particular, Frenzel glasses are convenient and even indispensable (7). Nystagmus that is more active without Frenzel glasses must be due to disturbances of the mechanism for fixation to the foveal image, whereas nystagmus that is clearer with Frenzel glasses is due to an imbalance of the vestibular system. Thus, spontaneous nystagmus should be tested both with and without Frenzel glasses.

The Frenzel glasses that are widely used in Japan have large lenses, 5 cm in diameter (Figure 1), enabling two or more persons to observe simultaneously, which is valuable for both clinical and teaching purposes.

OBSERVATION AND EVALUATION OF POSITIONAL AND POSITIONING NYSTAGMUS WITH FRENZEL GLASSES

It is widely accepted in Japan that observation and evaluation of positional and positioning nystagmus comprise one of the most informative clinical tests for the diagnosis of vestibular disorders (9, 17). Observation is carefully made behind Frenzel glasses. Characteristics of nystagmus, such as amplitude, frequency, direction, rotation component, position effect, and positioning effect, are carefully described.

The existence of spontaneous or positional nystagmus, even of small amplitude, may be regarded as pathological. Identification of the character of the nystagmus may help to localize lesions in the labyrinth. Each of the three semicircular canals has the capacity to produce specific nystagmus (11), whereas the otolithic organs appear to produce a greater variety of nystagmus. Careful observation can thus correlate a spontaneous nystagmus with a specific end organ in the labyrinth (Figure 2).

The direction-changing type of positional nystagmus can originate either from the

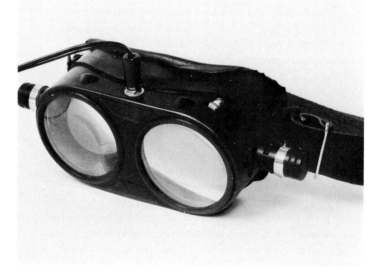

Figure 1. Frenzel glasses with large lenses.

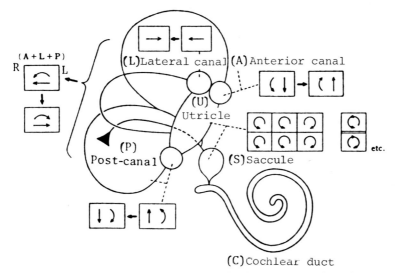

Figure 2.   Diagram of spontaneous nystagmus from localized lesions in the labyrinth. Spontaneous nystagmus from the right lateral canal is directed to the right (irritated state) and then to the left (paralytic state), as shown here: → ← ← Spontaneous nystagmus from other canals is shown in a similar fashion. When the three canals on the right side are involved, the induced nystagmus is horizontal, rotating to the right and then to the left. Nystagmus from the otolithic organs is mainly rotating and direction-changing, depending on positions and positionings.

labyrinth or from the central nervous system. For example, after almost every stapes operation, positional nystagmus of varying intensity, which is frequently direction-changing, appears. There have been discussions on the origin and mechanism of alcohol-induced positional nystagmus, which is direction-changing. It is accepted, however, that healthy labyrinths are necessary for this condition to appear.

EXAMINATION OF OPTOKINETIC NYSTAGMUS: OPTOKINETIC PATTERN TEST AND COMPUTERIZED OPTOKINETIC NYSTAGMUS EVALUATION

Optokinetic nystagmus (OKN) is especially useful for differentiating peripheral and central lesions. In 1962, an optokinetic pattern (OKP) test was reported by the authors (12). This is widely used in Japan as one of the most convenient clinical tests. In this test, an Ohm-type drum is used, and the rotation is constantly accelerated from 0 to approximately 150 deg/sec and then to 0 deg/sec at an acceleration of ± V4 deg/sec². The velocity of induced OKN is recorded with a slow chart speed of 1 mm/sec. The eye speed recording is thus condensed on the chart and forms a characteristic pattern, which is utilized for diagnostic assessment (Figure 3). As demonstrated, typical patterns from lesions in the peripheral and central systems can be easily distinguished. Recent investigations on OKP's from cortical lesions have revealed responsible areas in both the parietal and occipital lobes. These results will be reported in a separate paper.

Another important approach to OKN is the use of computers. Tokita *et al.* (16) reported on this in Japan in 1975. It has been shown to be useful, particularly since it provides digitalized data that can be used for an objective analysis of the results. We expect that the computerized OKN test will become more popular, especially when less expensive hardware and less complicated software are available.

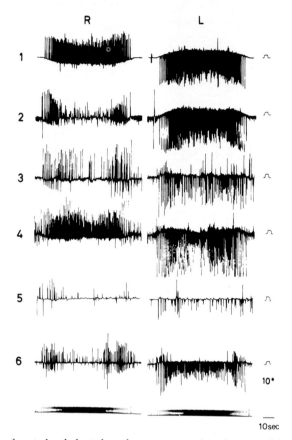

Figure 3.   Normal and typical pathological optokinetic patterns (OKP). A pair of the OKP's (right and left) from a normal subject (1), right Ménière's disease (2), right acoustic tumor (3), right Wallenberg syndrome (4), pons glioma (5), and cerebellar degeneration (6). The letter "R" indicates the OKP from clockwise drum rotation and "L," the OKP from counterclockwise rotation. The trace at the bottom is a recording of the stripes of the drum, indicating acceleratory and deceleratory drum rotation. Calibrations are for an eye speed of 10 deg/sec and for a chart feeding speed of 1 cm per 10 sec.

Eye Tracking Test: Linear and Circular Tracking Tests

Electronystagmographic recording of eye tracking is one of the simplest and most useful tests for differentiating peripheral and central lesions. Uyeda (19) first de-scribed this in 1967 in Japan.

In 1975, Umeda reported on the test procedure using a revolving target—in other words, a target that moves in a circular path (18). In addition to being convenient for simultaneous recording of both horizontal and vertical eye tracking motions, recordings by this method have fewer blink artifacts than do those with a target oscillating in a linear path.

Quantitative Evaluation of Caloric Nystagmus: Simple Calorimetry and the Visual Suppression Test

In Japan, the alternating bithermal test, or microcalorimetry, is not as popular as it was 15 years ago. In most institutions and clinics, simpler methods of cold calorimetry are usually applied. The interpretation of results obtained from the simple caloric test, therefore, is somewhat limited. However, caloric tests are at least semiquantitative, and their significance is that they can evaluate only one lateral canal.

Aside from the caloric test, which is useful in evaluating the responsiveness of the lateral canal, a so-called visual suppression test has proved to be a valuable method for localizing lesions in some parts of the brainstem and the flocculus (14). Electronystagmographically, a simplified eye speed recording system is used to measure the suppression of caloric nystagmus by visual stimulation (13) (Figure 4).

VERTICAL WRITING AND STEPPING TESTS

A vertical writing test and a stepping test are used to evaluate vestibular deviation (1). The writing test is based on the fact that Japanese is often written in vertical columns rather than in horizontal lines and the columns may deviate to the right or to the left in some equilibrium disorders (Figure 5). Since, however, the arms are largely under voluntary control, the test results are not always consistent; that is, they do not always indicate vestibular asymmetry. The writing test is believed to be more useful for detecting neurological conditions, such as cerebellar ataxia.

The stepping test (?) has received a similar evaluation from vestibular clinicians. Accordingly, the test may not be reliable clinically for showing slight lateral deviations, but it may be more useful for detecting ataxia. It is noted, however, that a

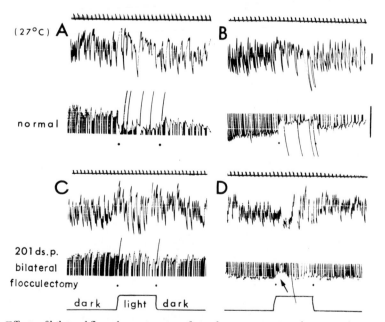

Figure 4. Effects of bilateral flocculus extirpation of visual suppression in a rhesus monkey. (A, C) Caloric nystagmus induced to the left by stimulation of the right ear with cold water (27°C). (B, D) Nystagmus induced to the right by stimulation of the left ear with cold water. (A, B) Normal visual suppression induced by the presence of fixation. (C, D) Decrease in visual suppression after bilateral flocculectomy. The top trace in each series is the time base; the second trace, the horizontal electrooculargraph (EOG). The bottom trace in A–D is the slow-phase velocity trace. Photocell recordings under C and D show the onset of light and darkness. Calibrations for the EOG traces in A–D are shown beside B and are 10 deg/sec for the EOG and 100 deg/sec for slow-phase velocity. Adapted from Takemori and Cohen (14).

Writing with
eyes open   Writing with eyes covered

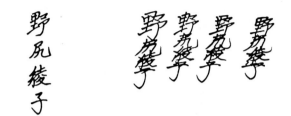

Figure 5.   Vertical writing in a case of the interval period of Ménière's disease. Left: A line of the patient's name written with the eyes open showing no deviation. Right: Four lines of the same letters written with the eyes covered, revealing left deviation in every case. From Fukuda (1) by permission.

staggering gait is closely related to the severity of vertiginous sensations. The stepping test still may not be dependable in some cases because it does not easily distinguish ataxia from other disturbances of gait as a result of malingering.

Computerized analysis of standing body sway is believed to be useful as a routine clinical test. In Japan, Tokita *et al.* reported on this in 1976 (15) and in 1981 as well (16). According to this report, the correlogram of sway of the center of gravity, especially if periodicity was demonstrated, had some correlation with the site of the lesion (Figure 6). The power spectrum of sway of the center of gravity—in other words, the distribution of frequencies—was also shown to be related to the site of the lesion.

ROTATION TESTS FOR CONGENITALLY DEAF CHILDREN

Rotation tests for clinical evaluation are no longer popular in Japan. In most institutions, they are used mainly for research purposes. A rotation test such as Bárány's using a simple chair may be very useful for the evaluation of labyrinthine responsivity in special cases such as that of congenitally deaf children (5).

Thus, the rotation test may be the only test by which evaluation of canal responses in patients with bilateral auditory atresia can be made. By means of this test, one can evaluate each of the three pairs of canals separately, corresponding to the three planes of rotation, by changing the position of the patient's head. In patients who have a unilaterally dead inner ear, single canal function can be evaluated by applying the above test procedures. Furthermore, patients who have disturbances of eye movements can be tested by observation of the response of vestibulospinal reflexes to rotation.

The clinical usefulness of rotation tests will be reevaluated when the tests are fully computerized.

INNER EAR ANESTHESIA IN DETECTING LABYRINTHINE LESIONS AND RESPONSIVITY

The normal inner ear can be easily anesthetized by the application of local anesthetics in the tympanic cavity through the eardrum. Lidocaine (2–4%) is effectively and safely used; the anesthetic condition usually disappears completely in 3 to 4 hours.

Long-lasting positional vertigo, for example, may arise from one or the other of the labyrinths, and this can be verified by applying inner ear anesthesia to the suspected side. The anesthetic may anesthetize both a vertigo-generating lesion and the end

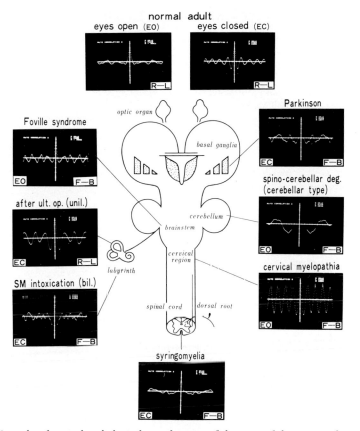

Figure 6. Normal and typical pathological correlograms of the sway of the center of gravity. Adapted from Tokita *et al.* (16).

organs. The former effect would suppress vertigo, but at the same time the latter would create new vertigo. In most instances, the latter effect does not last as long as the former. This procedure, then, can be useful for detecting a vertigo lesion or a tinnitus lesion in the labyrinth; the latter effect can be a test only for verifying the existence of functioning sensory portions in the labyrinth.

Thus, the test is used for two purposes: (1) to test pathological lesions in the labyrinth that generate vertigo or tinnitus and (b) to verify the existence of functioning vestibular end organs in the labyrinth (4, 10).

The effects of the anesthetic sometimes persist, and the original vertigo disappears. In other words, inner ear anesthesia can sometimes be therapeutic as well.

Furosemide Test for the Evaluation of Labyrinthine Conditions

The glycerol test for Ménière's disease is utilized to verify diagnosis. In 1975, Futaki and his colleagues (3) developed another test for Ménière's disease using furosemide, which has a different kind of diuretic action. According to the reports, furosemide produced an improved caloric response in cases of hydrops. This test may enable us to evaluate the vestibular component of the disease and the glycerol test, the cochlear component.

REFERENCES

1. Fukuda, T., Vertical writing with eyes covered: A new test of vestibulo-spinal reaction. *Acta Oto-Laryngol.*, 1959, **50**:26–36.
2. Fukuda, T., The stepping test: Two phases of the labyrinthine reflex. *Acta Oto-Laryngol.*, 1959, **50**:95–108.
3. Futaki, T., Kitahara, M., and Morimoto, M., A comparative study of the furosemide test and the glycerol test in patients with Ménière's disease. In: *Proceedings of the Fifth Extraordinary Meeting of the Bárány Society* (M. Morimoto, ed.). Bárány Society and Japan Society for Equilibrium Research, Kyoto, 1975:322–326.
4. Hughes, D. W., Yagi, T., and Suzuki, J.; Lidocaine depression of labyrinthine function. *Equilib. Res., Suppl.*, 1973:222–227.
5. Kaga, K., Suzuki, J. I., Marsh, R. R., and Tanaka, Y., Influence of labyrinthine hypoactivity on gross motor development of infants: Conference on vestibular and oculomotor physiology. *Ann. N.Y. Acad. Sci.*, 1981, **374**:412–420.
6. Kirikae, I., ed., *International Symposium on Vestibular and Oculomotor Problems*. Extraordinary Meeting of the Japan Society of Vestibular Research, Tokyo, 1965.
7. Kirikae, I., Suzuki, J., and Tokumasu, K., Spontaneous nystagmus as a sign of clinical significance. *Acta Oto-Laryngol.*, 1963, **179**:86–95.
8. Morimoto, M., ed., *Proceedings of the Fifth Extraordinary Meeting of the Bárány Society*. Bárány Society and Japan Society for Equilibrium Research, Kyoto, 1975.
9. Sakata, E., *Introduction to Clinical Neuro-otology*. Ishiyaku-shuppan, Tokyo, 1980 (in Japanese).
10. Suzuki, J., Inner ear anesthesia and inner ear surgery. *Clin. Physiol.* 1973, **3**:388–393 (in Japanese).
11. Suzuki, J., Cohen, B., and Bender, M. B., Compensatory eye movements induced by vertical semicircular canal stimulation. *Exp. Neurol.*, 1964, **9**:137–160.
12. Suzuki, J., and Komatsuzaki, A., Clinical application of optokinetic nystagmus-optokinetic pattern test. *Acta Oto-Laryngol.*, 1962, **51**:49–55.
13. Takemori, S., Visual suppression test. *Clin. Otolaryngol.*, 1978, **3**:145–153.
14. Takemori, S., and Cohen, B., Loss of visual suppression of vestibular nystagmus after flocculus lesions. *Brain Res.*, 1974, **72**:213–224.
15. Tokita, T., Maeda, M. and Miyata, H., The role of the labyrinth in standing posture regulation. *Acta Otolaryngol.*, 1981, **91**:521–527.
16. Tokita, T., Suzuki, T., Hibi, T., and Tomita, T., A quantitative test of optokinetic nystagmus and its data processing by computer. *Acta Oto-Laryngol., Suppl.*, 1975, **330**:159–168.
17. Uemura, T., Suzuki, J., Hozawa, J., and Highstein, S. M., *Neuro-otological Examination with Special Reference to Equilibrium Function Tests*. Igaku Shoin, Tokyo, 1977.
18. Umeda, Y., The standardization of eye-tracking test. *Ann. Otol., Rhinol., Laryngol., Suppl.*, 1980, **71**:7–12.
19. Uyeda, R., Eye tracking test in labyrinthine, cerebellar and brainstem lesions. *Pract. Otol. (Kyoto)*, 1967, **60**:918–925.

A Report from Europe

W. J. OOSTERVELD

E.N.T. Clinic, Wilhelmina Gasthuis
Amsterdam, The Netherlands

Introduction

Until recently, electronystagmography (ENG) was concerned mainly with the diagnosis of peripheral vestibular disorders. However, the increasing sophistication of the vestibular tests opened possibilities for detecting disorders of the central nervous system as well. This means that a larger variety of neurological disorders are found in the records of centers for vestibulometry. This fact immediately raises the question of whether the whole area of vestibulometry belongs to otorhinolaryngology or to neurology. Historic lines connect it to otorhinolaryngology, but, in general, the interest of neurologists in vestibulometry is gradually increasing, whereas that of many otologists is on the decline. In addition, since electroencephalography is becoming less prominent, clinical neurophysiologists are anxious to find new fields of interest.

It appears that in many European countries vestibular examinations with the aid of ENG are usually conducted in special centers, large hospitals, and university clinics. In The Netherlands the financial aspect plays an important role. Only recently have medical insurance companies agreed to pay for vestibular examinations done with the aid of ENG. However, the rather small amount of money paid for the time-consuming vestibular tests does not make this subspecialty very attractive to ear, nose, and throat physicians.

No large differences exist between American and European centers for vestibulometry. The equipment shows a rather high grade of standardization. However, clinical test programs differ among laboratories all over the world, although these differences are showing a tendency to decrease.

Vertigo

Vertigo is the sensation of movements that one knows do not actually exist. Vertigo is a symptom and not a disease; it is an illusion. In patients with vertigo one has to evaluate carefully what exactly is covered by this complaint, for sometimes signs that

NYSTAGMUS AND VERTIGO: CLINICAL
APPROACHES TO THE PATIENT WITH DIZZINESS

have nothing to do with vertigo, such as fear of height or claustrophobia, are labeled "vertigo."

Every vestibular laboratory has its own list of questions to ask of patients. These lists range from one to six pages and sometimes cover the entire field of internal medicine as well as that of neurology. Basically they have a similar framework, and the questions concern signs and symptoms in the fields of otology, neurology, ophthalmology, blood dynamics, metabolism, odontology, psychiatry, and toxicology.

Vertigo can be divided, according to its appearance, into five types: paroxysmal vertigo, chronic vertigo, vertigo with a sudden onset, positional vertigo, and dizziness spells. According to its origin, vertigo has three main sources: vestibular (central or peripheral), nonvestibular, and epileptic. By means of a questionnaire, the investigator is sometimes able to distinguish between the different origins. Signs and symptoms besides vertigo are of course very important. A loss of consciousness always points to a central lesion. The type of vertigo does not give decisive informa-

TABLE 1
CENTRAL VESTIBULAR VERTIGO

Diagnosis	Duration	Characteristics	Cause
Multiple sclerosis	Days to months	Positional vertigo and disturbance of equilibrium	Sclerotic patches in brain and spinal cord
Tumors fossa posterior	Minutes	Central positional vertigo, moderated	Pressure on brainstem
Apoplexia cerebelli	Weeks	Very acute, serious vertigo, accompanied by symptoms of cerebellar paralysis	Lesion arteria cerebelli
Acute vermis syndrome	Minutes to hours	Paroxysmal vertigo, vegetative symptoms, neurological disorders	Pressure on arteria vertebralis
Wallenberg's syndrome	Days to weeks	Acute rotatory vertigo with vegetative symptoms, homolateral paralysis of the palate, trigeminus paralysis, contralateral sensibility disturbance	Ischemia arteria cerebelli posterior inferior
Arteria cerebelli superior syndrome	Weeks	Acute vertigo, vegetative symptoms, cerebellar hemiataxia, hypotonia, intention tremor, disturbances in speech	Obstruction arteria cerebelli superior
Cerebral sclerosis	Long-lasting	Giddiness, unsteadiness, sway movements	Diminished cerebral blood flow
Arachnoiditis pontocerebellaris (Bárány syndrome)	Hours	Attacks of rotatory vertigo, occipital headache, vegetative symptoms, lesion of the n. vestibularis, n. cochlearis, n. trigeminus, n. abducens, n. facialis, and cerebellum	Arachnoiditis fossa posterior
Migraine equivalent	Hours	Vertigo by unilateral headache, vegetative symptoms	Migraine
Intoxication			
Barbiturates		Positional vertigo and positional nystagmus	Disinhibition
Alcohol		Positional vertigo and positional nystagmus	
Opiates		Vertical spontaneous nystagmus	

TABLE 2
PERIPHERAL VESTIBULAR VERTIGO

Diagnosis	Duration	Characteristics	Cause
Ménière's disease	Minutes to days	Irregular attacks of vertigo with tinnitus, hearing disorder, and vegetative symptoms	Endolymphatic hydrops
Labyrinthine vascular accident	Weeks	Sudden vertigo, with or without hearing disorder	Ischemia labyrinthii
Acute labyrinthitis	Days to weeks	Acute vertigo, vegetative symptoms, hearing impairment, and tinnitus	Otitis media
Serous labyrinthitis	Chronic	Rotatory vertigo	Chronic otitis media, sometimes fistula horizontal canal
Neuronitis vestibularis	Days to weeks	Acute rotatory vertigo, vegetative symptoms	Viral infection nervus vestibularis
Neuritis vestibularis	Days to weeks	Acute rotatory vertigo, vegetative symptoms, hearing disorder	Viral infection nervus octavus
Vestibular encephalitis	Days	Acute rotatory vertigo, vegetative symptoms, eye muscle disorders, pyramid track disorders	Viral infection
Herpes zoster oticus	Weeks	Rotatory vertigo, vegetative symptoms, earache, vesicular eruptions external ear canal and concha, sometimes paresis n facialis	Viral infection
Paroxysmal positional vertigo	Less than 30 sec	Positional vertigo	Disorder canal system
Childhood vertigo	Minutes	Paroxysmal vertigo in children up to 12 years, no vegetative symptoms, no hearing disorder	Unknown
Motion sickness	Days to weeks	Rotatory vertigo and vegetative symptoms	Linear accelerations, Coriolis effects

tion on the cause. Paroxysmal vertigo can be a sign of a peripheral vestibular disease such as Ménière's disease; however, a cerebellar infarction gives a similar attack, usually very severe. In the last case, vertigo contributes very little to the diagnosis because of other signs and symptoms. Vertigo appears as one symptom in many different diseases. An overview of these diseases is given in Tables 1–3.

TABLE 3
EPILEPTIC VERTIGO

Diagnosis	Duration	Characteristics	Cause
Temporal lobe epilepsy	Seconds	Acute attacks of vertigo, gastric aura, followed by diminished consciousness or unconsciousness	Focus temporal lobe
Vestibular epilepsy	Seconds	Absences, dizziness spells, no vestibular symptoms, EEG disturbances, nonprovokable	Focus gyrus temporalis superior
Vestibulogenic epilepsy	Minutes	Unconsciousness, dizziness spells, vestibular symptoms, no EEG disturbances, provokable	Low epileptic stimulation threshold

Vestibular Examination with the Use of Electronystagmography

Routinely, two electrodes are mounted beside the eyes at the canthae and one at the forehead. Horizontal eye movements are recorded for both eyes together. Only in cases in which central nervous system lesions are suspected are electrodes mounted on both sides of each eye. The main tests can be divided into static tests, dynamic tests, and oculomotor tests. These tests are outlined in the following tabulation:

Static tests
  1. Spontaneous nystagmus
  2. Positional nystagmus: supine, right lateral, left lateral, prone
  3. Cervical tests: head left, head right, head extension, head flexion
Dynamic tests
  1. Rotation test
  2. Caloric test
  3. Otolith test (parallel swing test)
Oculomotor tests
  1. Pursuit eye movements
     a. Pendular test
     b. Optokinetic nystagmus test
     c. Saccade test
  2. Gaze test

Interpretation of Findings

STATIC TESTS

Spontaneous and Positional Nystagmus

The presence of a spontaneous or positional nystagmus can be a sign of central as well as of peripheral disorders. Spontaneous nystagmus has five parameters on the basis of which one can differentiate between central and peripheral vestibular origin:

Central lesion	Peripheral lesion
Horizontal, vertical, oblique, or rotatory	Horizontal–rotatory
Non-direction-fixed	Direction-fixed
Enhanced by visual fixation	Suppressed by visual fixation
Strongest by gaze in direction fast phase	Strongest in direction of gaze
Does not change	Diminishes in weeks

About 1% of the population has a congenital nystagmus without any pathological implications (4). Because of its form, a spontaneous nystagmus can sometimes be rather easily interpreted as congenital. Several types of nystagmus are significant in identifying a congenital nystagmus (Figure 1). A finding that is less rare than previously considered is periodic alternating nystagmus, which consists of a horizontal–rotatory movement that alternates with intervals. This nystagmus can be present with eyes open or closed. Two types are known: the congenital form and the acquired form. The acquired form is caused (in most cases reported) by lesions in the cerebellomedullary region (6).

A positional nystagmus is regarded as pathological when present in any one of the

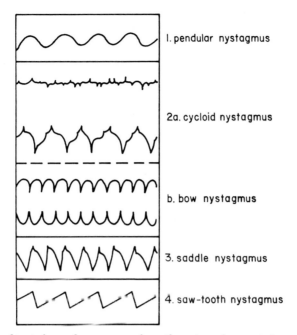

1. pendular nystagmus

2a. cycloid nystagmus

b. bow nystagmus

3. saddle nystagmus

4. saw-tooth nystagmus

Figure 1. Sample of typical waveforms among the wide variety of congenital spontaneous nystagmus. Adapted from Oosterveld and Rademakers (6).

following conditions: (a) direction-changing in any head position, (b) persistent in three or more head positions, (c) intermittent in four or more head positions, and (d) speed of slow component exceeds 7 deg/sec. In order to differentiate between central and peripheral origin of a positional nystagmus the following tabulation is helpful:

Abnormality	Significance
Nystagmus with eyes open	
Direction-fixed	Central lesion (usually)
Direction-changing	Central lesion
Nystagmus with eyes closed	
Direction-fixed	Peripheral vestibular lesion (usually)
Direction-changing	Central lesion (usually)
Nystagmus, direction-changing	
in one head position	Central lesion

Generally speaking, the differentiation between central and peripheral causes depends on four tests: position test, caloric test, pursuit movements test, and gaze test.

Cervical Tests

Extensive head movements cause a torsion of the cervical vertebral column (Figure 2). In patients with cervical pathology a cervical nystagmus accompanied by vertiginous sensations can be provoked. Cervical pathology has a variety of origins.

1. *Cervical spine arthrosis.* Degenerative and traumatically induced changes of the intravertebral joints are responsible.

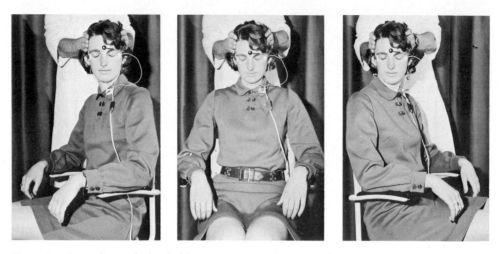

Figure 2. Cervical test. The head of the patient is rotated successively into the following positions: to the right, to the left, in flexion, and in extension.

2. *Vertebral artery obstruction.* Atherosclerosis, degenerative changes in the foramina costotransversaria are responsible.

3. *Irritation of cervical nerve roots.* Caused by afferent stimulation of the vestibular nuclei.

4. *Cervical migraine.* Due to osteochondrotic changes around the processus uncinatus.

DYNAMIC TESTS

Rotation Test

Rotation chairs are popular tools in vestibular laboratories. They provide angular accelerations in the horizontal plane, which result in a nystagmus when the horizontal canals on one or both sides are functional. When the nystagmus during clockwise rotation differs from that after counterclockwise rotation, there is a preponderance of nystagmus for a certain direction. This phenomenon is rather difficult to interpret since central as well as peripheral disorders can cause it. In my department a torsion swing is used, which is a rotation chair that provides an oscillating angular acceleration. For the routine vestibular examination, the rotation test does not give very helpful information.

Caloric Test

The caloric test provides information on the excitability of one horizontal semicircular canal. It is still regarded as the most important of the peripheral vestibular tests. The devices used to conduct the caloric test are currently much simpler than they were some years ago. Most European laboratories use the wet type of test device, providing water with a temperature of 30° and 44°C. The air caloric devices are much less popular because they cannot give so strong a stimulus. In most laboratories a program is used with stimulation periods of 30 sec. The parameters used for interpreting the caloric tests are the speed of the slow component and the frequency of the nystagmus. The first gives the most useful information, i.e., on the actual excitability of each labyrinth separately, on the existence of pathological differences in excitability between the labyrinths, and on the existence of a nystagmus preponderance. The visual suppression test must always be added to the caloric test. That is, 60 and 90 sec after the start of the irrigation the patient has to open his eyes for periods of 10 sec in order to fixate visually a target on the ceiling. If the speed of the caloric nystagmus does not decrease in these periods, the central pathology is obvious.

Otolith Test (Parallel Swing)

There are few tests that give adequate information on the functioning of the otolithic system. Ocular counterrolling measurements are regarded as too difficult, too costly, and too time-consuming to be part of a regular test battery. Positional alcoholic nystagmus may depend on the presence of a functional otolithic system, but this test is also too time-consuming. The otolith test used in some European laboratories is the parallel swing test. However, in most laboratories no tests of the otoliths are done.

The parallel swing provokes a linear acceleration of an oscillating type. This results in sinusoidal eye movements in the plane of movement (Figures 3 and 4). These eye movements are due to otolith stimulation. Sideways movements stimulate the utricle; movements in the lengthwise axis of the body stimulate the saccules and provoke vertical sinusoidal eye movements. Even information on the side of a utricular lesion can be found, as when a subject is swung sideways while lying in a lateral position; the underlying utricle seems to provoke the eye movements. Because of the space that a parallel swing device occupies, the device is present only in special vestibular departments. Also, its use is restricted to a rather limited number of patients. A parallel swing test is indicated when (a) there is no caloric response of one labyrinth, (b) there is no caloric response of both labyrinths, or (c) there are complaints of floating sensations without rotational vertigo.

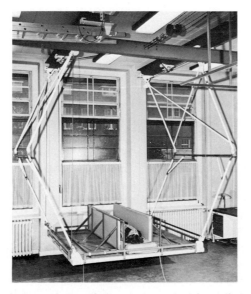

Figure 3. Parallel swing device in the Vestibular Department of the Wilhelmina Gasthuis, University Clinic of the University of Amsterdam.

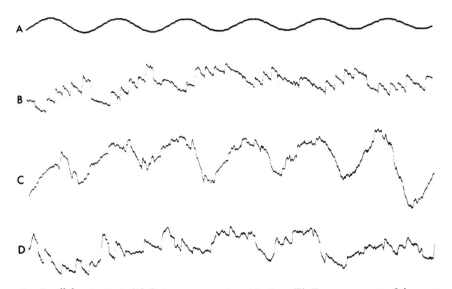

Figure 4. Parallel swing test. (A) Swing movement registration. (B) Eye movements of the patient in supine position. (C) Eye movements of the patient in right lateral position. (D) Eye movements of the patient in left lateral position. The diminished amplitude of the eye movements in the left lateral position points to an utricular lesion in the left labyrinth.

OCULOMOTOR TESTS

Pursuit Eye Movements

The task of the visual pursuit system is to keep the target on the fovea. This system is utilized when the eyes track targets that move rather smoothly and relatively slowly. A fixed relationship is maintained between the movements of the target and the eyes. Because the smooth pursuit movements directly relate the eye position to the target position, they are commonly termed "tracking movements."

Pursuit movements are characterized by a short latency time since eye and target movements must be matched continuously. The feedback control for the system seems to be continuous. The latency from the presentation of the target to the onset of the pursuit movement is approximately 125 msec. The maximum velocity of the pursuit movement is about 30 deg/sec. In many vestibular laboratories these tests are not a regular part of the test battery, the main reasons being the high cost of an optokinetic nystagmus (OKN) device and the lack of experience in interpreting the results.

Three main tests are available for the pursuit mechanism:

1. Pendular test. The patient visually tracks an oscillating target in the horizontal plane, with a sideways excursion of 15 deg and an oscillation time of 2.5 sec. A normal individual is able to follow the target with a tracing that resembles a perfect image of the target motion. The following abnormalities may be found: *saccadic pursuits,* in which the smooth pursuit pattern is interrupted by saccades and which suggests cerebellar or brainstem lesions, and *disorganized or disconjugate pursuits,* suggestive of cerebellar lesions.

2. Optokinetic nystagmus test. The patient is instructed to watch a visual stimulus that moves in the horizontal plane. The stimulus velocity used is between 40 and 120

deg of visual angle per second. In a normal person, the speed of the eye movement matches the speed of the stimulus up to 40 deg, with individual differences up to 60 deg. When the stimulus speed increases, the eye speed falls progressively below target speed. The maximum eye speed differs individually, but ranks between 40 and 90 deg. The following abnormalities may be found: *unilateral diminishing*, which points to hemispheric lesions; *bilateral diminishing*, which indicates brainstem lesions; *optokinetic disorganization*, which is characterized by the appearance of quick reversed jerks in the direction of the slow phases and is found in intoxication and symmetric hemispheric lesions. Inversion is found in patients with a congenital nystagmus and means that the OKN beats in a direction inappropriate to the stimulus. The OKN test is time-consuming, for both the patient and the investigator. Moreover, the equipment is rather expensive. However, for a complete otoneurological examination the test cannot be omitted.

3. Saccade test. In this test the patient looks back and forth between two dots on the wall, which register as square waves (saccades) on the recordings. One abnormality that may be found is *ocular dysmetria*, which means an overshoot or undershoot. Another is *saccadic slowing*, found in basal ganglia disorders. *Internuclear ophthalmoplegia* can be detected rather easily with this test. It is caused by a lesion of the medial longitudinal fasciculus between the third and the sixth nerve nuclei. The syndrome consists of an apparent medial rectus paresis in the eye on the side of the lesion, nystagmus of the abducting eye on lateral gaze to the side opposite to the lesion, and normal rectus activity on convergence.

The saccadic pursuits are caused by lesions in the occipitomesencephalic pathways. Unfortunately, they are not specific for damage to the oculomotor system, so they cannot be used as a reliable sign localizing an occipitomesencephalic lesion. (Pathology of the cerebellar pathways, conditions of a decreased state of alertness, or the effects of sedative drugs may also produce abnormal saccadics. However, in these cases the pursuit is affected bilaterally.) Abnormality in the pursuit in one direction indicates a probable lesion in the oculomotor pathways.

Gaze Test

In the gaze test, the patient looks straight ahead, then with an angle of 30 deg to the right, to the left, up, and down. The purpose of this test is to detect a nystagmus provoked by this off-centerline visual fixation. Several abnormalities can be encountered. *Bilateral horizontal gaze nystagmus* means a nystagmus beating to the right on rightward gaze and to the left on leftward gaze. The presence of brainstem lesions is suggested by these findings. *Unilateral horizontal gaze nystagmus* means that the nystagmus appears only by gaze in one direction. This is found in afferent vestibular nerve lesions. The gaze test has to be conducted with the patient's eyes open and then closed. Eye closure abolishes a gaze nystagmus of central origin. *Vertical nystagmus* can be found by upward and downward gaze. Upbeating gaze nystagmus is reported in patients with posterior fossa pathology. *Downbeating nystagmus* suggests pathology with medullary or medullocervical localization.

Currently, nystagmography means more than conducting positional, rotation, and caloric tests. The eye movement tests have become more and more important. For the investigator this implies that much knowledge of neurology and neurophysiology is necessary. Recently some very practical publications have appeared in this field (1–3, 5).

I have encountered two disappointing aspects of vestibular testing. The first is that, in the battery of vestibular tests, the functioning of two out of three semicircular canals is not evaluated. Also, information on utricle and saccule function is derived from relatively poor tests. The tabulation below summarizes the use of these tests to identify the location of pathology (i.e., the location of lesion after testing):

| | Peripheral vestibular organ | | | | | Central nervous system |
| | Canals | | | Otoliths | | |
Vestibular tests	Horizontal	Anterior	Posterior	Utricle	Saccule	
Spontaneous and positional nystagmus	X			X	X	X
Caloric test	X					
Rotation test	X					
Parallel swing test				X	X	
Pursuit movement tests						X
Fixation nystagmus						X
Gaze nystagmus						X

My second disappointment is that for several years no new test providing more insight into the function of the peripheral vestibular organ has been developed. This is the situation in spite of the tremendous efforts the aeronautical and space sciences have made to solve vestibular problems.

REFERENCES

1. Baloh, R. W., and Honrubia, V., *Clinical Neuro-physiology of the Vestibular System*. Davis, Philadelphia, Pennsylvania, 1979.
2. Barber, U. O., and Stockwell, C. W., *Manual of Electronystagmography*. Mosby, St. Louis, Missouri, 1976.
3. Gay, A. J., Newman, N., Keltner, J. L., and Stroud, M. H., (eds.), *Eye Movement Disorders*. Mosby, St. Louis, Missouri, 1974.
4. Knapp, H., *Kommt Spontannystagmus bei Gesunden vor?* H.N.O., 1950:2:17–19.
5. Kornhuber, H. H., ed., *Handbook of Sensory Physiology*, Vol. 6, Part 2. Springer-Verlag, Berlin and New York, 1974.
6. Oosterveld, W. J., and Rademakers, W. J. A. C., Nystagmus alternans. *Acta Oto-Laryngol.*, 1979, **87**:404–409.

Auditory Evaluation of Vestibular Patients

DOUGLAS NOFFSINGER,[1] DONALD E. MORGAN,[2] and DAVID G. HANSON[1]

[1]VA Wadsworth Medical Center, Los Angeles, and Division of Head and Neck Surgery, School of Medicine, University of California Los Angeles, Los Angeles, California
[2]Division of Head and Neck Surgery, School of Medicine, University of California Los Angeles, Los Angeles, California

Patients who present with evidence of vestibular system involvement may or may not report problems with hearing. Regardless of the presenting complaints, the evaluation of such patients should include a battery of auditory tests to rule out the presence of a hearing loss or to provide information regarding the site of any apparent auditory system lesion. The purpose of this chapter is to (a) identify the test procedures to be applied routinely to rule out the presence of a hearing loss of peripheral origin; (b) identify those test procedures that are available for the evaluation of patients presenting with possible or probable retrocochlear or central auditory system disorder; and (c) briefly describe the characteristic manifestations of lesions within the auditory system.

STANDARD AUDITORY TESTS

PURE-TONE STUDIES

Hearing sensitivity is evaluated at selected frequencies using short-duration (> 250 msec) pure-tone stimuli. Air conduction sensitivity is reported for pure tones from 250 Hz through 8,000 to 10,000 Hz in decibels (dB) relative to the sensitivity of normal-hearing persons. Air conduction stimuli are presented via earphones. Each ear is tested independently. Likewise, bone conduction sensitivity is tested across the frequency range from 250 to 4000 Hz and plotted in decibels relative to normal-hearing sensitivity (for bone-conducted stimuli). The results of air and bone conduction testing are plotted on an audiogram, from which the magnitude (in decibels) and configuration (sensitivity loss as a function of frequency) of the hearing loss can be determined.

Figure 1 is an example of an audiogram form on which the threshold sensitivity for air conduction and bone conduction is recorded for each ear individually. The results from the right ear reveal a mild hearing loss for air conduction, with normal bone

145

NYSTAGMUS AND VERTIGO: CLINICAL
APPROACHES TO THE PATIENT WITH DIZZINESS

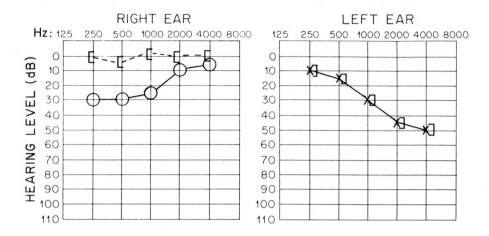

Figure 1. Audiogram used to summarize the results of pure-tone air conduction and bone conduction hearing tests. The right ear results represent an example of conductive hearing loss. The left ear results are an example of a sensorineural hearing loss. Right ear: ○, air conduction sensitivity; ⌈, bone conduction. Left ear: **x**, air conduction sensitivity;], bone conduction.

conduction sensitivity. The left ear is characterized by a sloping loss of hearing sensitivity for air conduction and bone conduction.

SPEECH STUDIES

Two types of tests are conducted to determine a person's ability to hear and understand speech. The speech reception threshold is the intensity (in decibels with reference to normal hearing sensitivity for speech) at which the patient can correctly recognize 50% of the words presented. The speech discrimination test is a measure of the patient's ability to understand speech accurately when it is presented at an intensity level well above threshold. Speech discrimination may be measured at a single preselected level above threshold or over a range of intensity levels. When speech discrimination is tested at several intensity levels, the results are referred to as a performance–intensity function.

IMPEDANCE STUDIES

"Acoustic impedance" refers to the opposition provided by a system to the flow of acoustic energy. In the auditory system, changes in acoustic impedance (from "normal" values) are almost always due to lesions of the middle ear system. The measurement is accomplished by obtaining an airtight seal of a probe tip in the ear canal. A "probe" tone is introduced into the ear canal. From the same probe tip, a microphone measures the sound pressure level of the tone in the ear canal. As changes occur in the mechanical properties of the middle ear, the resultant changes in acoustic impedance at the plane of the tympanic membrane are reflected as changes in the sound pressure level of the probe tone in the external ear canal. From such measures, the acoustic impedance of the middle ear can be inferred.

Two types of acoustic impedance measures are commonly employed: tympanometry and stapedius muscle reflex measurement. *Tympanometry* is a measure of relative impedance change with changes of air pressure in the ear canal. Air pressure changes in the external ear canal are introduced (via an opening in the probe tip); the resultant changes in acoustic impedance are recorded as the air pressure is changed from high positive values (with reference to atmospheric pressure) to high negative values. The graph, i.e., representation of change in acoustic impedance with change in ear canal air pressure, is referred to as a tympanogram. A tympanogram provides the information from which middle ear impedance can be determined. Tympanometry is especially useful in the detection of and differentiation among various middle ear disorders.

The *stapedius muscle reflex* is measured by monitoring acoustic impedance over time while inducing a contraction of the stapedius muscle. The contraction may be induced by tactile (6) or acoustic (4) stimulation, although acoustic stimulation is by far the most commonly used activating signal. The "acoustic" reflex threshold is determined by increasing the intensity of an acoustic signal until a change in impedance is observed coincidental with the onset of the activating stimulus. The magnitude of the impedance change induced by an acoustic signal of specified intensity is an indirect measure of the strength of the contraction of the stapedius muscle (4). By observing the time course of the impedance changes resulting from a continuous, constant-level stimulus, one can obtain an estimate of reflex adaptation (10).

DIFFERENTIAL DIAGNOSTIC PERIPHERAL AUDITORY SYSTEM MEASURES

AUDITORY ADAPTATION

Several procedures have been employed for the measurement of auditory adaptation, or "tone decay." Originally, the procedures were conducted at, or near, auditory threshold (5); more recently, suprathreshold levels have been employed (8, 12). The measure of adaptation may be accomplished by manual presentation of a signal from a conventional clinical audiometer or by using a continuously variable or automatic (Békésy-type) audiometer. In either case, a stimulus is presented continuously at the starting intensity level, and the examiner records the length of time the stimulus is audible to the patient. With the manual presentation methods, the examiner increases the intensity of the signal until the patient can perceive the tone for 60 sec at a constant intensity level. Using Békésy audiometer methods, a graphic representation is obtained of the intensity level required for the patient to maintain audibility of the signal. Abnormal adaptation is evident if increasing intensity (over time) is required for the patient to maintain the audibility of a continuous tonal stimulus.

LOUDNESS BALANCE MEASURES

The alternate binaural loudness balance test is the direct measurement of loudness recruitment (7). A short-duration (about 250 msec) tone is presented alternately to each ear. The intensity of the tone to one ear is fixed, while the intensity to the other ear is adjusted until the listener perceives the loudness of the two tones to be equal. Recruitment of loudness is present if the patient requires a smaller intensity increase (above threshold) in the hearing impaired ear than in the better-hearing (usually "normal") ear to achieve equal loudness between the two ears.

ACOUSTIC REFLEX MEASURES

The reflexive contraction of the stapedius muscle in response to acoustic stimulation is bilateral, requiring synaptic continuity of the eighth nerve (afferent neuron), the ventral cochlear nucleus, the superior olivary complex (contralateral and/or ipsilateral), the seventh nerve (efferent), and the stapedius muscle (3). Because of the bilateral contraction, an activating acoustic stimulus may be presented in the same ear as the probe tone or in the ear opposite the probe. By varying the intensity, spectrum, and duration of the activating acoustic signal, one can quantify several aspects of the acoustic reflex.

The threshold of the reflex may be defined for pure tones and/or bands of noise. Depending on pure-tone hearing sensitivity, there is a predictable threshold relationship for the various reflex-activating signals (15). Adaptation of the reflex is evidenced when an initial impedance change is not maintained throughout the time course of a continuous acoustic signal presented to the contralateral ear (1).

DIFFERENTIAL DIAGNOSTIC CENTRAL AUDITORY SYSTEM MEASURES

There are many ways to evaluate the functional status of the central auditory nervous system (CANS) in patients manifesting vestibular system symptomatology. Behavioral tests that require subjects to respond to various configurations of acoustic signals are a common approach. Two types of procedures are particularly valuable in evaluating CANS integrity: (a) tests that examine the capacity of the auditory brainstem to use binaural interaction cues, such as binaural masking level differences (13); and (b) tests that evaluate the capacity of the auditory cortex to comprehend difficult monotic and dichotic speech signals, such as time-compressed monotic speech (11) or dichotically presented nonsense syllables (2).

Objective procedures, i.e., those not requiring active participation by the subject, are also helpful in CANS probes. Three classes of procedures are useful: (a) acoustic reflex studies of the sort discussed earlier in this chapter (a combination of ipsilateral and contralateral acoustic reflex studies provides important clues to the seventh nerve, eighth nerve, and low brainstem function); (b) auditory brainstem response (ABR) studies to evaluate brainstem function; and (c) auditory cortical response (middle and late component) studies to evaluate cortical function. The remainder of this section concentrates on the use of ABR techniques and results as indicators of the

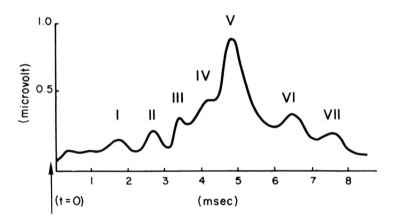

Figure 2. Schematic representation of auditory brainstem potentials obtained from human subjects, adapted from the report of Jewett and Williston (9). Latencies are given in milliseconds after stimulus onset. Stimuli were clicks. Upward-going events in this and all subsequent figures are those seen positive by a vertex electrode.

status of peripheral auditory structures and of auditory centers and pathways in the brainstem.

To review briefly, the term "auditory brainstem response" is used to describe five to seven electrical events that occur in fast succession following presentation of an acoustic signal to the ear. The events are time-locked to the signal onset. The signals are characteristically brief, rapid-onset, high-intensity clicks or tone pips. Although the amplitudes of the electric potentials are minute, a surface-electrode array featuring an active electrode on the vertex can detect the electrical events. Repetitive signal presentation and careful amplification and filtering of the electrical activity allow an averaging computer to separate any time-locked potentials from background "noise" with sufficient definition to enable one to measure the latency, amplitude, and waveform of the potentials.

A schematic representation of the potentials, adapted from the pioneering work with ABR by Jewett and Williston (9), is given in Figure 2. The immediacy and small magnitude of the events shown are typical. Although the issue is still debated, a number of studies (14, 16–18) suggest the following generator (origination) sites for the potentials: I. eighth nerve action potential; II. area of cochlear nucleus and/or second firing of eighth nerve; III. area of superior olivary complex, IV.–V. area of lateral lemniscus and inferior colliculus; VI.–VII. thalamic sites.

Research using normal human individuals has demonstrated that, although ABR

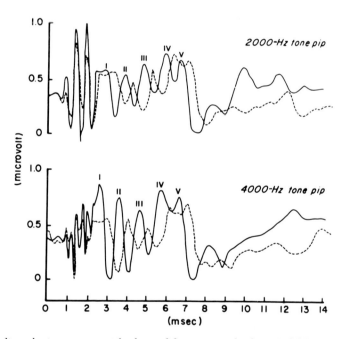

Figure 3. Auditory brainstem potentials obtained from a normal subject (solid line) and from a patient with a unilateral conductive hearing loss (dashed line). The patient was a 14-year-old boy. The tympanogram in the affected ear was flat (no point of maximum compliance). Speech discrimination via the affected ear was excellent at high intensity levels. Contralateral acoustic reflexes were absent bilaterally. Ipsilateral acoustic reflexes were present in the normal ear, absent in the conductive-loss ear. The medical diagnosis was acute otitis media. Auditory brainstem potentials were elicited by 2000- and 4000-Hz tone pips. Although their absolute latencies were delayed due to the middle ear conductive blockage, interpotential latencies (central conduction times) were normal.

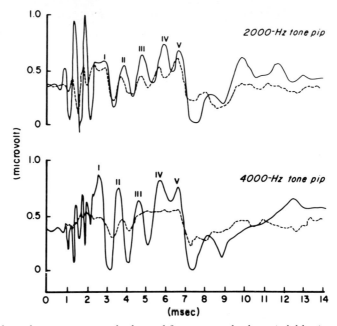

Figure 4. Auditory brainstem potentials obtained from a normal subject (solid line) and from a patient with Ménière's disease affecting the ear portrayed (dashed line). The patient was a 48-year-old woman. The affected ear had a moderate to severe sensorineural hearing loss and poor ability to understand speech. Tympanometry and acoustic reflex tests were normal. The brainstem potentials aroused by 2000-Hz tone pips were normal. The 4000-Hz tone pips elicited little activity. This was not surprising since there was a severe hearing loss at 4000 Hz. However, the (characteristic) negative shift following wave V occurred with the expected latency at 4000 Hz. These ABR results point to sensory rather than neural insult.

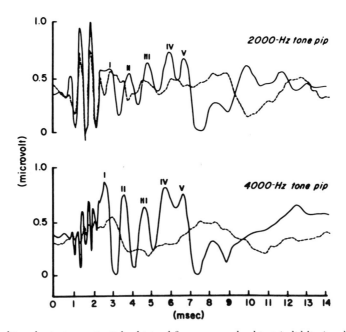

Figure 5. Auditory brainstem potentials obtained from a normal subject (solid line) and from a patient with von Recklinghausen's syndrome (dashed line). The patient was a 21-year-old woman. Both ears had mild sensorineural hearing losses. Speech discrimination was poor bilaterally. Tympanograms were normal for both ears. Neither contralateral nor ipsilateral acoustic reflexes were arousable. Radiographically confirmed masses were appended to each eighth nerve. Brainstem potentials were absent bilaterally. Recordings from one ear to 2000- and 4000-Hz tone pips are shown.

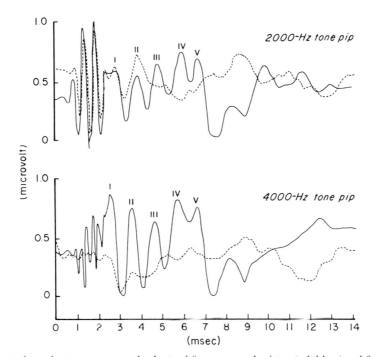

Figure 6. Auditory brainstem potentials obtained from a normal subject (solid line) and from a patient with multiple sclerosis (dashed line). The patient was a 42-year-old man. Hearing sensitivity and speech discrimination were excellent bilaterally. Tympanograms were normal. Although ipsilateral acoustic reflexes were present, contralateral reflexes were absent or decayed rapidly in amplitude over time. The sclerotic disease was in exacerbation at the time of these tests. Brainstem potentials I and II were elicited by 2000- and 4000-Hz tone pips, but later potentials were not present in either ear. CANS disease affecting the low brainstem often produces the pattern of auditory behavior exhibited by this patient: normal hearing sensitivity, normal speech discrimination, and normal ipsilateral acoustic reflexes but absent contralateral reflexes (requiring trans-brainstem transmission) and brainstem potential abnormalities appearing first in Jewett wave I, II, or III. Further evaluation of this patient demonstrated two other expected abnormalities: an inability to fuse binaurally presented signals and absent masking level differences. Both of these tasks are thought to require normally functioning auditory areas in the low brainstem. In contrast, patients whose brainstem potentials first became abnormal at Jewett peak IV or V usually have normal hearing, normal speech discrimination, normal ipsilateral and contralateral acoustic reflexes, and normal binaural fusion and masking level difference abilities. Such findings support the theory that the eighth nerve and the low brainstem produce the early auditory brainstem potentials and are critical for use of binaural auditory cues.

waveforms and amplitudes may vary among subjects, latencies of the brainstem potentials among subjects are sufficiently similar for identical signal parameters to make ABR useful in two ways. First, since potential V, particularly, can be elicited near a subject's behavioral threshold for the signals used, ABR studies can yield information that is helpful in assessing hearing sensitivity in subjects who cannot or will not participate in behavioral evaluations. Second, and more important to the focus of this chapter, inability to elicit the potentials or delay in one or more of the potential latencies provides evidence of diagnostic significance for the clinician.

The clinical diagnostic use of ABR can be illustrated by the case studies illustrated in Figures 3 to 8. These cases were chosen because they illustrate circumstances in which ABR suggested a locus of lesion in a dizzy patient. All the patients involved had a common complaint: vertigo, if that term is used to describe (a) the illusion of self in motion, turning, or spinning within the context of a stable environment; or (b) the illusion of a moving, turning, or spinning environment enveloping a stable self. The vertigo was described as episodic in both duration and intensity by all persons.

The patients gave different responses to the various basic audiometric tests described earlier in this chapter. For that reason, the legend to each figure showing ABR results includes comments on the patient's hearing sensitivity, speech discrimination ability, tympanometric results, acoustic reflex results, medical diagnosis, and a comment on the ABR findings.

The ABR results shown in Figures 3 to 8 were those elicited in response to 2000- and/or 4000-Hz tone pips of 2 msec total duration. The presentation level was 75 dB re threshold for the pips as established from a control group of normal listeners. An arbitrarily chosen normal ABR result is shown for comparison purposes in each figure. (The short period of synchronized activity beginning almost at stimulus onset in these figures is stimulus artifact.) Each trial run represents the activity averaged over 2000 signal presentations.

These case studies were carefully chosen to illustrate how combinations or batteries of auditory tests can assist one in evaluating vestibular patients. The importance of a combined vestibular–auditory system evaluation is not limited to a small number of selected patients, however. The authors reviewed a series of 85 patients with auditory complaints and subsequently confirmed eighth nerve tumors by surgery. Sixty-two percent complained of episodic or constant vertigo. In a similar series of patients with brainstem lesions ($N = 95$), 66 had vertigo, and 60% of these pronounced vertigo their chief complaint.

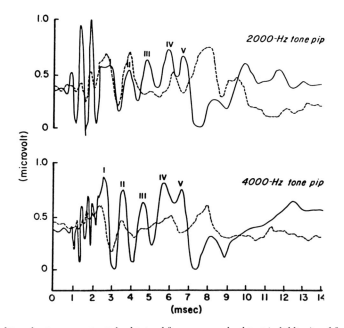

Figure 7.   Auditory brainstem potentials obtained from a normal subject (solid line) and from the multiple sclerotic patient (dashed line) also shown in Figure 6. These potentials were obtained following 2 weeks of intensive adrenocorticotropic hormone therapy, which produced or coincided with a partial remission of symptoms. Despite the remission, only brainstem potentials I and II were consistently present on repeated trials.

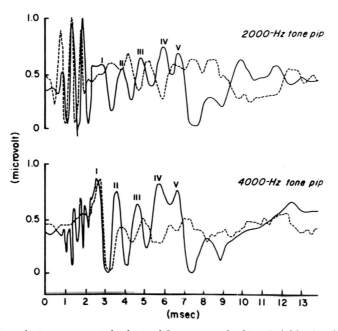

Figure 8. Auditory brainstem potentials obtained from a normal subject (solid line) and from a patient with widespread central nervous system (CNS) damage (dashed line). The patient was a 21-year-old woman. Both ears had a mild sensorineural hearing loss. However, speech discrimination (for meaningful words) was 0% bilaterally. Tympanograms were normal. Ipsilateral acoustic reflexes were normal. Contralateral acoustic reflexes were absent or rapidly decayed over time. The medical history reported widespread CNS lesion due to air embolitic damage secondary to cerebellar astrocytoma surgery. Auditory brainstem potential studies revealed dysynchronous or delayed potentials for both ears. Averaged electric activity obtained from one ear is shown.

CLASSIFICATION OF AUDITORY DISORDERS

The complexity of the auditory system precludes identification of the site of auditory lesion on the basis of cursory physical examination or a single auditory test. Disorders of the auditory system are commonly classified as conductive, sensorineural, or central. In this section, typical audiological manifestations of these classifications are summarized.

CONDUCTIVE DISORDERS

Conductive hearing loss occurs when a lesion involves the external or middle ear structures or both. The hearing is typically characterized by a loss in air conduction sensitivity, abnormal impedance studies, and increased latencies on ABR measures. Otherwise, "normal" auditory test findings are observed.

SENSORINEURAL DISORDERS

Sensorineural disorders are caused by lesions of the cochlea or eighth nerve or both. Lesions involving only the sensory structures of the inner ear are described as cochlear, and those affecting the function of the eighth nerve as retrocochlear.

The hearing in *cochlear* lesions typically includes a loss of air and bone conduction sensitivity but normal tympanometric findings. Auditory adaptation is minimal, and recruitment is present. The ABR measures and modified speech measures are all reasonably predictable on the basis of the magnitude of the pure-tone hearing loss, but in each case deviate from normal auditory system findings.

Retrocochlear lesions may or may not include a significant loss of pure-tone hearing sensitivity. Tympanometric studies are normal. Auditory adaptation is typically significant, recruitment is absent, and acoustic reflex studies are characterized by an elevated or absent acoustic reflex. When the reflex is present, adaptation throughout a 10-sec continuous stimulation period is predictable. The ABR measures and modified speech measures usually show evidence of problems in auditory encoding and processing beyond what might be expected on the basis of the magnitude of the pure-tone hearing sensitivity loss.

CENTRAL DISORDERS

Central disorders usually do not affect pure-tone or speech sensitivity. Speech discrimination for unmodified materials is good. Tympanometric studies reveal normal results. Auditory adaptation is usually not marked, but, when present, it is often seen bilaterally. Decruitment (opposite of loudness recruitment) is sometimes seen. Acoustic reflex studies are often abnormal in brainstem lesion patients, but normal for cortical lesion patients. Auditory brainstem potentials are absent or delayed for brainstem cases but normal for cortical cases. On the other hand, difficult speech tests are more useful in detecting lesions in the cortex than in the brainstem.

THE "TEST BATTERY" APPROACH

This discussion of auditory test measures illustrates that the complexity of the auditory system defies any simplistic diagnostic approach to the identification of auditory lesion site. In fact, a review of the manifestations of auditory lesions at specific points within the system reveals that any single auditory test result, when viewed in isolation, invariably leads to ambiguous conclusions regarding the possible site of the auditory lesion. For example, an absent (or elevated) acoustic reflex threshold may be observed with any one of the following conditions: middle ear lesion, severe cochlear hearing loss, eighth nerve lesion, seventh nerve lesion, or brainstem level lesion affecting ipsilateral, contralateral, or bilateral innervation of the stapedius muscle. Only when the examiner has access to other auditory test results can an accurate prediction of the site of lesion be made.

In principle, the more central the auditory lesion, the more complex the auditory task required to identify the lesion. However, any peripheral auditory lesion may affect the patient's performance on complex tasks designed to identify central auditory dysfunction. Therefore, the diagnostic evaluation of the patient presenting with a neurotological complaint should proceed systematically so that the integrity of the auditory system from periphery to cortex can be determined. The sequential progression of auditory test measures should include the following:

1. Pure-tone air and bone conduction studies to determine the magnitude and configuration of pure-tone hearing loss.

2. Standard speech tests to determine speech recognition performance in each ear under ideal (quiet) conditions.

3. Impedance studies to determine the integrity of the middle ear mechanism and the integrity of the acoustic reflex arc.

4. Differential auditory test measures, as indicated, to delineate the site of lesion in cases of apparent sensorineural loss.

5. Tests for central auditory system function even when the results of standard test measures reveal normal peripheral system function but other indications suggest the possibility of a central auditory system disorder.

ACKNOWLEDGMENTS

The support of NIH/NINCDS via NS17115 grant is gratefully acknowledged. Case studies were assembled with the assistance of Mr. Charles D. Martinez, Research Audiologist at VA Wadsworth Medical Center, Los Angeles.

REFERENCES

1. Anderson, H., Barr, B., and Wedenberg, E., Intra-aural reflexes in retrocochlear lesions. In: *Disorders of the Skull Base Region* (C. A. Hamberger and J. Wersall, eds.). Almquist & Wiksell, Stockholm, 1969:49–55.
2. Berlin, C. I., Lowe-Bell, S. S., Janetta, P. J., and Kline, D. G., Central auditory deficits after temporal lobectomy. *Arch. Otolaryngol.*, 1972, **96**:5–10.
3. Borg, E., On the neuronal organization of the acoustic middle ear reflex: A physiological and anatomical study. *Brain Res.*, 1973, **49**:101–123.
4. Borg, E., Dynamic characteristics of the intra-aural muscle reflex. In: *Acoustic Impedance and Admittance* (A. S. Feldman and L. A. Wilber, eds.). Williams & Wilkins, Baltimore, Maryland, 1976:236–299.
5. Carhart, R., Clinical determination of abnormal auditory adaptation. *Arch. Otolaryngol.*, 1957, **65**:32–39.
6. Djupesland, G., Nonacoustic reflex measurement procedures. In: *Acoustic Impedance and Admittance* (A. S. Feldman and L. A. Wilber, eds.). Williams & Wilkins, Baltimore, Maryland, 1976:217–235.
7. Fowler, F., The diagnosis of diseases of the neural mechanism of hearing by the aid of sounds well above threshold. *Trans. Am. Otol. Soc.*, 1937, **27**:209–219.
8. Jerger, J., A simplified tone decay test. *Arch. Otolaryngol.*, 1975, **102**:403–407.
9. Jewett, D. L., and Williston, J. S., Auditory-evoked far fields averaged from the scalp of humans. *Brain*, 1971, **94**:681–696.
10. Kaplan, H., Gilman, S., and Dirks, D., Properties of acoustic reflex adaptation. *Ann. Otol., Rhinol., Laryngol.*, 1977, **86**:348–356.
11. Kurdziel, S., Noffsinger, D., and Olsen, W., Performance by cortical lesion patients on 40 and 60% time-compressed materials. *J. Am. Audiol. Soc.*, 1976, **2**:3–7.
12. Olsen, W., and Noffsinger, D., Comparison of one new and three old tests of auditory adaptation. *Arch. Otolaryngol.*, 1974, **99**:94–99.
13. Olsen, W., Noffsinger, D., and Carhart, R., Masking level differences encountered in clinical populations. *Audiology*, 1976, **15**:287–301.
14. Picton, T. W., Hillyard, S. A., Krausz, H. I., and Galambos, R., Human auditory evoked potentials. I. Evaluation of components. *Electroencephalogr. Clin. Neurophysiol.*, 1974, **36**:179–190.
15. Popelka, G., Margolis, R., and Wiley, T., Effect of activating signal bandwidth on acoustic-reflex thresholds. *J. Acoust. Soc. Am.*, 1976, **59**:153–159.
16. Sohmer, H., Feinmesser, M., and Szabo, G., Sources of electrocochleographic responses as studied in patients with brain damage. *Electroencephalogr. Clin. Neurophysiol.*, 1974, **37**:663–669.
17. Starr, A., and Hamilton, A. E., Correlation between confirmed sites of neurological lesions and abnormalities of far field auditory brainstem responses. *Electroencephalogr. Clin. Neurophysiol.*, 1976, **41**:595–608.
18. Stockard, J. J., and Rossiter, V. S., Clinical and pathological correlates of brainstem auditory response abnormalities. *Neurology*, 1977, **27**:316–325.

Atypical Cogan's Syndrome: A Case Report

ROBERT D. YEE

Department of Ophthalmology
School of Medicine, University of California Los Angeles
Los Angeles, California

A 21-year-old man was admitted to the UCLA Medical Center for evaluation of pain and redness of both eyes and severe loss of hearing in both ears. Eight months earlier he had developed aching, redness, and photophobia of both eyes. An ophthalmologist had diagnosed iritis of both eyes. Topical steroids relieved the ocular symptoms in a few weeks. Six months later the patient suddenly developed vertigo, nausea, vomiting, and ringing in the left ear. At that time he also noted a progressive, severe loss of hearing in the left ear over a period of 1 week. Two weeks later a second episode of vertigo, nausea, and vomiting occurred, and a progressive loss of hearing in the right ear was noted. An otolaryngologist diagnosed Cogan's syndrome (interstitial keratitis and vestibuloauditory loss). The patient was treated with prednisone, 50 mg po QD. Although the vertigo, nausea, and vomiting resolved, hearing remained impaired in both ears. One month before admission the patient developed mild aching of the calves and ankles of both legs.

The patient had been previously healthy. There was no history of other ophthalmological, otolaryngological, or neurological disorders or of syphilis. The patient had not shown other significant symptoms, such as fever, rash, hematuria, or weight loss.

Physical examinations at UCLA were unremarkable, except for the neurootological and ophthalmological examinations. Audiological testing demonstrated a severe sensorineural hearing loss in both ears. Hearing loss by air conduction was more severely impaired in the left ear than in the right ear (left ear: 250 Hz, −60 dB; 500 Hz, −80 dB; 1000 Hz, −100 dB; right ear: 250 Hz, −50 dB; 500 Hz, −60 dB; 1000 Hz, −50 dB; 3000 Hz, −80 dB). Results from tests of air conduction, bone conduction, speech reception and discrimination, acoustic impedance, and acoustic reflex were consistent with a cochlear disorder. Electrooculography demonstrated a spontaneous, vestibular nystagmus with fast components to the left and a slow-component velocity of less than 5 deg/sec with eyes open in the dark. The vestibuloocular response to sinusoidal rotation in the dark (0.05 Hz, 60 deg/sec) was markedly decreased, but optokinetic nystagmus in response to similar sinusoidal drum rotation

NYSTAGMUS AND VERTIGO: CLINICAL
APPROACHES TO THE PATIENT WITH DIZZINESS

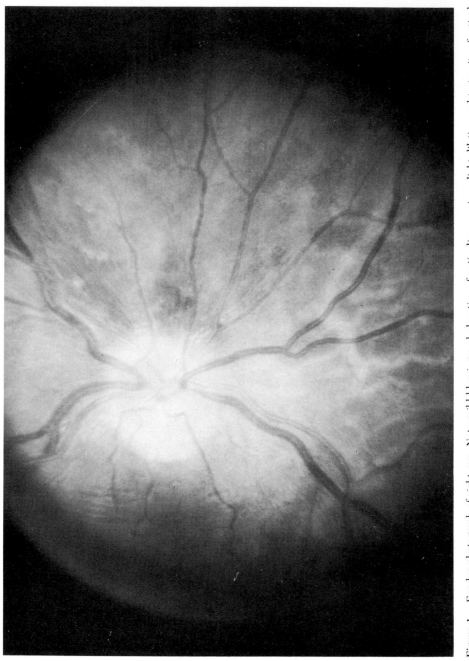

Figure 1. Fundus photograph of right eye. Note mild blurring and elevation of optic disc margins, slight dilation and tortuosity of retinal veins, and small, superficial retinal hemorrhages with white centers at the nasal and superonasal margins of the optic disc.

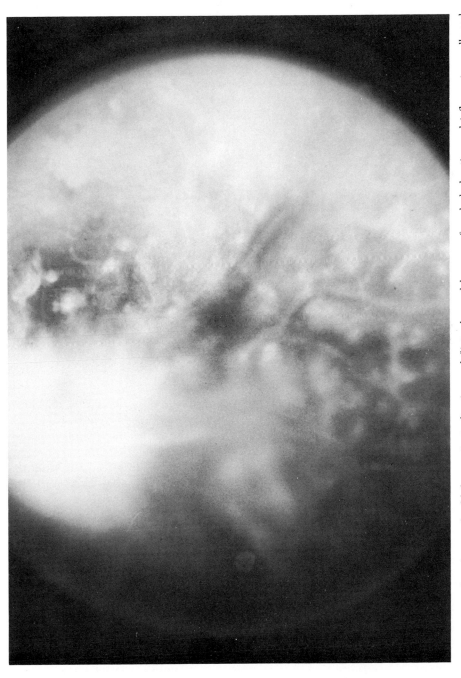

Figure 2. Fundus photograph of left eye. Optic disc (upper left) is obscured because of marked elevation and inflammatory cells and hemorrhage in the vitreous humor overlying the disc. Note sheathing of retinal vessels; marked dilation of retinal vein, and exudation in retina. There is a large retinal hemorrhage at the temporal margin of the disc.

and constant-velocity drum rotation was normal. The vestibuloocular response to bithermal, caloric testing of both ears was greatly diminished. Saccadic and smooth pursuit were normal. These findings were consistent with severe, bilateral, peripheral vestibular system lesions.

Ophthalmological examination revealed visual acuity of 20/20 in both eyes. Slit lamp biomicroscopy did not reveal opacities or blood vessels in the corneas, which have been described in patients with Cogan's syndrome. Dilated fundus examination of the right eye demonstrated slight blurring of the optic disc margins, small peripapillary hemorrhages in the nerve fiber layer with white centers (Roth spots), and slight dilation and tortuosity of the retinal veins (Figure 1). The appearance of the left fundus was normal.

The complete blood count was normal, except for elevation of the white blood cell count to 17,200 (normal differential). The Wintrobe sedimentation rate was abnormally increased to 39 mm/hr. The venereal disease research laboratory test and fluorescent treponemal antibody-absorption test were nonreactive, and antinuclear antibody titers and lupus erythemotosis cell preparation were negative. Other routine laboratory tests, such as chest x-ray and EKG, were normal.

Two days after admission the patient noted a sudden, painless, marked loss of vision in the left eye. Visual acuity had decreased to counting fingers at 2 ft. Fundus examination of the left eye revealed findings consistent with a central retinal vein occlusion (Figure 2). Extensive superficial and deep retinal hemorrhages surrounded the optic disc and extended into the macula; numerous cotton-wool spots and hard, retinal exudates were present throughout the posterior pole; retinal veins were tortuous and dilated; and retinal arteries and veins demonstrated yellow-white sheathing. Peripapillary hemorrhages had increased slightly in the right eye, but visual acuity was unchanged.

Nerve conduction studies in the legs demonstrated slightly decreased velocities, which were thought to be consistent with a polyneuropathy. Muscle biopsy of the legs showed mild infiltration of the walls and adventitia of arterioles by inflammatory cells, consistent with a periarteritis. A diagnosis of systemic vasculitis was made. Treatment was initiated with prednisone and immuran. Three months later the retinal hemorrhages had resolved and visual acuity had returned to 20/30 in the left eye, but cochlear and vestibular functions had not improved.

DISCUSSION

Dr. Yee: We are particularly fortunate to have Dr. David Cogan from the National Eye Institute to comment upon this case report. At one point in our patient's clinical course he was thought to have Cogan's syndrome. Dr. Cogan, what is the relationship between the disorder in our patient and that in patients with nonluetic, interstitial keratitis and vestibuloauditory loss, and what are your thoughts concerning the etiology of Cogan's syndrome?

Dr. Cogan: I wince a little every time I hear reference to Cogan's syndrome because it implies that I have some inside information. It is true that the eponymic designation has given me the opportunity to see a large number of relevant patients—35 at the last count—but that does not necessarily guarantee greater knowledge. In fact, I have to admit that I have little understanding of the pathogenesis of this curious combination of signs. Referring physicians and their patients find this out. One patient candidly said, "If you don't understand Cogan's syndrome, would you refer me to someone who does?"

Fortunately, a few years ago I joined forces with a physician, Dr. Barton Haynes, interested in immunology and vascular disease. To my great relief, he undertook a comprehensive study of all the patients referred to me and has written a definitive report.* Reviewing 13 patients whom he examined personally and the 111 cases reported in the literature, he concluded that there were two types of disease that have been called Cogan's syndrome: (a) typical cases, or those causing a chronic form of interstitial keratitis with a Ménière's-like complex leading to deafness; and (b) atypical cases with conjunctivitis, scleritis, retinal vascular disease, or other eye signs with or without keratitis. In the former cases there is some risk (10%) of developing an aortitis, whereas in the latter there is somewhat greater risk of developing a systemic necrotizing vasculitis. It is unfortunate that the two types have been confused under one eponym. The present patient clearly represents the latter type.

Dr. Yee: What treatment would you recommend?

Dr. Cogan: The treatment is outlined in Dr. Hayne's report. Prompt administration of systemic steroids prevents progression of the deafness, and topical steroids benefit the interstitial keratitis. For the atypical case, such as the one under discussion, I believe Dr. Haynes might suggest cytotoxic agents.

Dr. Yee: What are your thoughts about the etiology of the typical Cogan's syndrome?

Dr. Cogan: An immunologic process is suspect with an antigen common to the cornea, inner ear, and aorta. This tissue triad also comprises the targets for congenital syphilis, but the nature of the antigen is unknown. In exploratory observations with Dr. Devron Char we were unable to demonstrate abnormal skin sensitivity to corneal extracts in several patients with the syndrome. On the other hand, a flu-like episode often precedes the onset by 2 to 3 weeks, suggesting a viral origin, yet no virus has been consistently demonstrated.

*Haynes, B. F., Kaiser-Kupper, M. I., Mason, P., and Fauci, A. S., Cogan Syndrome: Studies in thirteen patients, long-term follow-up, and a review of the literature. *Medicine (Baltimore),* 1980, **59:**426–441.

CLINICAL TESTING OF VESTIBULOSPINAL FUNCTION

Equilibrium Testing of the Disoriented Patient

LEWIS M. NASHNER

Neurological Sciences Institute
Good Samaritan Hospital & Medical Center
Portland, Oregon

INTRODUCTION

Observing the upright balance of patients standing in various fixed configurations is not a new facet in the examination of the disoriented patient; Romberg (20) described this approach over a century ago. However, as observed by Graybiel and Fregly (5), available equilibrium tests are useful only during the rough, initial screening of patients, since patients gradually adapt their strategy of control after exposure to test environments. Because adaptive processes are crucial in enabling normal individuals, and to a more limited extent disoriented patients, to maintain balance under a wide variety of conditions, these authors suggest that quantitative measures of adaptive capability are necessary to make equilibrium tests clinically more useful. The aim of the study described in this chapter is therefore in keeping with Graybiel and Fregly's assessments: A hypothesis of adaptive equilibrium control based on theoretical arguments was advanced and experimentally tested. Experimental techniques were then applied to selected groups of disoriented patients to characterize the role played by adaptive processes in the impairment of orientation controls.

Two characteristics of the equilibrium control system collectively enable an individual to stand and walk under a variety of support-surface and visual conditions: (a) Redundant information related to orientation is provided by three sensory modalities (somatosensation derived principally from the forces and motions exerted by the feet on the support surface, vestibular inputs derived from head motions related to body sway, and visual inputs derived from sway-dependent motions of the head relative to objects in the visual surrounds), and (b) the system can adaptively modify the relative importance given to each of the sensory modalities in the control process. Because the three sensory modalities provide orientational information with respect to different frames of reference, each provides redundant information that is influenced differently by a change in support-surface or visual conditions. To illus-

NYSTAGMUS AND VERTIGO: CLINICAL
APPROACHES TO THE PATIENT WITH DIZZINESS

trate this principle with an example, standing or walking on a compliant foam rubber surface alters the accuracy of somatosensory inputs. Because the foam surface yields to the forces exerted by the feet, the orientation of the feet on the surface is no longer fixed with respect to the vertical. However, the vestibular and visual inputs received under this condition are not disturbed. Presumably, a normal individual does not fall or become disoriented while supported by such a surface, because his strategy of control is focused on vestibular and visual inputs.

The ability of the individual to modify his strategy of equilibrium control adaptively in response to changes in environmental conditions is one of the characteristics that makes this system so difficult to assess quantitatively. Selectively perturbing one of the three inputs in order to measure its influence on equilibrium control, the experimental approach utilized commonly in laboratory and clinical tests, may not accurately define the relation between the input and resulting muscular activity. Because awake, functioning individuals quickly modify their control strategy to minimize the effect of environmental perturbations, the relative weight given to the perturbed input may be reduced in favor of other unperturbed inputs. Thus, experimental and clinical tests of this kind can significantly underrate the influence of the component being selectively tested.

The ability to reorganize the strategy of equilibrium control adaptively makes the diagnosis of the disoriented patient equally difficult. The abnormal controls of the disoriented patient can be a complex superposition of impaired and other normal components that have been adaptively modified to compensate for the disability. As long as the impairment is sufficiently limited so as not to eliminate redundancy completely, the orientational deficit may be completely compensated for by adaptive reorganization of normal controls. The mildly impaired patient may become disoriented only when confronted with unusual or unexpected support-surface and/or visual conditions that also disturb the redundant, normal sensory inputs.

The above arguments help to explain the difficulties associated with equilibrium testing and to justify the conclusions of Graybiel and Fregly (5) that techniques to quantify adaptive controls are in part what is lacking in current clinical equilibrium tests. These arguments also suggest ways in which difficulties associated with equilibrium assessment can be surmounted; tests must be carried out while a variety of support-surface and visual conditions are successively imposed. In this way, controls mediated by each sensory input can be reassessed as the subject adopts a number of different control strategies, each focusing on a different combination of sensory inputs.

The hierarchical system is a useful model with which to describe the equilibrium control system, because it is a theoretical construct that embodies many of the adaptive processes mentioned above. The experimental approach to equilibrium control advanced in this chapter has therefore been developed using this concept.

HIERARCHICAL ORGANIZATION OF EQUILIBRIUM CONTROLS

A hierarchical system is one in which simple, stereotyped functions are mediated at the lowest levels. Reflex movements elicited by local stimuli in the absence of central inputs are examples of low-level "automatic" motor behavior, for which stimulus and response are relatively fixed. Higher levels coordinate and modify simple reflex behaviors. For example, extension and flexion movements of the leg of an animal in response to cutaneous stimulation of the foot are simple reflex behaviors that are probably involved in supporting the animal and in protecting its limbs from noxious stimuli. However, a relative balance between the two reflex behaviors must be established in the intact animal to prevent inappropriate limb flexion when support is necessary. Experiments indicate that coordination of these reflex behaviors is carried out by more centralized processes, presumably those involved in establishing the overall strategy of control relative to environmental conditions.

What are the advantages of a hierarchically organized equilibrium control system? Reflexlike equilibrium adjustments stereotyped with respect to the stimulus and responding quickly to local stimuli minimize the time required to compensate for perturbations and also reduce the requirements for centrally mediated equilibrium controls. The risk of using these automatized equilibrium controls is similar to that described for the extensor and flexor reflex behaviors; automatized equilibrium adjustments may be inappropriate under some environmental conditions. A critically important function of higher-level controls is therefore to minimize the occurrence of inappropriate equilibrium adjustments. Unfortunately, the hierarchical model does not describe a mechanism by which changes in environmental conditions are detected and the appropriate control strategies determined.

The hypothesis to be scrutinized in this chapter divides the adaptive process into two separate functions: (a) Changes in support-surface and visual conditions are detected and conflicts between them resolved by distinguishing those externally referenced modalities that transmit useful information about orientation from those disturbed by the surface and/or visual changes. (b) The strategy of equilibrium control is modified to rely more heavily on useful sensory inputs and to suppress the influence of those disturbed by the conditions. According to this hypothesis, adaptive reorganization is initiated after unexpected conflicts in the information transmitted by somatosensation and vision. Because vestibular inputs are, in contrast, relatively insensitive to environmental disruption, they provide the internal orientational reference used to resolve conflicts. The characteristics that render the vestibular input most useful in supplying the internal frame of reference for adaptation also make it difficult to assess directly the role played by these inputs in adaptation; it is not possible to alter the "vestibular" conditions of the task selectively. For this reason, much of the emphasis in this chapter is on defining the relationship between vestibular abnormalities and dysequilibrium. A patient with a clinically well defined vestibular deficit provides an opportunity to test adaptive changes in control strategy under selectively altered "vestibular" conditions.

The most conclusive evidence in favor of hierarchical organization of movement controls has been obtained from spinalized cat preparations (6). When the isolated circuits of the cord were tonically activated (by means of drugs or electrical or cutaneous stimuli), these preparations walked, trotted, and even galloped when suspended above a moving treadmill. The patterns of interlimb coordination, individual leg movements, and electromyographic (EMG) activities of individual muscles associated with leg movements were all similar to those of the intact animal. In addition, spinal preparations responded very rapidly to external perturbations by producing EMG adjustments organized in phase with the stepping of the perturbed limb (3, 4). However, despite the coordination of reflex adjustments into the walking movements, spinal preparations were unable to maintain equilibrium while walking on the treadmill. Presumably, the lack of a centrally mediated control strategy left the organization of these adjustments in a state inappropriate for balance.

Experimental Approach to Equilibrium Assessment

Two basic principles of experimental design emerge from the application of hierarchical concepts: (a) The conditions under which equilibrium controls are measured must be carefully controlled to ensure that control strategy does not change during sequences of tests. (b) Because the ability to assume different strategies of control is a highly important characteristic of the system, unexpected changes in conditions must be imposed to observe the ways in which adaptive changes in strategy alter the relative selection among the three sensory inputs. Establishing careful controls over the conditions of the task has been achieved utilizing a platform system that permits full control by the experimenter over the support-surface and visual conditions under which the subject stands.

The platform system illustrated schematically in Figure 1 assesses the anteroposterior (AP) component of equilibrium control. The support surfaces of the platform (one for each foot) are designed to measure the forces exerted by the feet and move in two directions: forward and backward translations, and "toes up" and "toes down" rotations about an axis collinear with the ankle joints. The subject stands within a rectangular enclosure that surrounds his field of view and that can be rotated forward or backward about an axis also collinear with the ankle joints.

The support-surface and visual conditions of the task are controlled by continuously moving these surfaces in relation to the AP sway movements of the subject. The somatosensory inputs derived from AP sway can be altered by a technique called "ankle stabilization" (Figure 2A); the support surfaces are rotated in direct proportion to the subject's AP sway orientation, thereby stabilizing the rotational position of the ankles with respect to the body and approximately eliminating somatosensory inputs derived from ankle joint rotations (10). The same stabilization procedure can also be applied to the visual system (Figure 2B); the enclosure is rotated in direct proportion to the AP sway rotations of the body, thereby eliminating any changes in the orientation of the visual environment relative to the subject (15).

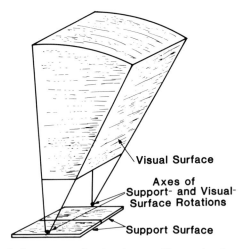

Figure 1.   Sketch of the platform system showing the movable visual and support surfaces. The subject stands with one foot on each support surface and faces the visual box. The subject's feet are positioned on the support surfaces so that the rotational axes of support and visual surfaces are collinear with that of the ankle joints.

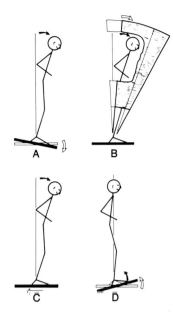

Figure 2.   Schematic representation of four platform techniques used to alter the conditions of the task (A and B) and to perturb orientation (C and D). Fine vertical lines indicate body orientation and outline the platform surface orientations before perturbation. Following perturbations, body orientations are outlined and platform surfaces indicated by heavy lines. (A) Rotational position of the ankle joints is stabilized with respect to AP sway motion (solid arrow) by rotating the platform surface (open arrow) in direct proportion to the AP sway angle. (B) Position of the visual surrounds is stabilized with respect to AP sway motion (solid arrow) by rotating the visual box (open arrow) in direct proportion to the AP sway angle. (C) Anteroposterior sway in one direction (solid arrow) is induced by translating the platform surfaces (open arrow) in the opposite direction. (D) Rotational orientation of the ankle joints is displaced (solid arrow), independent of the AP sway motions of the body, by rotating the platform surfaces (open arrow).

Brief displacements of the support surfaces or enclosure can be used to perturb different combinations of somatosensory, vestibular, and visual inputs. Translating the support surfaces either forward or backward induces AP sway in the opposite direction, with the axis of sway rotation centered at the ankle joints (Figure 2C). Under this condition, all three sensory modalities are affected in a way similar to that occurring during spontaneous AP sway. The ankle joints rotate, the head rotates and accelerates forward, and the visual surround is translated backward and rotated. "Toes up" or "toes down" rotation of the support surfaces rotates only the ankle joints; under this condition there are no correlated vestibular or visual inputs (Figure 2D). Now somatosensory inputs are in conflict with the others. Similarly, the visual enclosure can be rotationally displaced forward or backward to produce a visual input very similar to that occurring during spontaneous sway but in conflict with somatosensory and vestibular inputs.

The above-described displacements can also be applied while the subject is standing under the altered support-surface or visual conditions shown in Figure 2A and B. In this way, the influence of each sensory input can be retested as the individual adaptively modifies his strategy of control.

In several experiments with normal subjects it was possible to distinguish the automatized equilibrium controls from those mediated directly by vestibular and visual inputs. Following brief transient movements of the support surfaces, freely standing subjects responded rapidly (95- to 110-msec latency) with the changes in EMG activities of leg muscles specified by the pattern of ankle and knee joint motions produced by the perturbation (14, 19). Support-surface translations, which caused AP sway principally about the ankle joints, activated the lengthening ankle muscles and the hip muscles on the same dorsal or ventral aspect of the leg (Figure 3A). These EMG adjustments resisted the ankle joint displacements and at the same time resisted mechanically coupled rotations of the hips. Under normal support-surface conditions this rapid adjustment of ankle and hip joint activities helped to compensate for AP sway motions about the ankles and hips. When horizontal and vertical perturbations were interposed at random with other forms of platform displacements, the resulting rapid EMG adjustments were always organized appropriately with respect to the unexpected displacement of the leg joints (18, 19). The lack-of-response errors under random platform stimulus conditions are one result that illustrates the automatized nature of rapid equilibrium adjustments. Were these ad-

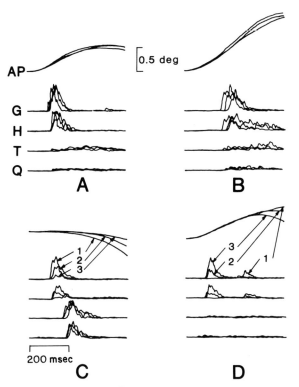

Figure 3.   Representative EMG responses and AP sway motions elicited by platform surface motions. AP indicates the anteroposterior sway orientation of the body; G, H, T, and Q respectively illustrate rectified and filtered EMG signals from the gastrocnemius, hamstrings, tibialis anterior, and quadriceps. (A) Coordinated activation of G and H muscles (95- to 110-msec latencies) following translation-induced forward AP sway (Figure 2C). (B) Delayed activation of G and H muscles (175- to 250-msec latencies) following forward AP sway under stabilized ankle conditions (Figure 2A). (C) Adaptive attenuation of rapid G and H adjustments (95- to 110-msec latencies) following unexpected imposition of platform surface rotations (Figure 2D). Amplitude of G and H EMG's and of AP sway perturbations are reduced in trial 3 compared to trial 1. (D) Lack of rapid EMG adjustments in G and H muscles during first translation-induced AP sway trial (Figure 2C) following subjects' adaptation to a sequence of platform surface rotations (Figure 2D). Rapid G and H adjustments, however, are progressively facilitated in trials 2 and 3.

justments "voluntary" reaction-time movements rather than automatized, executional errors would have been expected to occur under stimulus conditions that required subjects to choose between two alternative modes of response (16)?

The automatization of rapid equilibrium adjustments was further demonstrated by exploiting the fact that these activities may be inappropriately organized after unexpected changes in support-surface conditions. Specifically, "toes up" and "toes down" changes in surface inclinations (ankle motions now uncorrelated with AP sway) were alternately imposed between horizontal translations (AP sway and ankle rotations directly correlated). The waveforms of both perturbations were scaled to produce the same rotational change about the ankle joints. The EMG adjustments elicited by the unexpected support-surface rotations illustrated in Figure 3C are organizationally and metrically similar to those produced by normal AP sway (13, 14). This result supports the hypothesis that rapid equilibrium adjustments are mediated primarily by somatosensory inputs derived from ankle joint rotations. However, under this test condition, rapid EMG adjustments were inappropriate and increased rather than compensated for AP sway. Inappropriate adjustments were followed at 150- to 175-msec latencies by activation of the antagonist distal and proximal leg muscles. These later adjustments, which compensated for the AP sway produced by the surface rotation and increased by the earlier inappropriate adjustments, were presumably mediated by more complex processes involving vestibular and visual inputs.

The role of the more temporally delayed equilibrium adjustments that were vestibularly and visually mediated was studied further by observing the EMG responses of subjects deprived of somatosensory inputs utilizing the ankle stabilization procedure illustrated in Figure 2A. Under this condition, the equilibrium adjustments illustrated in Figure 3B were considerably more delayed (175 to 250 msec), and subjects swayed a good deal more (10). This observation has since been supported by another group of investigators, who applied pressure cuffs to block selectively somatosensory inputs derived from the lower leg musculature and from the feet (9). They also reported that the interruption of local somatosensory inputs resulted in a significant delay of equilibrium adjustments.

Presumably, the generation of equilibrium activities is delayed following the disruption of somatosensory inputs because subjects are forced to rely on controls mediated directly by vestibular inputs (12). Equilibrium activities generated with eyes closed and ankle joints stabilized are therefore believed to be a direct measure of vestibularly mediated EMG adjustments. This hypothesis is supported by the observation that patients with complete disruption of vestibular inputs could not maintain balance under this condition (1).* In fact, when perturbed while standing under this condition, these patients often fell until stabilized by a restraint without ever having responded to the motion.

Subjects were exposed to different support-surface and visual conditions in order to quantify the changes in rapid adjustments that parallel adaptation to altered environments. When somatosensory information derived from the leg musculature was repeatedly disturbed by rotational motions of the support surface, the amplitude of these rapid adjustments was progressively attenuated until all EMG activity corre-

*A study of patients with selected vestibular deficits was conducted in collaboration with F. O. Black and C. Wall III (18a).

lated with ankle joint motions was abolished (7, 13). Figure 3C shows that the amplitude of activity was progressively reduced from trial 1 to trial 3, whereas the later functionally useful component remained equally strong. Note that this change in strategy also progressively reduced the effect of the platform disturbance on the body. However, when subjects adopted a control strategy in which somatosensory inputs were suppressed, they also responded more slowly and with longer sway deviations following AP sway perturbations, as illustrated in Figure 3D. In the first trial, the stimulus paradigm had just been changed from a series of platform rotations to a platform translation. Now the subject responded to this AP sway perturbation with a latency of approximately 200 msec, as slowly as he did when somatosensory inputs were eliminated by the experimenter in Figure 3B. Thus, adaptive reorganization can suppress a component of equilibrium control so that the subject performs as if this input were absent. However, when several more platform translations are imposed, the subject quickly restores the use of automatized equilibrium controls.

The same kind of results were obtained by imposing unexpected enclosure rather than support-surface rotations. While subjects stood under the influence of occasional support-surface translations, the motions of the visual surround were unexpectedly stabilized (15). Automatized EMG adjustments elicited by translations during the first trials after unexpected visual stabilization were significantly attenuated in amplitude, and the sway deviations of the subjects were therefore larger. The unexpected nature of this visual perturbation was clearly the critical factor causing attenuation, since subjects who voluntarily closed their eyes did not demonstrate this phenomenon. When visual stabilization was maintained over sequences of five trials, the amplitudes of subsequent EMG adjustments became nearly equal to those observed under normal (or eyes closed) visual conditions. These observations indicate that under normal conditions visual inputs modulate automatized equilibrium activities according to relationships that are also fixed in advance. However, these fixed relationships are adaptively modified following the imposition of conditions that reduce the efficacy of visual inputs.

A study of equilibrium controls in young children has also helped to selectively observe automatized and adaptive components of equilibrium control. When children as young as 1.5 years were exposed to unexpected platform perturbations, the temporal and spatial organization of automatized EMG activities was similar to that observed in adults.* Also similar was the ability of young children to stand with eyes closed and the ankle joints stabilized continuously, presumably the test of direct vestibular mediation of equilibrium activities. However, there were dramatic differences between children below 6 to 8 years and older children whenever support- and visual-surface conflicts were imposed unexpectedly. Those below 6 to 8 years could not perform certain tasks with vision stabilized, although they could perform the same task with their eyes closed. Thus, instability was caused not by the lack of visual control but by an inability to suppress visual inputs when they transmitted conflicting information. Children below 6 to 8 years also did not adaptively attenuate automatic adjustments during sequences of rotational support-surface displacements.

In summary, the series of platform tests illustrated in Figure 2 enable one to make a selective evaluation of automatized equilibrium adjustments, vestibularly and

---

*This study of normal young children was conducted in collaboration with H. Forssberg (4a).

visually mediated adjustments, and the adaptive changes in the selection among these inputs. Automatized adjustments elicited by brief motions of the platform support surfaces are characterized by the latency and directional specificity of EMG activities. Selective deprivation of local somatosensory and visual inputs is achieved by stabilization of the platform and the visual enclosure surfaces with respect to the AP sway motions of the subject. Depriving the subject of both somatosensory and visual inputs (eye closure) provides a method for measuring vestibularly mediated adjustments, again by characterizing the latency and directional specificity of EMG activities. Finally, unexpected changes in surface conditions can be used to force the individual to alter adaptively the priority given to each of the three sensory modalities. Because this adaptive process is carried out more slowly than the execution of individual automatized adjustments, a series of perturbations imposed immediately after changes in surface conditions can be used to assess adaptive changes in the selection of inputs quantitatively.

AUTOMATIZED CONTROLS AND ADAPTIVE CHANGES IN THE STRATEGY OF PATIENTS WITH VESTIBULAR LESIONS

The equilibrium controls of selected patients with vestibular deficit were examined in order to test the hypothesis that vestibular inputs provide the internal reference with which conflicts between externally referenced (somatosensory and visual) inputs are resolved. According to this hypothesis selective vestibular lesions should not directly disrupt somatosensory and visual equilibrium controls. Hence, these patients may perform quite normally as long as the support-surface and visual conditions of the task are unaltered. More subtle equilibrium impairments may be expressed only as the inability to adopt the appropriate strategy of somatosensory and visual control under altered conditions.

The equilibrium of seven patients with vestibular deficits was studied using the techniques described in the previous section (1). The patients, whose vestibular deficits ranged in severity from complete disruption to nearly normal function, were independently evaluated by quantitatively measuring postural sway under static conditions (2) and vestibuloocular reflex (VOR) gains (21). In addition, two age-matched normal subjects were included in the study. The nine participants were then tested using a protocol that evaluated (a) overall performance under a variety of support- and visual-surface conditions, (b) automatized equilibrium adjustments under fixed surface conditions, (c) vestibularly mediated adjustments elicited under somatosensory and visually deprived conditions, and (d) ability to modify adjustments adaptively following unexpected altered support- and visual-surface conditions.

The results of this study are briefly summarized in Table 1. The nine participants are ranked numerically in order of overall performance; participant 1 swayed the most and 9 the least during continuous performance tests. The overall performance indices quantify the mean amplitude of swaying over 50-sec test intervals (0 indicates no swaying, and 100 indicates the limits of stability). Automatic adjustments are classified as normal or abnormal on the basis of their latency (N = 100 ± 25 msec) and the activation of appropriate muscle groups. Vestibular adjustments are also classified as normal or abnormal on the basis of latency (N = 175 to 300 msec). Adaptation is classified as normal if the adaptation ratio (AR) is less than 0.25. The AR quantifies the relative amplitude of last as compared to first responses in sequences of five trials

TABLE 1
EVALUATION OF PATIENTS WITH VESTIBULAR DEFICITS[a]

	Clinical test summary[c]			Platform test summary		
Participant[b]	VOR gain	VOR symmetry	Static posture	Automatic adjustments	"Vestibular" adjustments	Adaptive adjustments
1	A	—	A	N	A (none)	A (both modalities)
2	N	A	A	N	N	A (visual only)
3	N	N	A	N	N	A (both modalities)
4	A (hyperactive)	A	N	N	N	A (somatosensory only)
5	A (hypoactive)	N	N	N	N	N
6	N	A	N	N	N	A (somatosensory only)
7	N	N	N	N	N	N
8	N	N	N	N	N	N
9	N	N	N	N	N	N

[a] Key: N indicates test results within the normal range (within ± 2 SD of the mean); A indicates test results falling outside the normal range.

[b] Clinical histories of the patients are the following; (1) postototoxicity, (2) right Ménière's disease (3) left labyrinthectomy (25 years before) and right Ménière's disease, (4) vestibular hydrops (presumed), (5) bilateral Ménière's disease, (6) right Ménière's disease, (7) left Ménière's disease, clinically in remission at time of platform testing, (8), (9) age-matched normal subjects.

[c] VOR test procedures have been reported by Wall (21). Static posturography test procedures have been reported by Black (2).

imposed following unexpected changes in support- or visual-surface conditions. The results of independent clinical tests are summarized as the gain and symmetry of VOR's and as the amount of sway measured during the static postural tests.

Table 1 shows good correspondence between the clinical assessment of equilibrium and the results of platform tests. Deficiencies in automatized or vestibularly mediated controls were evident only in the most severely afflicted patient (number 1). The other participants experienced equilibrium difficulties only when the environmental conditions placed somatosensory and visual inputs in conflict with one another. These difficulties were correlated with abnormal adaptive controls. Following unexpected changes in the conditions of the task, mildly impaired patients focused inappropriately on the disturbed rather than the useful sensory stimuli. Some of these patients randomly changed the focus of control from trial to trial, providing a highly erratic level of performance. Others were able to converge slowly on the appropriate control strategy, but only after 5 to 10 times as many trials as required by normal subjects. Vestibular deficit patients seemed unable to adapt their control strategy to the environmental conditions. This observation is consistent with the hypothesis that vestibular inputs provide the internal reference frame within which conflicts are resolved. The two patients (numbers 5 and 7) and the two normal subjects (numbers 8 and 9) who reported no equilibrium difficulties in the clinical examination were also normal on all platform tests. Patient 7 suffered unilateral Ménière's disease, which was clinically in a state of remission at the time of testing. Patient 5 was unusual inasmuch as equilibrium control was normal despite a relatively severe VOR deficit.

Table 1 shows clear differences between equilibrium and eye movement (VOR) assessments of orientational control. Among the patients with milder (adaptive) equilibrium deficits (numbers 3 to 6), performance under all predictable conditions was normal. The only abnormal characteristic of these patients was in their ability to adapt quickly following unexpected changes in surface conditions. Despite the consistent findings in relation to equilibrium tests, the VOR test results of this group ranged from normal to deficient in gain and/or symmetry. This finding suggests that VOR and equilibrium tests assess different subprocesses related to orientation within the central nervous system (CNS).

The results of patient studies help to explain the deficiencies associated with tests conducted under fixed environmental conditions. Because the automatic equilibrium controls of vestibular patients are not directly impaired, even those suffering severe vestibular deficits can use these to stand and walk quite normally under normal conditions. Testing patients under fixed condition, therefore, maximizes the ability to compensate adaptively for their impairment. This is why some severely impaired patients must be subjected to additional stress—for example, standing with feet placed in heel-to-toe positions with the eyes closed. Unfortunately, the emergence of an equilibrium deficit under these stressed conditions does not by itself help to localize the cause of the patient's instability. In contrast, using the approach advanced here, one can selectively assess automatic controls and their adaptive reorganization. For example, a patient who is stable under a given set of conditions with eyes closed and yet is unstable under the same set of conditions when opening his eyes in the presence of a conflicting visual stimulus is clearly suffering from the inability to suppress visual inputs adaptively rather than from the inability to perform in the absence of this input.

EQUILIBRIUM ASSESSMENT OF THE DISORIENTED PATIENT

An experimental technique based on principles of hierarchical organization has made it possible to measure quantitatively several components of equilibrium control: automatic adjustments, vestibularly mediated adjustments, and adaptive modification of automatized controls. Theoretical concepts and experimental results based on a study of normal subjects and a very limited number of disoriented patients has advanced the understanding of disorientation. Specifically, disorientation may evolve from vestibular lesions either through the loss of vestibularly mediated adjustments or (more likely) through impairment of the ability to adapt to altered environmental conditions. Because the vestibular system may provide inputs critical to the adaptive process, patients with vestibular lesions are unable to interpret appropriately sensations of orientation derived from other externally referenced somatosensory and visual inputs. Because automatic adjustments initiated by local somatosensory inputs and modulated by vision are sufficiently effective to maintain equilibrium under normal conditions, disorientation occurs in these patients only when automatized and visually mediated controls are disorganized by conditions that bring these two important inputs into conflict. Thus, the independent assessment of lower-level automatic and higher-level adaptive components is essential in the evaluation of the patient with dysequilibrium.

Whereas equilibrium testing of this kind may significantly improve the ability to diagnose certain subpopulations of disoriented patients, this form of assessment cannot replace the information provided by other procedures such as VOR testing.

Because preliminary results suggest that visual and postural orientation can be selectively impaired by vestibular lesions, these two approaches should be complementary rather than exclusive facets of the clinical assessment.

Although the platform studies described here demonstrate the potential role of equilibrium tests in the comprehensive assessment of disorientation, a host of questions are left unanswered regarding the clinical application of this technique. The most important question is whether platform assessment can differentiate between vestibularly derived equilibrium disorders and those arising from other types of CNS lesions. In this regard, a good deal of additional work is necessary.

The platform evaluation of a select group of cerebellar deficit patients whose primary sysmptom was gait ataxia revealed impaired functions that were qualitatively similar to thsoe exhibited by vestibular deficit patients (17). The two most commonly observed equilibrium deficits among the cerebellar patients were the inability to maintain balance with ankles stabilized and eyes closed (presumably the direct test of vestibularly mediated control) and a lack of adaptation following the imposition of support-surface rotations. However, there were important quantitative differences in performance between cerebellar and vestibular deficit patients. Whereas ataxic cerebellar patients showed few if any adaptive changes in control strategy, the vestibular patients showed inappropriate adaptive changes. There were also important differences in the ways cerebellar and vestibular patients lost their balance when concurrently deprived of somatosensory and visual inputs. Whereas only the more severely impaired vestibular patients lost their balance (through a loss of low-threshold activity, i.e., increased response latencies), most of the ataxic cerebellar patients responded as rapidly as normal subjects but nevertheless drifed slowly toward an unstable orientation, usually within 5–10 sec.

The above-described differences between vestibular and cerebellar disorientation conform to current theories about the functional role of these two organs. Extensive animal studies have shown cerebellar circuits to be essential in mediating adaptive changes in the gain and phase of vestibuloocular reflexes (8). The review of McKay and Murphy (8) together with that of Wilson (22), which emphasizes the rich interrelations among cerebellar, vestibular, and spinal motor centers, indicates that vestibular inputs and cerebellar circuits are collectively involved in the adaptive reorganization of spinal motor activities. Hence, adaptive reorganization is ambiguous without essential vestibular inputs and altogether absent without the essential mediating circuitry.

Differences in the way vestibular and cerebellar patients lose balance when concurrently deprived of somatosensory and visual inputs poses another problem; to date there are no practical clinical tests that selectively assess semicircular canal (rotational) and utricular otolith (linear) functions. However, a theoretical model of equilibrium control suggests that the differences in balance between the cerebellar and vestibular subpopulations of patients relates to selective impairment of rotational and linear acceleration inputs (11). According to this model, steady-state orientation and rapid changes in orientation are mediated by different subcomponents of the vestibular system. Although studies of vertical semicircular canal inputs are most appropriate for detecting rapid (sway) rotational motions, only the utricular otoliths provide information relating the steady-state orientation of the subject to the gravitational vertical. It is therefore possible that cerebellar lesions leading primarily to ataxic gait selectively affect those cerebellar circuits mediating the control of steady-state orientation. However, because there are no practical clinical techniques for evaluating otolithic impairment, the question of selective impairment of static and dynamic equilibrium controls must await further study.

Another issue requiring considerable effort is that disturbances in vestibular inputs can assume a variety of forms. Primarily on the basis of VOR assessments of patients (21), it has been found that vestibular lesions can result in (a) increases or decreases in VOR gain, (b) directional asymmetries, (c) activity uncorrelated with motion inputs, (d) random changes in transduction characteristics over time, and (e) various combinations of the aforementioned categories. How each kind of functional deficit selectively affects the control of equilibrium is not understood, although the hierarchical model of equilibrium control predicts some of the ways. For example, adaptive control requires an internal orientation reference that is both accurate and consistent. Any of the above functional alterations might therefore equally impair adaptive control but have very different effects on direct vestibular controls. For example, a patient suffering only occasional attacks, in learning to suppress vestibular conflicts caused by the disease, might also (inappropriately) suppress vestibular inputs when the conflict results from the external perturbation of other sensory inputs. In other words, faced with the possibility that any of the three sensory modalities may be disturbed during a conflict situation, a patient has no reliable way of resolving the conflict.

Another issue that may be addressed is the practicality of clinical platform testing in the form suggested in this chapter. Are all of the complex platform movements necessary for assessment of equilibrium controls, or could the procedure be reduced to a few easily implemented tests that would provide the most essential information?

In summary, dynamic equilibrium testing may contribute a new facet to the array of clinical tests for the disoriented patient. However, it is clearly not a panacea. Because equilibrium controls, eye movement controls, and the conscious perception of orientation may be selectively impaired by different CNS disorders, tests are needed that examine each of these functions. Equilibrium testing based on hierarchical concepts may be most valuable in assessing the patient with subtle equilibrium deficits. Further effort is therefore most appropriate to understand more fully the complex, integrative functions of the equilibrium control system and to quantify the ways in which different types of CNS lesions alter specific subfunctions of this system.

ACKNOWLEDGMENTS

The author wishes to acknowledge the contributions made by F. O. Black and C. Wall III to the studies of vestibular deficit patients, R. J. Grimm to studies of cerebellar deficit patients, and H. Forssberg to the studies of young children. This work has been supported by NINCDS grants NS00148 and NS12661.

REFERENCES

1. Black, F. O., Nashner, L. M., and Wall, C., III, What is the role of vestibular inputs in positive control. *Soc. Neurosci. Abstr.*, 1980, **6**:676.
2. Black, F. O., Wall, C., III, and O'Leary, D., Computerized screening of the human vestibulospinal system. *Ann. Otol., Rhinol. Laryngol.*, 1978, **87**:853–864.
3. Duysens, J., and Pearson, K. G., The role of cutaneous afferents from the distal hindlimb in the regulation of the step cycle in thalamic cats. *Exp. Brain Res.*, 1976, **24**:245–255.

4. Forssberg, H., Grillner, S., and Rossignol, S., Phasic gain control of reflexes from the dorsum of the paw during spinal locomotion. *Brain Res.*, 1977, **132**:121–139.

4a. Forssberg, H., and Nashner, L. M., Ontogenetic development of postural control in man: Adaptation to altered support and visual conditions during stance. *J. Neurosci.* (in press).

5. Graybiel, A., and Fregly, A. R., A new quantitative ataxia test battery. *Acta Oto-Laryngol.* (Stockh.), 1966, **61**:292–312.

6. Grillner, S., Locomotion in vertebrates: Central mechanisms and reflex interaction. *Physiol. Rev.*, 1975, **55**:247–304.

7. Gurfinkel, V. S., Lipshits, M. J., and Popov, K. E., Is the stretch reflex the main mechanism in the system of regulation of the vertical posture of man? *Biophysics*, 1974, **19**:744–48.

8. MacKay, W. A., and Murphy, J. T., Cerebellar modulation of reflex gains. *Prog. Neurobiol.* 1979, **13**:361–417.

9. Mauritz, K. H., and Dietz, V., Characteristics of postural instability induced by ischemic blocking of leg afferents. *Exp. Brain Res.*, 1980, **38**:117–119.

10. Nashner, L. M., A model describing the vestibular detection of body sway motion. *Acta Oto-Laryngol.*, 1971, **72**:429–436.

11. Nashner, L. M., Vestibular posture control model. *Kybernetik*, 1972, **10**:106–110.

12. Nashner, L. M., Vestibular and reflex control of normal standing. In: *Control of Posture and Locomotion* (R. B. Stein, K. B. Pearson, R. S. Smith, and J. B. Redford, eds.). Plenum, New York, 1973:291–308.

13. Nashner, L. M., Adapting reflexes controlling the human posture. *Exp. Brain Res.*, 1976, **26**:59–72.

14. Nashner, L. M., Fixed patterns of rapid postural responses among leg muscles during stance. *Exp. Brain Res.*, 1977, **30**:13–24.

15. Nashner, L. M., and Berthoz, A., Visual contribution to rapid motor responses during posture control. *Brain Res.*, 1978, **150**:403–407.

16. Nashner, L. M., and Cordo, P. J., Relation of postural responses and reaction-time voluntary movements in human leg muscles. *Exp. Brain Res.*, 1982, **43**:395–405.

17. Nashner, L. M., and Grimm, R. J., Analysis of multiloop dyscontrols in standing cerebellar patients. *Prog. Clin. Neurophysiol.*, 1977, **4**:300–319.

18. Nashner, L. M., and Woollacott, M., The organization of rapid postural adjustments of standing humans: An experimental-conceptual model. In: *Posture and Movement* (R. E. Talbott and D. R. Humphrey, eds.). Raven, New York, 1979:243–257.

18a. Nashner, L. M., Black, F. O., Wall, C., III, Adaptation to altered support and visual conditions during stance: Patients with vestibular deficits. *J. Neurosci.* (in press).

19. Nashner, L. M., Woolacott, M., and Tuma, G., Organization of rapid responses to postural and locomotor-like perturbations of standing man. *Exp. Brain Res.*, 1979, **36**:463–476.

20. Romberg, M. H., *A Manual of the Nervous Diseases of Man*, (E. H. Siereking, ed. and trans.). Sydenham Society, London, 1853:396.

21. Wall, C., III, Black, F. O., and O'Leary, D., Clinical use of pseudo random, binary sequence white noise in assessment of the human vestibulo-ocular system. *Ann. Otol., Rhinol., Laryngol.*, 1978, **87**:845–852.

22. Wilson, V. J., Physiological pathways through the vestibular nuclei. *Int. Rev. Neurobiol.*, 1972, **15**:27–81.

The Pathophysiology of Postural Imbalance in Cerebellar Patients

JOHANNES DICHGANS[1] and KARL-HEINZ MAURITZ[2]

[1]*Department of Neurology, University of Tübingen, Federal Republic of Germany*
[2]*Department of Neurology, University of Freiburg, Federal Republic of Germany*

INTRODUCTION

The recently developed methods for measuring the displacement of the body's center of force* allow for a rather detailed analysis of postural sway. A computational treatment of the data obtained by the use of a force-measuring platform results in parametric documentation of sway area and sway path per unit time, mean amplitude of sway, and histograms of sway direction as well as sway position (16). These and power spectral density analysis of the anteroposterior and lateral sway components (2) help to distinguish several kinds of postural ataxia in human beings.

Special techniques, such as sudden displacement of the platform (1, 15, 19, 21, 28), displacement of the subject's visual surround (7, 16, 17), or vestibular stimulation (6, 24), can be used to test the function of the three main control loops involved in the stabilization of posture (23).

Key patterns of disturbance emerge that make it possible to distinguish three kinds of postural ataxia in cerebellar patients (21). These will be briefly described. Following this, some physiological studies will be reported that have been performed in order to investigate the pathophysiological mechanisms of postural tremor in patients with cerebellar ataxia. The latter studies have been published elsewhere in more detail (22).

---

*Displacement of the body's center of force is not identical to displacement of the center of gravity since, except for the static condition, dynamic forces due to body inertia contribute. Their proportional amount increases with increasing frequency (14, 36).

NYSTAGMUS AND VERTIGO: CLINICAL
APPROACHES TO THE PATIENT WITH DIZZINESS

Types of Postural Ataxia in Patients with Cerebellar Disorders

LATE CORTICAL CEREBELLAR ATROPHY OF THE ANTERIOR LOBE (THE SPINOCEREBELLUM) (37)

This disease probably results from nutritional deficiencies in alcoholics and from other forms of malnutrition (38). Mean amplitudes of sway and sway path are significantly increased without exception in these patients. More specific is a 3-Hz postural tremor in the anteroposterior direction (7, 21, 33, 34). The 3-Hz sway component can easily be differentiated from the postural tremor in a patient with Parkinson's disease (Figure 1B). The frequency of the anteroposterior component in the patient with anterior lobe atrophy decreases with progression of the disease (Figure 1C). In incipient cases, when the tremor cannot be detected clinically, it can be evoked by sudden mechanical destabilization of the body.

Less characteristic and smaller in amplitude is a 0.5- to 0.7-Hz frequency peak mainly within the spectrum of the lateral sway component (Figure 1A). This points to an independent control of body equilibrium in the anteroposterior and lateral directions. The low-frequency peak is also seen with other kinds of postural disequilibrium, as in visually destabilized normal subjects (7) and in patients with spinal ataxia, as with tabes dorsalis.

Visual stabilization of posture is frequently preserved in patients with cortical cerebellar atrophy. The degree of visual stabilization does not correlate with the general instability of posture. Intersegmental movements between head, hips, and legs are characteristically exaggerated, each being roughly 180 deg out of phase with respect to the other, and they participate in the 3-Hz sway. Normally, each of these intersegmental movements automatically compensates for the displacement of their adjacent segment. They belong to the group of fixed intersegmental reaction patterns, the importance of which has been stressed by Bernstein (3), Gurfinkel *et al.* (13), and Nashner (27).

One of the key features of these patients that distinguishes them from patients with ataxia due to neocerebellar and vestibulocerebellar lesions is the prevalence of the anteroposterior sway component. This is most easily evidenced by histograms of sway direction or sway position (Figure 2). Although stance is very unstable in patients with late anterior lobe atrophy, falling rarely occurs.

LESIONS OF THE CEREBELLAR HEMISPHERES

If these lesions disturb stance at all, they cause only slight postural instability without directional preference and without a special frequency peak within their sway (Figure 2). Sway parameters with eyes open are within the 2σ range of normal values, and there is no significant difference in these parameters from normal values even when the eyes are closed. The 3-Hz tremor may never be provoked, either by pushing the body or by suddenly tilting the platform. The cerebellar hemispheres interact with the neocerebral cortex and are concerned mainly with the temporospatial organization of goal-directed movements of the limbs and with speech but not with body posture.

LESIONS OF THE VESTIBULOCEREBELLUM (THE POSTERIOR VERMIS, INCLUDING FLOCCULUS AND NODULUS)

Such lesions cause extreme instability of stance without preferred axis or frequency (Figure 2). The average amplitude of sway is unusually large. Sway on the average is

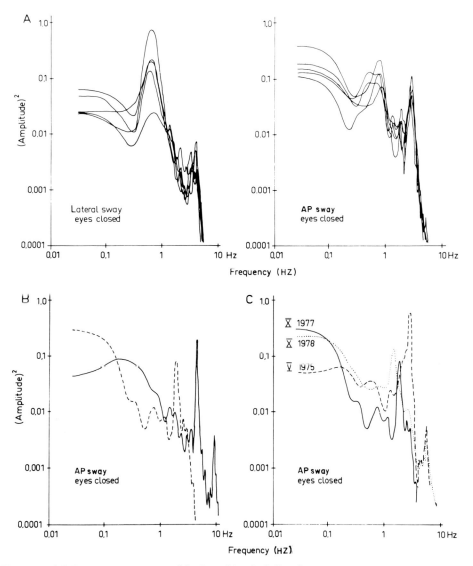

Figure 1. (A) Fourier power spectra of the lateral (on the left) and anteroposterior (AP) body sway (on the right) in a patient with late cortical cerebellar atrophy. The five spectra represent measurements on five consecutive days. Note the high reproducibility of the 3-Hz peak in the anteroposterior direction and a 0.7-Hz peak mainly in the lateral component. (B) Comparison of Fourier power spectrum of a patient with Parkinsonism (solid line) with that of a patient with late cortical cerebellar atrophy (dashed line). The prominent tremor frequency is clearly separate in the two syndromes. (C) The dominant tremor frequency shifts to lower frequencies with progressive cerebellar atrophy, as seen in one typical patient studied repeatedly for 3.5 years.

definitely slower than in patients with spinocerebellar atrophy. In contrast to patients with anterior lobe lesions, these patients, suffering mainly from a medulloblastoma, are characterized by the absence of intersegmental movements and the lack of a set value determining the upright position (21). Thus, they may fall even when sitting. Neocerebellar functions, such as pointing, may be intact.

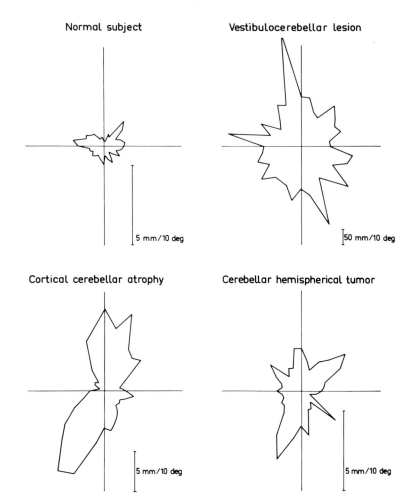

Figure 2. Comparison of position histograms (eccentricities summed within every 10-deg polar bin, sampling interval 30 msec, integration over 1 min) of a typical normal subject, a patient with a vestibulocerebellar medulloblastoma, a patient with late cortical cerebellar atrophy, and a patient with a cerebellar hemispheric lesion. The patient with the hemispheric lesion has only a slightly increased instability compared to the other two patients. The patient with the anterior lobe atrophy has a predominant (high-frequency, low-amplitude) anteroposterior instability, which would be even more impressive in the direction histogram (not shown). The patient with the vestibulocerebellar lesion exhibits omnidirectional sway of an extremely large amplitude. His low-frequency, high-amplitude instability is more pronounced in the position histogram presented here. Note the different scaling, which was necessary for technical reasons.

LABYRINTHINE LESIONS

If unilateral, these lesions may cause the classical falling or a lateral deviation of the center of force toward the side of the lesion. In later stages, sway amplitude and sway area, the two most significant parameters in patients with labyrinthine lesions, are not necessarily higher than normal when the eyes are open. With the eyes closed, however, even the sway path is significantly higher than in normal subjects. The sway in patients with vestibular lesions is slow in comparison to that in patients with spinocerebellar atrophy (16).

ALTERED REFLEX RESPONSES AS THE POSSIBLE CAUSE OF POSTURAL TREMOR IN SPINOCEREBELLAR ATROPHY

Recent evidence from normal subjects suggests that myotatic reflexes at 40- to 50-msec latencies are seen only with a very sudden angular displacement of the ankle joint and are of little functional significance (1, 4, 15, 26). Functional stretch reflexes occurring after latencies of between 100 and 120 msec in normal subjects are the first to be mechanically effective. They are probably mediated by suprasegmental and central structures (9, 31), although an observation by Ghez and Shinoda (12) in the cat suggests that the spinal cord itself may produce these so-called long-loop reflexes. Responses occurring later than 180 msec after body displacement may be vestibularly elicited (25).

Reflex responses obviously are stereotypically organized into a pattern of fixed synergisms of multiple leg muscles structured as a preprogrammed subroutine (11) that is controlled by the pattern of movement inputs from the entire leg. Reflex responses are also selected according to the environmental conditions and their behavioral significance to the subject. According to Nashner (28), "the adjustments are too complexly interwoven into an organizational structure involving many leg muscles to be characterized simply as the response of each individual muscle to its own stretch input." It may then be investigated whether the spinocerebellum, which is intensely supplied by proprioceptive afference from the legs (30), is in the long loop of the functional stretch reflex and/or plays any role in organizing motor patterns for postural stabilization.

We tested more than 30 patients with late cortical cerebellar atrophy of the anterior lobe by using a platform that could be rapidly tilted in pitch about an axis aligned to the ankle joint, or by applying a current to the tibial nerve in order to stimulate afferent fibers from muscle spindles directly. Stimulus efficiency was directly monitored by recording the H reflex while the patient was standing on the platform. Surface electrodes recorded electromyographic (EMG) activity over the gastrocnemius and tibial muscles. The EMG was then fully wave-rectified and filtered. Displacement of the center of foot pressure was recorded by strain gauges connected to the four corners of the platform. Also recorded were the angular displacements of ankle angle, hip, and head. Recordings were frequently averaged to eliminate noise. Electrical stimuli to the tibial nerve were applied in the popliteal fossa. Stimulus intensity was usually adjusted to 50% of that necessary to evoke a maximal H-reflex response (and rarely an M response). We could thus assume that mainly Ia afferents were excited and that subsequent mechanical effects were due to reflex responses only. Electrical stimulation was preferred to mechanical tilting of the platform since the latter per se displaces the body, possibly excites reflex responses, and by the displacement of the ankle joint involves viscoelastic forces of the stretched muscle and inertial reaction forces of the body. The methods used have been extensively described by Mauritz *et al.* (22).

In contrast to Nashner and Grimm (29), who in a pilot study of the posture of patients with cerebellar atrophy found little alteration in functional stretch responses, mainly in terms of a deficit in adaptation, we observed an increased gain and delayed appearance of postural long-loop reflexes. These and increased intersegmental reflexes were shown to be the most likely cause of the 3-Hz tremor observed in these patients.

SHORT-LATENCY, SEGMENTAL STRETCH REFLEX RESPONSES

Electrical stimulation in normal subjects and patients with anterior lobe atrophy (usually without demyelinizing neuropathy) similarly elicits the H reflex after a normal latency of about 30 msec. This response exerts a forward torque on the platform starting 45 to 50 msec after the onset of the stimulus. Although the center of force is still displaced forward, the ankle joint is extended and the tibial muscle is stretched. This stretch starts 80 msec (with maximal stimulation arousing an M response 50 msec) after the stimulus is applied. Stretch of the tibial muscle after another 30 to 40 msec (total latency 120 and 90 msec, respectively) results in a short-latency response of this muscle termed tib_1 (Figure 3). As a result of the reaction force a more tonic backward sway of the center of foot pressure follows. This is automatically compensated for by an intersegmental flexing forward of the trunk (and head), thereby stabilizing posture (Figure 4). The amplitude of tib_1 frequently increases with eye closure. As advocated by Taborikova (35) and Allum and Büdingen (1), tib_1 could in principle also be a long-loop response to tibial nerve stimulation directly. We argue that this is not the case, stressing the following evidence:

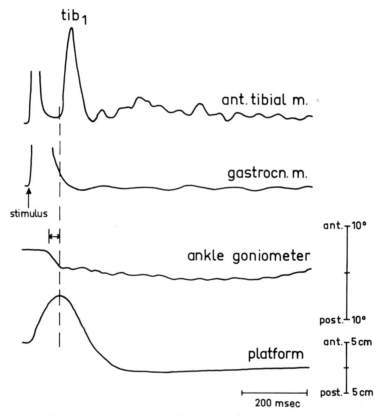

Figure 3.   Averaged stimulus responses ($n = 16$) in a normal subject after electrical stimulation of both tibial nerves. Rectified recordings of the surface EMG of the anterior tibial and gastrocnemius muscles, of the ankle angle, and of the displacement of the center of force. The initial gap in the recording includes the high-amplitude stimulus artifact and, in the gastrocnemius muscle, the H reflex and the direct response of the muscle to stimulation. The latter two responses cause an ankle angle displacement, which is followed by a discharge of the stretched anterior tibial muscle within 40 msec (dashed line).

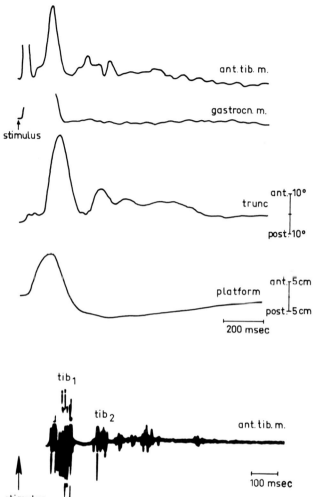

Figure 4. Typical stimulus response in a normal subject (average of rectified EMG responses, $n = 16$). Note the large tib_1 and the smaller tib_2 discharge in the anterior tibial muscle. This is also seen in the original recording below.

1. The amplitude of tib_1 depends on the rate and amplitude of the forward displacement of foot pressure (32).

2. If body displacement and tibialis stretch are reduced by inertial loading of the trunk with 30 kg, an identical stimulation of Ia fibers cause a smaller tib_1 potential.

3. With supramaximal stimuli, when M responses occur exclusively and H responses are occluded by antidromic collision, tib_1 latencies are shortened by an amount roughly equal to the time interval between M and H responses (24 to 35 msec).

If one considers the mechanical delays due to body inertia and striction and takes into account a certain threshold for exciting the muscle receptors, the 120-msec latency seems to be compatible with the assumption of a spinal stretch reflex causing tib_1.

The assumption that Ia afferents are involved is supported by an experiment with ischemic blockage of Ia afferents (8) but preserved motor innervation. This occurs 20 to 25 min after cuff insufflation, when H reflexes are minimized and tib_1 is equally reduced, although with higher stimulus intensities M responses are preserved.

The possibility that late EMG responses are flexor reflexes triggered by the painful stimulation of cutaneous receptors was ruled out by displacing the stimulating electrodes a few centimeters in the popliteal fossa or by applying the stimulation to several places on the leg and foot. Even if stimulus strength was increased until it was almost intolerable, no motor reactions in tibialis anterior were indicated by EMG. The possibility that tib_1 was a long-loop response to direct electrical costimulation of the peroneal nerve was ruled out by the lack of M and H responses in the tibial muscle.

The fact that tib_1 does not change in gain and loop time in cerebellar patients compared to normal subjects shows that tib_1 does not depend on intact cerebellar function.

LONG-LATENCY, SUPRASEGMENTAL REFLEX RESPONSES

In contrast to short-latency responses (tib_1), long-latency responses show very marked differences in normal subjects and patients with cerebellar anterior lobe atrophy. Whereas normal subjects may, or more frequently may not, show a second discharge in tibialis anterior (tib_2), this is regularly the case in patients with the anterior lobe disease. Normal subjects exhibit an interpeak ($tib_1 - tib_2$) interval of 90 to 120 msec, whereas in patients with the anterior lobe syndrome this interval is increased by an average of 80 msec (compare Figures 4 and 5). We suggest that tib_2 in normal subjects (and in patients) is a long-loop reflex response to the stretch of the tibial muscle. This assumption is based on its latency, which seems appropriate when one considers the rather low velocity of stretch (5, 26). The delay of tib_2 increases with progression of the disease and reached 350 msec in one rare exception. Whereas a third discharge is very exceptional in normal subjects, this and later discharges, frequently a sustained sequence of tibial muscle discharges, occur in these patients. They parallel the postural tremor regularly evoked or synchronized by this stimulation. The tremor has the same frequency as the spontaneous oscillations, repeatedly occurring in clusters in advanced cases. The increased delay in interpeak latency of the long-loop reflexes coincides with the decrease in tremor frequency (Figure 1C). Both long-loop reflexes and tremor are inhibited by visual stabilization of posture with the eyes open (Figure 5).

Long-latency responses in triceps surae are inconsistent in normal subjects, occurring simultaneously with tib_1 or 30 to 60 msec later. In patients with anterior lobe atrophy, there is an alternating discharge of the tibial and gastrocnemius muscle, which is not seen in normal subjects. We think that the alternation of discharges in flexors and extensors constitutes and sustains the tremor. So far we have not been able to synchronize postural tremor in patients with Parkinson's disease when using this stimulation technique.

The tremor seems to be the consequence of reflex facilitation increasing the gain of long-latency responses and their loop time. This is not the case with segmental reflex responses. The tremor also results from the temporal coincidence of segmental stretch reflexes, with exaggerated and delayed suprasegmental responses adding to each other. This conforms with the results of Vilis and Cooke (39), who observed

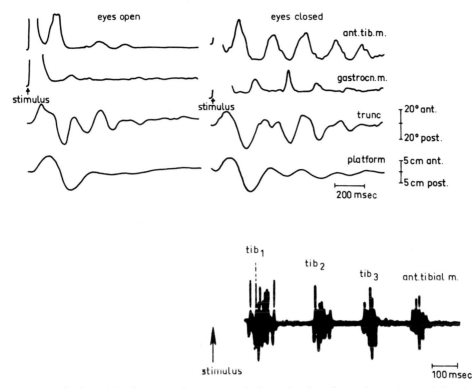

Figure 5. Rhythmical discharges in the anterior tibial muscle after electrical stimulation of the tibial nerve are evoked in a patient with incipient anterior lobe atrophy only with the eyes closed. Correspondingly, a damped oscillation is seen in the platform and trunc (angle) recording. The original recording of poststimulus tibialis activity with eyes closed is shown below.

large M_2 responses only if motor activity over short and long pathways coincided in time. The schematic drawing in Figure 6 illustrates the hypothetical mechanism of the postural tremor in our patients.

Stretch of the gastrocnemius or electrical stimulation elicits an H reflex, which in turn elicits a stretch response in the antagonist, and so on. Stretch responses in agonist and antagonist then coincide with the long-loop response following a previous stretch of the same muscle. In addition, it seems possible (but so far has not adequately been tested) that the hypotonia observed in some cases also contributes to the tremor in that the mechanical damping of possible oscillations by visoelastic forces is decreased in these patients.

The pathways responsible for tib_1, which is not delayed in patients with anterior lobe lesions, cannot be responsible for tib_2 and later responses. The latter obviously depend on intact cerebellar function. The former are independent and segmental. Despite the evidence from the cat presented by Ghez and Shinoda (12), a transcortical loop for these reflexes must be assumed in man (5, 18, 20). That the loop depends on intact cerebellar function is further evidenced by the observation of delayed long-loop reflexes in the arm in patients with cerebellar lesions (20) and by the publication of Vilis and Hore (40). Vilis and Hore found normal short-latency but delayed long-latency responses (of the antagonist) in animals with reversible cooling

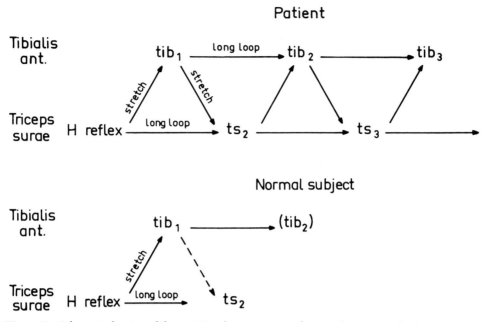

Figure 6. Schematic drawing of the poststimulus responses and postural tremor mechanism in patients with cerebellar cortical atrophy. By the electrical stimulation of the tibial nerves the H reflex is evoked in the triceps surae muscle, exerting a stretch of the anterior tibial muscle. This stretch causes a segmental stretch response in the tibial muscle (tib_1). Simultaneously, the stimulated Ia afferents are responsible for a long-loop response in the triceps surae (ts_2) and the tibialis anterior (tib_2). Whereas in the normal subject the segmental response (occasionally elicited by tib_1) and the long-loop reflex (in response to the stimulus) arrive at different times in the triceps surae, they coincide in the patient as the result of a delay in the long-loop reflex time. Due to the consequently powerful contraction of ts_2, postural tremor is induced and by way of the same mechanism is sustained, since ts_2 stretches the tibialis with a subsequent synchronous arrival of both reflex components forming the delayed tib_2, etc.

of the cerebellar nuclei. Tremor frequency decreased with progressive cooling, just as it did in our patients with progression of the disease.

Vilis and Hore (40) assume that the reflex is delayed by the lack of a predictive input from the cerebellum to precental motor cortex, from which the long-loop reflex response of the antagonist [the intended cortical response of Evarts and Tanji (10)] originates. Rather than being preprogrammed on the basis of prior stretch information from the agonist by the cerebellum, the reflex now corresponds to a suprasegmental response of the antagonist to its own stretch. The reflex in the paradigm of Vilas and Hore (40) normally occurs together with the end of the long-latency response in the agonist and breaks its action, terminating the movement. Cooling due to the delayed antagonist response causes an initial overshoot of the agonist movement and, by way of the delayed activity of the antagonist, an oscillatory rebound. According to our own experiments this explanation does not hold for tib_1, since tib_1 is not delayed in our patients with anterior lobe atrophy. The explanation of Vilis and Hore, however, may be valid for the subsequent EMG bursts. Our model clearly does not advocate the assumption of abnormal fixed patterns of rapid postural responses (27) as the basis for tremor but rather the "falling back" into having to use the reflex response of each individual muscle to its own stretch input after a lesion, possibly damaging the predictive capabilities of the spinocerebellum.

Our understanding of the postural disorders in patients with cerebellar lesions is still incomplete, and the challenge to clinical neurophysiologists is demanding. We believe that the methods developed for analysis and documentation help to differentiate and classify certain groups of patients and are promising enough to justify future research.

REFERENCES

1. Allum, J. H. J., and Büdingen, H. J., Coupled stretch reflexes in ankle muscles: An evaluation of the contributions of active muscle mechanisms to human posture stability. *Prog. Brain Res.*, 1979, **50**:185–196.
2. Bensel, C. K., and Dzendolet, E., Power spectral density analysis of the standing sway of males. *Percept. Psychophys.*, 1968, **4**:285–288.
3. Bernstein, N., *Coordination and Regulation of Movements, Part 1.* Pergamon, Oxford, 1967:66–100.
4. Burke, D., and Eklund, G., Muscle spindle activity in man during standing. *Acta Physiol. Scand.*, 1977, **100**:187–199.
5. Chan, C. W. Y., Melvill-Jones, G., and Watt, D. G. D., The "late" electromyographic response to limb displacement in man. I. Evidence for supraspinal contribution. *Electroencephalogr. Clin. Neurophysiol.*, 1070, **16**:173–181.
6. De Wit, G., Optic versus vestibular and proprioceptive impulses measured by posturometry. *Agressologie*, 1972, **13B**:75–79.
7. Dichgans, J., Mauritz, K. H., Allum, J. H., and Brandt, T., Postural sway in normals and atactic patients. Analysis of the stabilizing and destabilizing effects of vision. *Agressologie*, 1976, **17C**:15–20.
8. Dietz, V., Analysis of the electrical muscle activity during maximal contraction and the influence of ischemia. *J. Neurol. Sci.*, 1978, **37**:187–197.
9. Evarts, E. V., and Tanji, J., Gating of motor cortex reflexes by prior instruction. *Brain Res.*, 1974, **71**:479–494.
10. Evarts, E. V., and Tanji, J., Reflex and intended responses in motor cortex pyramidal tract neurons of monkey. *J. Neurophysiol.*, 1976, **39**:1069–1080.
11. Gelfand, J. M., Gurfinkel, V. S., Tsetlin, M. L., and Shik, M. L., Problems in the analysis of movements. In: *Models of the Structural-Functional Organization of Certain Biological Systems* (V. S. Gurfinkel, S. V. Fomin, and M. L. Tsetlin, eds.). MIT Press, Cambridge, Massachusetts, 1971:330–345.
12. Ghez, C., and Shinoda, Y., Spinal mechanisms of the functional stretch reflex. *Exp. Brain Res.*, 1978, **32**:55–68.
13. Gurfinkel, E. V., Kots, Y. M., Pal'Tsev, Y. J., and Feldmann, A. G., The compensation of respiratory disturbances of the erect posture of man as an example of the organization of inter-articular interaction. In: *Models of the Structural-Functional Organization of Certain Biological Systems* (V. S. Gurfinkel, S. V. Fomin, and M. L. Tsetlin, eds.). MIT Press, Cambridge, Massachusetts, 1971:382–395.
14. Gurfinkel, V. S., Physical foundations of the stabilography. *Agressologie*, 1973, **14C**:9–14.
15. Gurfinkel, V. S., Lipshits, M. I., Mori, S., and Popov, K. E., The state of stretch reflex during quiet standing in man. *Prog. Brain Res.*, 1976, **44**:473–486.
16. Hufschmidt, A., Dichgans, J., Mauritz, K. H., and Hufschmidt, M., Some methods and parameters of body sway quantification and their neurological applications. *Arch. Psychiatr. Nervenkr.*, 1980, **228**:135–150.
17. Lee, D. N., and Lishman, J. R., Visual proprioceptive control of stance. *J. Hum. Movement Stud.*, 1975, **1**:87–95.
18. Lee, R. G., and Tatton, W. G., Motor responses to sudden limb displacements in primates with specific CNS lesions and in human patients with motor system disorders. *Can. J. Neurol. Sci.*, 1975, **2**:285–293.
19. Lestienne, F., Soechting, J., and Berthoz, A., Postural readjustments induced by linear motion of visual scenes. *Exp. Brain Res.*, 1977, **28**:363–384.
20. Marsden, C. D., Merton, P. A., Morton, H. B., and Adam, J., The effect of lesions of the central nervous system on long-latency-stretch reflexes in the human thumb. *Prog. Clin. Neurophysiol.*, 1978, **4**:334–342.

Diagnostic Implications of Induced Body Sway

ROBERT O. ANDRES *

Kresge Hearing Research Institute
Ann Arbor, Michigan

INTRODUCTION

The analysis of the posturally impaired patient is continuously evolving in a variety of clinical and laboratory settings. Our efforts toward this development have centered on studies with a moving-platform posture test in which the subject is confronted by several types of stimuli that are closely related to everyday experiences. We control the motion of the platform and record the displacement of hips and shoulders with respect to the platform. The procedure is noninvasive and reveals interesting characteristics of the patient's whole-body neurological function. Most of our early efforts were devoted to studying the responses of normal subjects to our moving-platform posture test, but more recently we have begun to study the postural responses of patients with neurological and/or otological problems. Two diagnostic approaches are under investigation: (a) a comparison of induced body sway responses of normal subjects with those of patients with known neuropathologies and (b) a comparison of induced body sway responses of patients before and throughout a treatment regimen; such treatment could consist of surgery, physical therapy, drug administration, or a combination of these.

Our technique for inducing and measuring postural sway is briefly explained, and then examples of responses from both normal subjects and various patient groups are shown. These comparisons highlight the implications of our technique for the diagnosis of the dizzy patient.

METHODS

Our research approach to the study of postural sway was initially to design a postural measurement system (5) and then to implement the system for preliminary experiments, verifying that the system performed according to specifications. We

---

*Present address: Center for Ergonomics, University of Michigan, Ann Arbor, Michigan.

NYSTAGMUS AND VERTIGO: CLINICAL
APPROACHES TO THE PATIENT WITH DIZZINESS

then designed a brief test battery for postural tracking to use on patients and assembled a data base management system to catalog the postural responses.

The system is illustrated in Figures 1 and 2. Figure 1 is a block diagram of the measurement system, showing the microcomputer that provides the motion commands to the moving platform through a D/A converter. Platform data in the form of platform velocity and position are fed back through A/D converters, as are the data gathered from the subject (3). Sway responses are measured by digital line scan cameras that sense the average position of the body silhouette in the sagittal plane at the hips and shoulders (1), as shown in Figure 2. The platform translates only front to back; the maximum translation is 1.5 ft, and the maximum peak velocity is 1 ft/sec (3,4).

Before we began the preliminary experiments, it was necessary to standardize the task in order to reduce the variability of response techniques. The following conditions were selected: arms folded across the chest, knees locked gently, feet with heels together, toes comfortably apart, and eyes open or closed as specified.

In the design of a brief test battery, it was necessary to consider the classes of stimuli possible with our platform. These included a static, or stationary, trial with no platform motion, a sinusoidal oscillation, a band-limited pseudorandom translation, and a transient of platform translation. The standard test battery that we use with patients includes a static trial followed by a sinusoidal trial (7.5 cm/sec peak velocity at 0.2 Hz), both with eyes closed, after which 16 trials selected in random order from a set of pseudorandom and transient step motions are presented to the platform rider. The pseudorandom platform motions are generated from all combinations of two peak velocities (4.0 and 7.5 cm/sec), two bandwidths (0.1 to 1.0 Hz and 0.2 to 2.0 Hz), and eyes closed versus eyes open. Transient, fast translation platform motions are generated from two durations (0.5 and 1.5 sec), two different peak velocities (7.5 and −7.5 cm/sec), and eyes closed versus eyes open. The final trial in the test battery is again a static trial with eyes closed. Each trial lasts 20 sec.

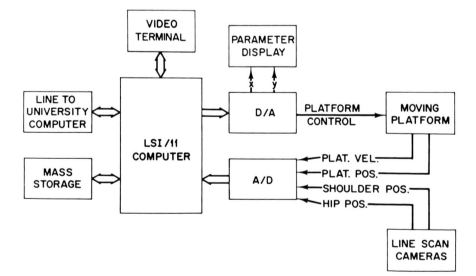

Figure 1.　Block diagram of the postural measurement system. Platform velocity is fed back from a tachometer on the shaft of the torque motor; platform position is fed back from a potentiometer geared to the platform.

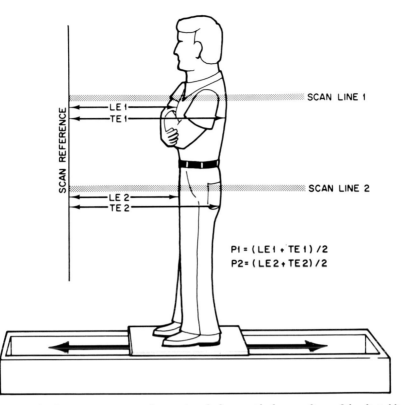

Figure 2.   Typical subject in position on the moving platform, with the scan lines of the digital line scan cameras shown at the hips and shoulders. Notice that the platform translates only fore to aft in the plane of the floor. LE, leading edge; TE, trailing edge; P, average position.

The remainder of this chapter focuses on sway responses to the three types of moving-platform stimuli and on examples of how these responses can be used for the diagnostic applications outlined earlier.

Sinusoidally Induced Sway

Several investigators have induced body sway with sinusoidal oscillations, either through fore-to-aft translations or rotations around the ankle joint (3,6–8). After a few cycles of a sinusoidal platform translation, the subjects have enough knowledge to predict future motion. At low frequencies with eyes closed, normal subjects ride the platform smoothly and comfortably with little change as a result of practice from session to session. A distinct advantage of the sinusoidal platform stimulus is the ease of analyzing the body sway responses. Parameters that are calculated with fast Fourier transform techniques at both the waist and the shoulders include the gain (where the input is the platform translation and the output is the shoulder or waist displacement), the phase lag, and the signal-to-noise (S/N) ratio. The signal is the squared magnitude of the response at the input frequency, and the noise is the sum of the squared magnitudes at all other frequencies.

The experimental results from three healthy male subjects, ages 20 to 25, who had undergone one session daily for 14 days [each session being composed of eight sinusoidal trials (eyes closed, four frequencies ranging from 0.2 to 0.8 Hz, and two peak velocities: 6 and 18 cm/sec)] can be summarized as follows. At low frequencies

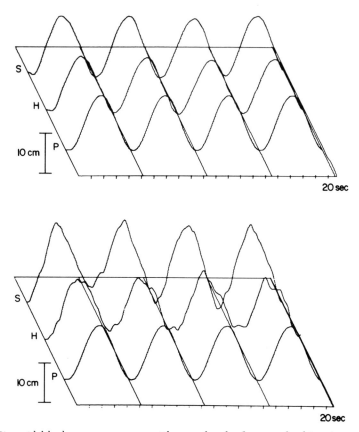

Figure 3. Sinusoidal body sway responses, with eyes closed, of a normal subject (upper graph) and a patient with multiple sclerosis (lower graph). Frequency, 0.2 Hz; peak velocity, 7.5 cm/sec; P, platform position data; H, average hip silhouette position; S, average shoulder silhouette position.

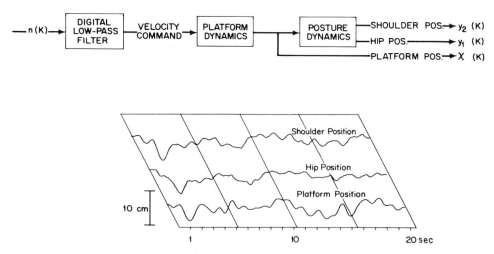

Figure 4. Top: Block diagram of the formation of the pseudorandom platform stimulus. Bottom: An example of the raw data from the platform, hips, and shoulders.

the S/N ratio was large and nonadaptive, whereas the gain and phase lag were consistent. However, at higher frequencies the S/N ratios were adaptive, whereas the gain and phase lag were inconsistent. We therefore selected a low-frequency sinusoid for use in our brief test battery, because normal, naive subjects did not adapt their sway responses. This is not to say that patients with central nervous system disturbances would not show adaptation to such a stimulus.

An example of the difference in smoothness of response between a normal subject and an ataxic patient is shown in Figure 3. The normal subject, whose responses are

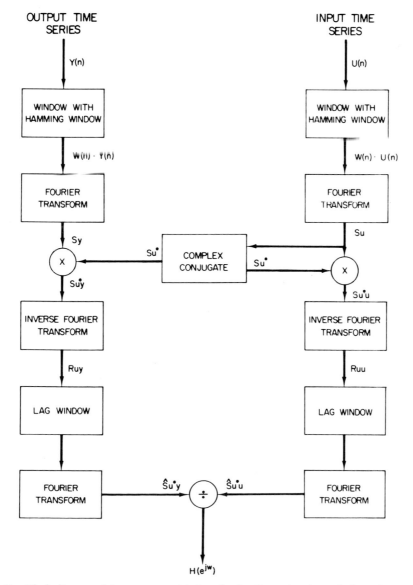

Figure 5. Block diagram of the nonparametric transfer function extraction technique. In our case the input time series is the platform motion, and the output time series is the record of either the hip or shoulder motion.

shown in the upper graph, was a 27-year-old man, and the patient, whose responses are shown in the lower graph, was an 18-year-old woman with a 1-year history of multiple sclerosis (MS). She had incoordination and gait difficulty, with findings referable to the brainstem (nystagmus and ataxia) and the spinal cord (spasticity and bladder dysfunction). Her gait was spastic and slightly ataxic. The plots in Figure 3 show platform, hip, and shoulder motion data for the last four cycles of a 0.2–Hz, 7.5 cm/sec sinusoid. Eyes were kept closed. The lack of smoothness in the patient's response implies a degree of spasticity, or hyperreflexia.

Pseudorandom Induced Sway

The next motion stimulus to be discussed is a pseudorandom translation. Meyer and Blum (8) used pseudorandom platform rotations around the ankle joint. Their measured responses were in the form of moments around the ankle joints, not actual body sway. These differences from our approach prevent us from directly comparing experimental results.

Figure 4 illustrates how we generate the pseudorandom motion. The velocity command is band-pass-filtered from either 0.1 to 1.0 Hz or 0.2 to 2.0 Hz. The plot of raw data at the bottom shows how difficult it would be to observe the sway responses empirically. However, one can derive nonparametric transfer functions for this type of stimulus, as shown in Figure 5, with signal processing techniques.

Figure 6 shows responses to four pseudorandom trials gathered from a healthy man. The peak velocity is 10 cm/sec for all of the cases; the upper two plots are for the narrow-bandwidth (0.1- to 1.0-Hz) stimulus, whereas the bottom plots are for the wide-bandwidth (0.2- to 2.0-Hz) platform translations. The left plots are from trials with eyes open, and the plots on the right are from trials with eyes closed. The raw time-domain data are difficult to interpret, but the transfer characteristics simplify interpretation. Figure 7 is from the same data as Figure 6, with the amplitude plot and phase plot of the transfer functions on the top and bottom, respectively. The top two trials are for the narrow-band (0.1- to 1.0-Hz) platform motions. The data outside

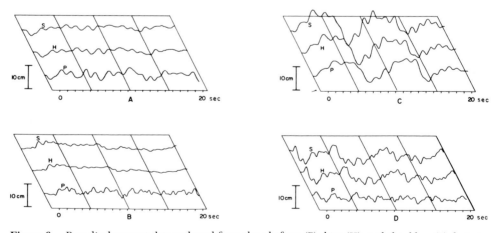

Figure 6. Raw displacement data gathered from the platform (P), hips (H), and shoulders (S) during a 20-sec pseudorandom platform translation with a peak velocity of 10 cm/sec. (A) Narrow-band (from 0.1 to 1.0 Hz) stimulus; eyes open and fixated. (B) Wide-band (from 0.2 to 2.0 Hz) stimulus; eyes open. (C) Narrow-band stimulus; eyes closed. (D) Wide-band stimulus; eyes closed.

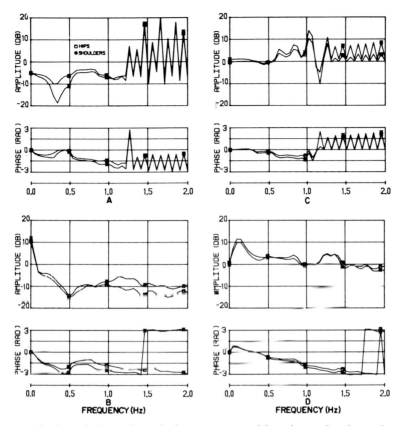

Figure 7. Amplitudes and phases of transfer functions extracted from the raw data depicted in Figure 6. (A) Narrow-band stimulus; eyes open. (B) Wide-band stimulus; eyes open. (C) Narrow-band stimulus; eyes closed. (D) Wide-band stimulus; eyes closed. □, hips; *, shoulders.

the input band are spurious, and the oscillatory results past 1.0 Hz can be ignored. It can be seen that for both the narrow- and wide-band trials the effect of closing the eyes is to increase the motion of the trunk and head, as shown by the larger amplitude, or gain, values. At zero decibels, the trunk moves exactly as far as the platform during translation, which is particularly the case with eyes closed. Visual stabilization is obvious in the decreased amplitudes of trunk motion in the left plots. Head position is being fixed relative to the visual target.

Diagnostically, pseudorandom sway responses can be used to quantify the degree of visual stabilization the patient uses. Statistical techniques can be applied to derive normative response bands for age, sex, height, and weight combinations, but this will require running posture tests on a large number of normal subjects. We are currently concerned with exploring the diagnostic possibilities of our technique instead.

Pseudorandom stimuli may be used to assess the pre- and posttreatment status of the patient or the daily variation of his or her symptoms. An example is the case of a female patient, age 25, with episodic dizziness and nausea. She was diagnosed in the ear, nose, and throat clinic as having bilateral Ménière's disease. The sway response of the patient before drug treatment (Figure 8) and on a difficult day can be compared with the response 1 week later, after treatment had begun and when the patient did

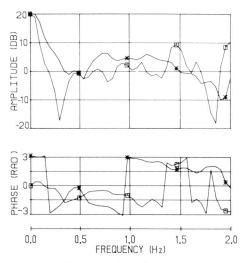

Figure 8.   Transfer functions extracted from pseudorandom sway responses of a female patient, age 25, with bilateral Ménière's disease before treatment, eyes closed. The upper plot is the amplitude, and the lower plot is the phase. Peak velocity, 7.5 cm/sec; □, hips, *, shoulders.

not feel sick (Figure 9). The trials are both wide band, eyes closed, at a peak velocity of 7.5 cm/sec. The transfer functions are much smoother in Figure 9, which implies that the patient reacted to all of the platform motions similarly across the frequency content of the input. Figure 8 shows her increased sensitivity to certain frequencies of randomly induced sway.

TRANSIENT-INDUCED SWAY

The transient step stimulus is unpredictable to the extent that the subject is not told either the exact time (within a few seconds) at which the motion will begin or the direction in which the platform will move. Nashner (9) used small step translations of

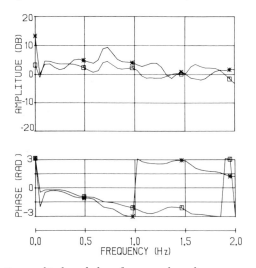

Figure 9.   Transfer function amplitude and phase from pseudorandom sway responses of the same female patient shown in Figure 8, but after 1 week of treatment. The notations are the same as those in Figure 8.

the subject's base of support in his experiments, but his platform tilted so that the ankle angle remained constant, resulting in a different sensory environment than that which our subjects and patients experienced. Parameters of sway responses induced by these steps are difficult to express because of nonlinearities, but observation of the responses can yield a wealth of information.

Figures 10 through 17 illustrate responses to all combinations of forward and backward steps with eyes open and eyes closed. Responses of a normal 19-year-old woman are shown in Figure 10. The two upper graphs are responses to forward steps, whereas the bottom plots are responses to backward steps, although they are shown with reversed polarity so that the same coordinate system could be used. The two plots on the left show responses with eyes open, and the plots on the right are for the eyes-closed condition. The responses here are generally underdamped, with overshoot of the trunk. Furthermore, after overshooting, the trunk moves smoothly to its new location without much wandering, or oscillation. This pattern is typical but not universal. We shall now compare the features of these normal responses with those of patients with various neurological findings.

The first example of a patient is a 36-year-old man with a long-standing history of seizures. He was found to be ataxic of speech and gait, which was thought to be the result of an excessive level of anticonvulsant drugs in the blood. Figure 11 shows his responses in the same format as Figure 10. His responses to the motion stimulus appear to be underdamped, but his trunk wanders unsteadily after the step, indicating that a noise process has been excited by the stimulus, particularly with the eyes closed. The plot on the lower right, a backward step with eyes closed, shows evidence of a stretch reflex response that jerked the body forward momentarily.

Figure 12 shows the responses of a 42-year-old woman with a 1-year history of double vision and right-sided ataxia localized to the brainstem. Spinal fluid analysis indicated a diagnosis of MS. The patient also had gait ataxia. Comparing her responses with those of the normal subject, the most notable difference is the larger

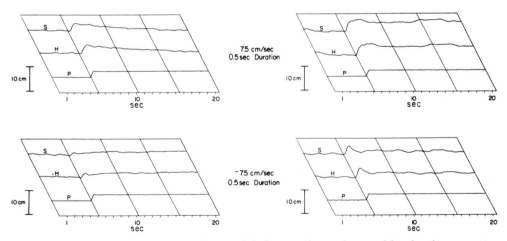

Figure 10. Body sway responses to small steps of platform translation of a normal female subject, age 19. The two upper plots are responses to forward steps of platform motion; the bottom plots are responses to backward steps of platform motion shown with their polarity reversed. The two plots on the left result from eyes-open trials, whereas the two plots on the right are from eyes-closed trials. P, platform; H, hips; S, shoulders.

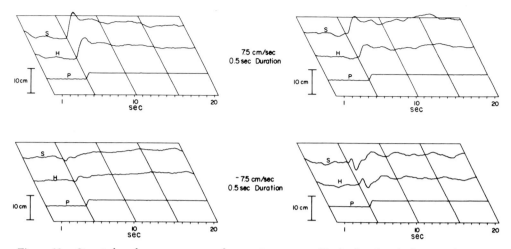

Figure 11.   Step-induced sway responses of an ataxic man, age 36, displayed with the same format as Figure 10.

overshoot for the trial with eyes closed and forward platform motion. The patient was also generally less steady when the platform was stationary. She demonstrated the variability of her disease, and how provocative these small steps can be, when she could not successfully complete the backward, eyes-closed trial in a session 3 days later (Figure 13). As shown in the upper right plot, on this day she had a stretch reflex response that jerked her trunk back after the step. Her other responses were also exaggerated.

Another example of a patient is a 30-year-old woman with MS and an 8-year history of migratory and transient neurological problems, including gait incoordination, decreased vision in the right eye, and urinary difficulty. She had gait ataxia, as well as spasticity in both lower extremities (Figure 14). The most striking observation here is how heavily the patient relied on her vision to stabilize her trunk. The upper right graph, showing the patient's responses with eyes closed and a forward platform

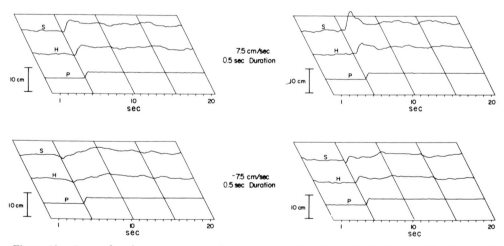

Figure 12.   Step-induced sway responses of a woman, age 42, with multiple sclerosis. The format of Figure 10 was used.

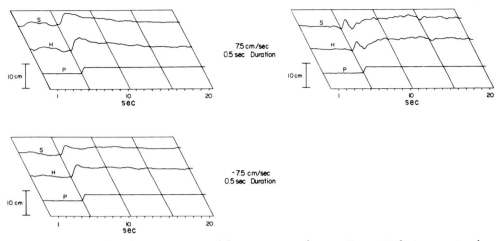

Figure 13. Step-induced sway responses of the same patient shown in Figure 12 during a session that took place 3 days later. The blank quadrant shows that the patient could not perform the balance task with eyes closed and the platform moving backward.

motion, shows exaggerated trunk overshoot, but the lower plot on the right for the eyes closed and backward step shows a great deal of trunk wandering, which never actually damps out.

Figure 15 is a dramatic demonstration of spastic responses. A 36-year-old man with a history of back and neck trauma secondary to over 200 parachute jumps had problems referable entirely to the cervical spinal cord due to degenerative disease and pressure on the cord at that level. He had severe lower extremity spasticity. All of his responses, as shown in the figure, have exaggerated overshoot compared to the normal subject. The upper right graph, showing the patient's responses when eyes were closed and the platform moved forward, shows a quick jerk of the trunk forward and back, followed by a drift in trunk position. The patient had problems settling on a final trunk position in three of the four trials shown.

A striking contrast to the normal subject response is seen in the data for a 48-year-

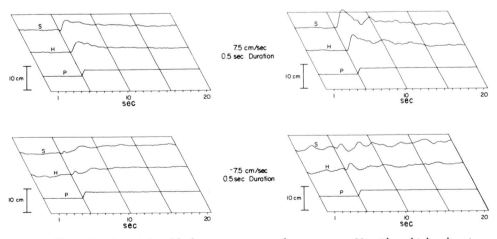

Figure 14. Step-induced body sway responses of a woman, age 30, with multiple sclerosis.

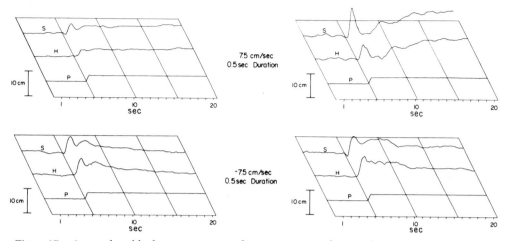

Figure 15. Step-induced body sway responses of a man, age 36, with cervical spine damage resulting in severe lower extremity spasticity.

old woman with a seizure disorder dating back to childhood. She had diffuse cerebellar dysfunction secondary to long-term anticonvulsant intake for her epilepsy (Figure 16). Her responses with eyes open show some trunk wandering, but when she closed her eyes the degree of instability increased. For the forward step, as shown in the upper right corner, her trunk jerked forward and back before beginning to drift. The backward step with eyes closed (lower right) shows marked overshoot and trunk oscillation. This woman was the most susceptible to eyes-closed transient trials of any patient in our series of tests.

These examples illustrate the potential for classifying patients by comparing their responses to the brief test battery with sway responses of normal subjects. Establishing the parameters of step responses will enable us to compare these responses statistically, so we are now actively pursuing this in our laboratory (2).

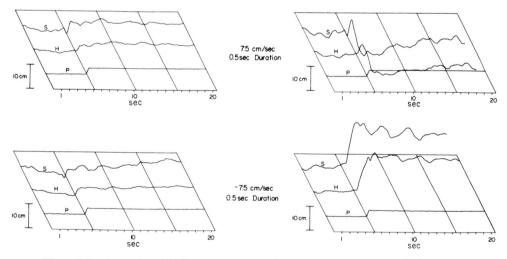

Figure 16. Step-induced body sway responses of a woman, age 48, with cerebellar ataxia.

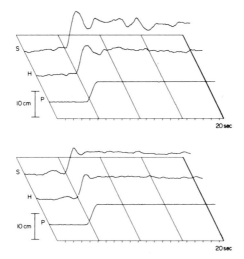

Figure 17.   Step-induced body sway responses, with eyes closed, before (upper graph) and after (lower graph) treatment of a woman with multiple sclerosis. Peak velocity, 7.5 cm/sec; 1.5 sec duration; P, platform motion; H, hip silhouette motion; S, shoulder silhouette motion.

An example of the capability of the moving-platform posture test for comparing responses in patients before and after treatment is that of an 18-year-old woman with MS. She was tested after she had treated herself with inhaled marijuana (Figure 17). The top trace is her response before inhalation of the drug, the stimulus being a forward step of 1.5 sec duration at a peak velocity of 7.5 cm/sec with eyes closed. The bottom trace is her response to the same stimulus approximately 15 min after inhaling the drug. The degree of overshoot is diminished, but even more noticeable is the smoothness of her response following treatment. This is just one example of differences in pre- and posttreatment sway response.

Conclusions

The diagnostic implications of induced body sway can be summarized as follows:

1. Low-frequency sinusoids and short steps of translation can document hyperreflexia or spasticity in patients.
2. Step stimuli elicit sway responses in patients that enable one to easily observe deviations from normal responses.
3. Pseudorandom stimuli enable one to quantify visual stabilization.
4. All of the induced body sway stimuli mentioned can be used to classify patients with respect to dysfunction in postural control systems, and they may be useful for chronicling changes in postural control status following a treatment regimen.

These preliminary data demonstrate the potential of this new technique for postural assessment. Further work must be done before it can be established as a routine clinical tool.

Acknowledgment

This research has been supported by NASA contract NAS 9-15244.

REFERENCES

1. Anderson, D. J., Homick, J. L., and Jones, K. W., Line scan cameras applied to posturography. *Proc. San Diego Biomed. Symp.*, 1977, **16**:35–40.
2. Anderson, D. J., and Werness, S., A systems identification approach to induced postural sway. Presented at a workshop entitled *Information Process in the Normal and Abnormal Human Postural Control Systems,* at the Third Midwinter Meeting of the Association for Research in Otolaryngology, St. Petersburg, Florida, January 1980.
3. Andres, R. O., *A Postural Measurement System for Induced Body Sway Assessment.* Ph.D. Thesis, University of Michigan, Ann Arbor, 1979.
4. Andres, R. O., and Anderson, D. J., A moving platform system for the study of induced body sway. *Proc. N. Engl. Bioeng. Conf.*, 1977, **5**:71–75.
5. Andres, R. O., and Anderson, D. J., Designing a better postural measurement system. *Am. J. Otolaryngol.*, 1980, **1**(3):197–206.
6. Gantchev, G., Dunev, S., and Draganova, N., On the spontaneous and induced body oscillations. In: *Second International Symposium on Motor Control* (A. A. Gydikov, N. T. Tankov, and D. S. Kosarov, eds.). Plenum, New York, 1973:179–194.
7. Gantchev, G., and Popov, V., Quantitative evaluation of induced body oscillations in man. *Agressologie,* 1973 **14**(C):91–94.
8. Meyer, M., and Blum, E., Quantitative analysis of postural reactions to induced body oscillations. *Agressologie,* 1978, **19**(A):30–31.
9. Nashner, L. M., *Sensory Feedback in Human Posture Control.* D.Sc. Thesis, Massachusetts Institute of Technology, Cambridge, 1970:MVT-70-3.

TESTING OF VISUAL-VESTIBULAR INTERACTION: CLINICAL APPLICATION

Applied and Clinical Aspects of Visual-Vestibular Interaction

THOMAS BRANDT

Neurological Clinic with Clinical Neurophysiology
Alfried Krupp Hospital
Essen, Federal Republic of Germany

Three main sensory systems (visual, vestibular, and somatosensory) subserve static and dynamic spatial orientation, and control posture and locomotion. Within this multiloop control the individual systems are mutually interactive and redundant in that the functional ranges overlap, enabling them to compensate partially for each other's deficiencies.

Under natural conditions with the eyes open, an individual adequately perceives active as well as passive body motion, whether of constant or varying velocity. When an individual is riding in a vehicle with the eyes closed, however, the deficiencies of the vestibular system become apparent. Vestibular information about motion is then evoked only through acceleration and deceleration and dies out as the cupulae in the semicircular canals or the otoliths progressively return to their resting position during constant velocity. Thus, at constant velocity, the sensation of self-motion is maintained almost entirely by the visual input deriving from attendant relative motion of the surroundings.

A mismatch among simultaneous inputs from the sensory systems may elicit either a displeasing distortion of static gravitational orientation or an erroneous perception of either self-motion or object motion: a multisensory vertigo syndrome (9). Vertigo may be induced by physiological but unusual (and therefore unadapted) stimulation (motion sickness) or pathological dysfunction of any of the stabilizing sensory systems (Figure 1). The symptoms of vertigo include sensory qualities identified as vestibular, visual, and somatosensory, involving perceptual, oculomotor, postural, and vegetative manifestations: vertigo, nystagmus, ataxia, and nausea, respectively. As distinct from one's perception of self-motion during natural locomotion, the vertigo experience is linked to an impaired mechanism for space constancy that contributes to the distressing admixture of both self-motion and surround motion. The intensity of vertigo is a function of the magnitude of the mismatch and increases if the intact

NYSTAGMUS AND VERTIGO: CLINICAL
APPROACHES TO THE PATIENT WITH DIZZINESS

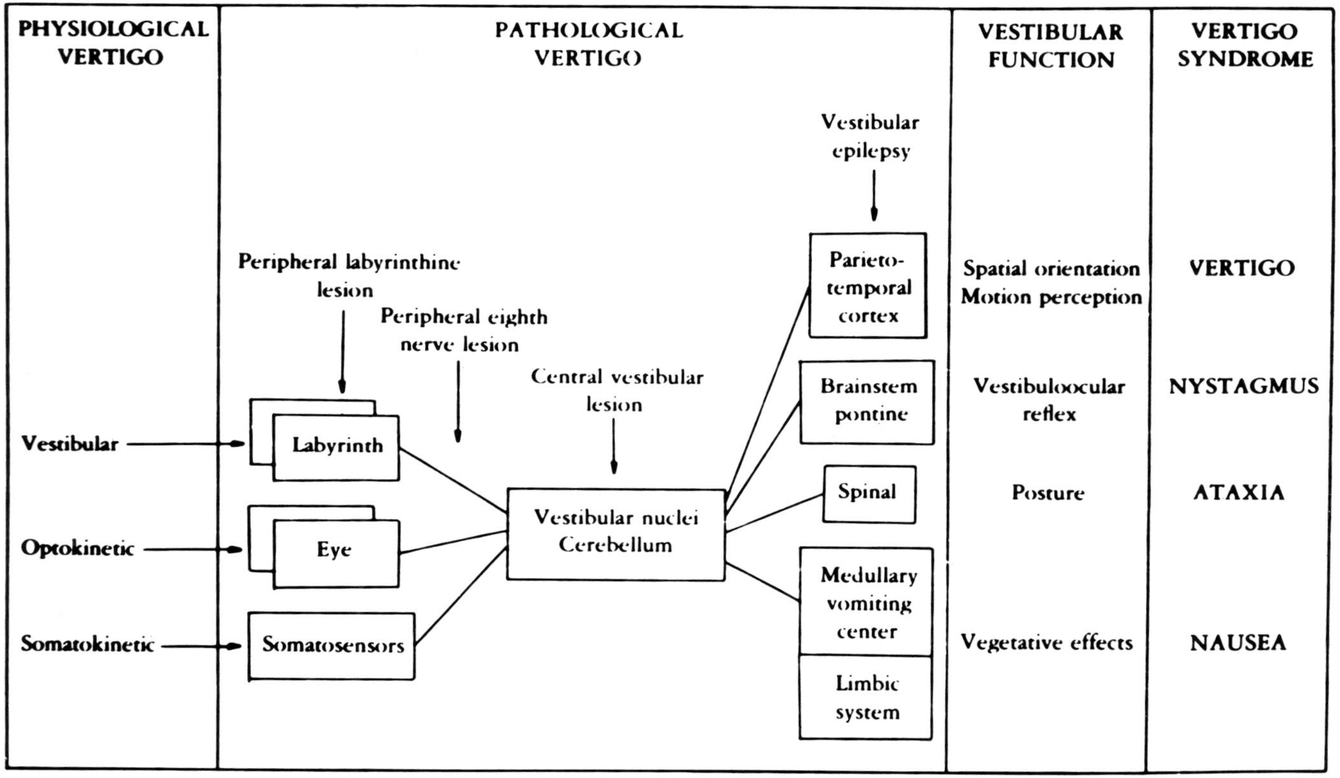

Figure 1.   Schematic classification and origin of different types of vertigo (9).

sensory systems are eliminated, such as with eye closure during pathological vestibular vertigo.

This chapter emphasizes the particular sensorial value of vision in dynamic spatial orientation, in postural control, as well as in motion sickness and clinical vertigo syndromes.

VISUAL PERCEPTION OF SELF-MOTION

Unlike vestibular stimuli, which invariably lead to the sensation of body motion, visual motion stimuli provide for two perceptual interpretations, either self-motion or object motion (Figure 2). The subject watching moving stimuli may perceive himself as being stationary in space (egocentric motion perception) or may experience the actually moving surroundings as being stable and himself as being moved (circularvection, linearvection). The latter illusion has been known for a long time (19,22,31) but has not been thoroughly studied under experimental conditions until recently [for a review, see Dichgans and Brandt (15)]. Figure 2 provides basic information about the features of visual stimuli that determine whether self-motion or object motion occurs. Uniform motion filling the entire visual field invariably leads to a self-motion sensation that is indistinguishable from an actual body movement. Following the onset of the stimulus, circularvection begins after a few seconds of latency and slowly increases in apparent velocity until saturation and may outlast the visual stimulus as an aftereffect. Concurrent body accelerations shorten latencies of circularvection and linearvection considerably, which is a necessary condition for appropriate

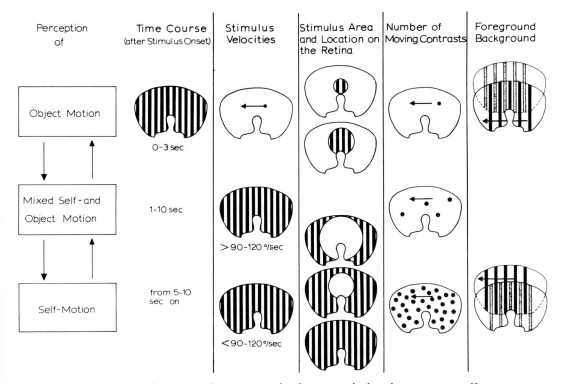

Figure 2. Critical optokinetic stimulus properties that determine whether object motion or self-motion is perceived (15).

visual control of posture. The velocity of apparent self-rotation in circularvection matches stimulus speed up to 90 to 120 deg/sec, but at higher speeds circularvection velocity lags behind, resulting in additional egocentric object-motion perception.

In a series of psychophysical experiments, we showed (15) that the visual perception of self-motion is dependent on the density of moving contrasts randomly distributed within the visual field and the total area of the coherent stimulus field. Using optokinetic patterns equal in area, we demonstrated that the peripheral retina dominates visually induced vection, whereas central vision (central visual field up to 30 deg in diameter) dominates pattern recognition and egocentric object-motion detection. On simultaneous presentation of conflicting central and peripheral, or foreground and background, optokinetic stimuli, dynamic visual spatial orientation relies mainly on the information from the seen periphery, both the retinal and the depth periphery. When an individual is riding in a car at constant velocity, self-motion sensation is produced by a relative backward motion of the surroundings, but, simultaneously, the driver looking in the rearview mirror is able to detect and pursue single objects moving with respect to himself and in relation to the environment.

Velocity and luminance thresholds for optokinetically induced vections are close to those for image-motion detection, even in low scotopic vision (4,29). Vections are independent of refractive errors up to 20 diopters, which cause a blurring of the image (29). This "immunity of vections" causes an overconfidence in car drivers under conditions of degraded focal vision.

Optokinetic Graviceptive Interaction

Gravitational orientation depends on two major sources of experience: the exteroceptive visual and the proprioceptive postural. A stationary observer, while viewing a large visual scene rotating around his line of sight, experiences a continuous sensation of self-motion (rollvection) but only a limited body tilt and displacement of visual vertical (17,21). Induced displacement can be measured in terms of tilt angles of *apparent visual and postural vertical* from gravitational upright and may be conceptualized as the result of a compromise weighing the different and, in part, contradictory sensory inputs for gravitational orientation. Tilt angles for pitch are smaller than those for roll and in addition exhibit asymmetry between the smaller pitch-up and larger pitch-down angles (40) that appear to be fixed with respect to the body (egocentric localization), rather than with the direction of down (absolute localization). A similar asymmetry is observed for postural reactions to a linearvection stimulus with the tendency to fall backward considerably stronger than the one to fall forward (30).

The apparent displacement of both visual and postural vertical has been explained as the result of a central recomputation of the orientation of the gravity vector based on vision (17). This is supported by the finding that the visually induced tilt markedly increases when the otoliths are placed in a less favorable position by lateral head tilt (16,40). The potentiation of the net visual effect on apparent vertical in an inclined head position is maximal if the visual stimulus is moving opposite to the head tilt (Figure 3). This asymmetry can be interpreted as the functional hypertrophy of a biologically adaptive mechanism that assists postural righting when the visually induced tilt perception adds to the otoliths' information. Under natural conditions body tilt causes relative motion of the visual scene that is opposite in direction to the body displacement. The induced relative motion of the visual environment, in this case, will correlate with the actual information from graviceptors for postural adjustment.

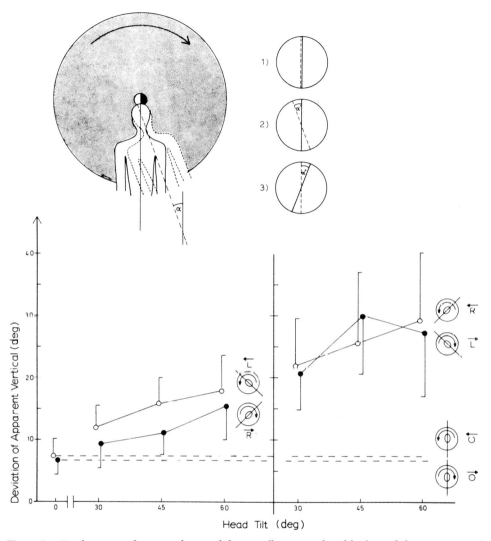

Figure 3. Displacement of perceived vertical during rollvection induced by large disk rotating around subject's line of sight. Clockwise rotation causes apparent counterclockwise tilt of the observer's body (dashed line in upper left drawing). Vertical edge (1) separating black and white halves of test target appears similarly tilted (2). Perceived tilt is measured by having subject adjust test edge to apparent vertical (3). Lower half of the figure depicts deviation of apparent vertical induced by rotating visual display with different angles of head inclination (abscissa) after subtracting corresponding "A" or "E" effects. Disk rotation and head inclination in the same direction (left panel) and in opposite directions (right panel) for deviations of apparent vertical to right (closed circles) or to left (open circles). Dashed lines depict deviation with head erect and only disk moving (15).

VISUAL STABILIZATION AND DESTABILIZATION OF POSTURE

Optimal balance requires the continuous central evaluation of the reafferent sensory consequences of self-generated body movements as an input for motor compensation of fore–aft and lateral body sway. Within this multiloop control, vision plays a major role for postural stabilization, which is well known to clinicians, particularly in patients with diseases involving proprioceptive joint and muscle afferents, as in tabes dorsalis or sensory polyneuropathy. Visual stabilization of posture can easily be dem-

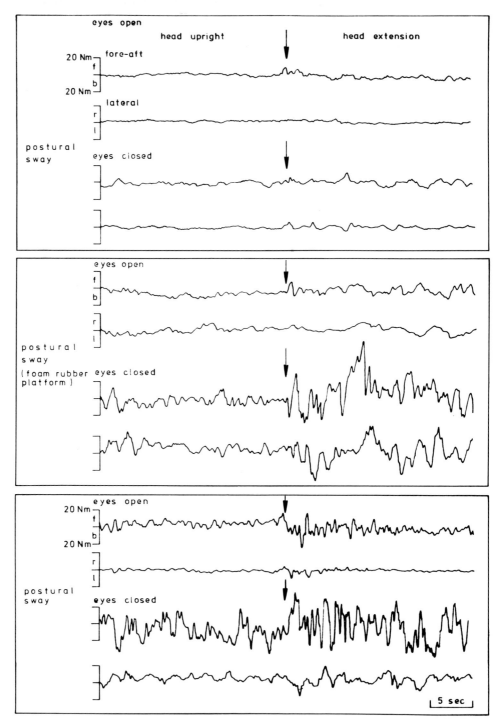

Figure 4. Differential effects of head extension and normal head position upon forward–backward and lateral body sway (original recordings, posturography) with the eyes open or closed. Top: Normal subject standing on a firm stabilometer platform; middle: normal subject standing on a piece of foam rubber; bottom: patient with sensory polyneuropathy standing on a firm platform. Postural imbalance is the most pronounced and similar for the normal subject standing on foam rubber and the patient during head extension with the eyes closed (11). Postural destabilization is due mainly to reduced accuracy of head and body sway information by the otoliths. Head extension brings the utricular otoliths out of optimal working range, and the input originating from the saccular otoliths as well as from the semicircular canals is not sufficient to make up this deficit.

onstrated by attempting to balance on one foot with the eyes closed and the head maximally extended (retroflexion) as compared with the eyes open and with vision widely compensating for the reduced gravitational information from the labyrinths. *Head extension* brings the utricular otoliths out of their optimal working range, and obviously the input originating from the saccular otoliths as well as from the semicircular canals is not sufficient to make up this deficit when the sensory input from other control loops, such as vision and somatosensory joint receptors, is largely eliminated (11). Thus, patients with sensory polyneuropathy who lack accurate positional sense in the legs exhibit a postural instability with head extension and eyes closed, similar to that shown by normal subjects standing on foam rubber, which also reduces the reliability of the somatosensory input (Figure 4).

In contrast to reports in some textbooks, most patients suffering from a *late cortical cerebellar atrophy* of the anterior lobe (spinocerebellar ataxia) still exhibit a very effective visual compensation of postural imbalance (18,31a),which may be absent in others, particularly in forms of vestibulocerebellar ataxia (Figure 5).

Visual stabilization of posture is dependent on the functional range of visual detection of motion. A head or body sway causes a shift of the visual surround on the retina

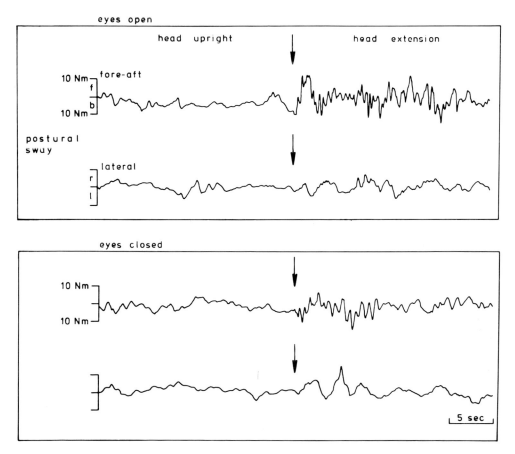

Figure 5. Differential effects of head extension and normal head position upon body sway with the eyes open or closed in a patient suffering from a vestibulocerebellar ataxia due to a demyelinizing disease. Vision is ineffective in compensating for postural imbalance as induced by head extension.

when the eyes are stationary in the head or an eye movement of an appropriate angle if the object is fixated, involving afferent or efferent motion perception, respectively. Simple geometric analysis indicates that, in order to be visually detected, body sway must increase with increasing distance between the observer's eyes and the nearest stationary contrasts (Figure 6). The greater the distance Y to the object becomes, the smaller is the angular displacement α on the retina. Since the natural lateral head sway is about 2 cm in amplitude (24), an important determination would be the specific eye–object distance at which this sway amplitude could not be visually detected. Since an angular displacement of the visual scene of 20 min of arc is necessary for detection by the paracentral and peripheral parts of the retina (2,28), a normal lateral head sway of 2 cm would be subthreshold at a distance of about 3 m. This leads to a perceptual conflict since the vestibular and somatosensory receptors sense a body shift which the visual system cannot detect. The conflict might be resolved by increasing the postural sway and thereby reactivating visual control. For a simple loop control, a relationship between distance and sway amplitude could be expected (tan $\alpha = x/y$), with the gain dependent on the retinal movement detection threshold. However, with the lower limbs close together at free stance, one falls over at a head sway of more than 10 cm. Thus, at an eye–object distance of 15 to 20 m, a "maximal body sway" would produce retinal angular deviations of less than 2 min of arc according to trigonometry. Since we are dealing with a multiloop control of postural balance, it can be assumed that, with increasing sway amplitudes, the particular sensory weight of somatosensory and vestibular afferences becomes greater, increasing their contribution to postural stabilization.

This simple geometric analysis served as a basis for an explanation of the *mechanism for physiological height vertigo* being a distance vertigo through visual destabilization of postural balance when the distance between the observer's eye and the nearest visible stationary contrasts becomes critically large (5,7). Although this physiological height vertigo may, without question, be contaminated by additional cognitive and psychological factors, it represents a sensory-motor mechanism distinct from psychopathological acrophobia.

To confirm the validity of this hypothesis a series of psychophysical and posturographic experiments was performed showing that (a) the occurrence of physiological height vertigo is clearly related to body position, being the strongest with the erect stance, while maintenance of balance is most difficult and minimal in the lying position; (b) height vertigo can be induced by either downward or upward gaze because it is the distance rather than the visual direction that is critical; (c) height vertigo appears at a distance of about 3 m, increases with increasing altitude, but saturates at less than 20 m; (d) lateral and fore–aft body sway (posturographic measurements, Figure 6) as well as head sway increases nonlinearly with increasing eye–object distance. Nearby stationary contrasts in the periphery of the visual field alleviate both subjective vertigo and measurable postural imbalance, which dictates practical advice for susceptible subjects. The significant increase in body sway amplitudes introduces a real danger of falling from a high position. The "static" stimulus condition of height or distance, however, will not per se destabilize posture, resulting in an unavoidable fall because of the redundancy in the control loops. But additional disturbances, such as wind or an unstable foot support, may result in serious problems in the maintenance of an upright position, for subjects are apt to use the "false" visual information in problematic circumstances. Therefore, patients with

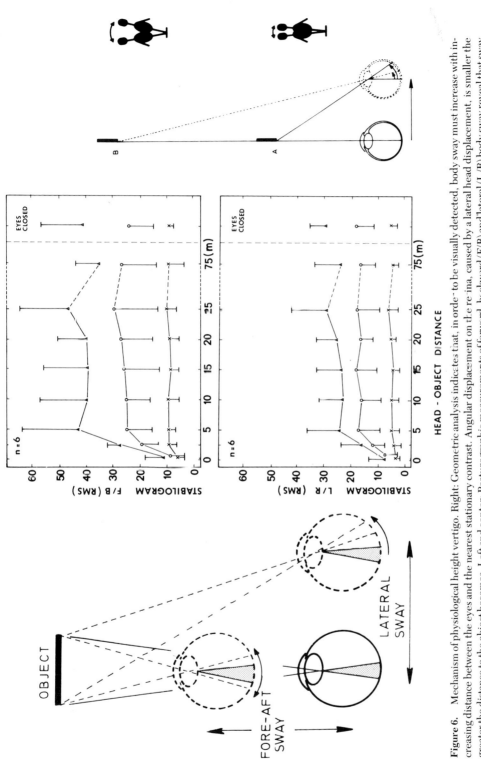

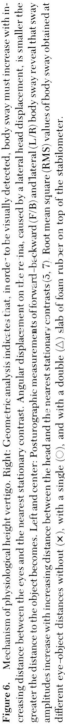

Figure 6. Mechanism of physiological height vertigo. Right: Geometric analysis indicates that, in order to be visually detected, body sway must increase with increasing distance between the eyes and the nearest stationary contrast. Angular displacement on the retina, caused by a lateral head displacement, is smaller the greater the distance to the object becomes. Left and center: Posturographic measurements of forward–backward (F/B) and lateral (L/R) body sway reveal that sway amplitudes increase with increasing distance between the head and the nearest stationary contrasts (5, 7). Root mean square (RMS) values of body sway obtained at different eye–object distances without (×), and with a single (○), and with a double (△) slab of foam rubber on top of the stabilometer.

vestibular or somatosensory dysfunctions are subject to a particularly greater risk when exposed to height vertigo situations.

Under experimental laboratory conditions, vision may have a strong destabilizing effect on posture, particularly when visually perceived motion does not adequately correspond to the actual body shift sensed by the vestibular and somatosensory systems. Observations of an *optokinetically induced body sway* were reported in the older literature (19). Extensive experiments on that phenomenon were performed with movements of an artificial surround as circular motion about the vertical Z axis (25), roll motion about the line of sight (18), a sinusoidally tilting room (6), and linear motion of the seen environment (4,27). In these instances there was an optokinetically induced perception of apparent self-motion opposite in direction to pattern motion. The postural reflexes compensate for this subjective body shift, resulting in a measurable body tilt in the direction of motion pattern. These optokinetically induced postural reactions require stimulation of the entire visual field or substantial portions of the periphery, which corresponds to the stimulus characteristics for visually induced vections. According to the vection data, visual input affects postural balance even under conditions of minimal illumination, increasing as a function of illumination level during the state of transition from scotopic to clear photopic vision (26). That continuous motion of the retinal image may be an important determinant of postural stabilization, although not a necessary condition, was shown by the use of stroboscopic illumination. In contrast to earlier results by others (1) who found that visual stabilization was absent at strobe frequencies of up to 6 Hz, it could be demonstrated by the use of the tilting room (26) that a sequential displacement of the room (1 to 4 Hz) without continuous retinal motion was sufficient to cause a continuous modulation of postural sway of the same periodicity rather than a kind of "photic driving" of body sway according to the flicker frequency.

The development of the *visual stabilization of free stance in infants* was tested by means of a large visual display rotating around the stationary subject's line of sight (12). In the adult this causes a marked optokinetic postural reaction, with the shift of the body center of gravity toward the direction of pattern motion. Scalings of the reactions in children revealed that 6 to 12-month-old infants show no or very little optokinetic disturbance of their newly acquired ability to sit whereas, with the development of upright stance and gait, optokinetic influences become progressively important (Figure 7). It may be concluded that the optokinetic loop participates rather late in the multisensory process of postural stabilization. The calibration of the three main loops, visual, vestibular, and proprioceptive, seems to be sequential and mutually interactive.

Visual vertigo and postural imbalance can also be observed in patients with *oculomotor disorders* that cause either involuntary eye movements or acute extraocular muscle paresis. Involuntary ocular oscillation that overrides fixation is a well-known cause of oscillopsia independent of head motion. Oscillopsia, the illusory movement of the viewed stationary scene, differs from perception of real motion in that it constitutes a disturbing experience of spatial disorientation affecting posture and locomotion (Figure 8). The spontaneous eye movements (e.g., acquired pendular nystagmus in demyelinating disease, downbeat nystagmus in flocculus or medullary brainstem lesions, and superior oblique myokymia in spontaneous discharges of the trochlear nucleus) reduce the ability to stabilize posture visually and induce apparent

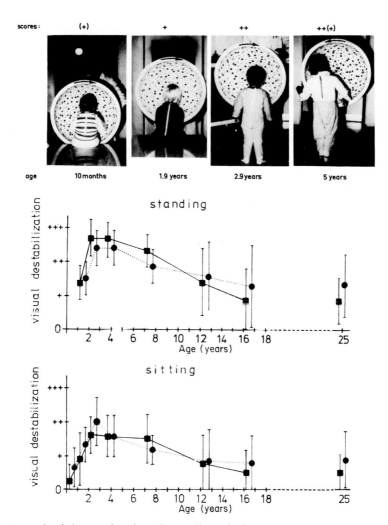

Figure 7. Postural imbalance induced optokinetically in children using a rotating half-spherical dome. Infants 6 to 12 months old show no or very little optokinetic disturbance whereas, with the development of upright stance and gait, optokinetic influences become increasingly important. Optokinetic loop participates rather late in the multisensory process of postural stabilization (12). Key: ■, males; ●, females.

motion because the eye movement is not associated with an appropriate corollary discharge signal. The sudden onset of an extraocular muscle paresis (e.g., in patients suffering from ocular myasthenia) may induce imbalance and vertigo during voluntary head or eye movements. Here, the lack of rather than an excess of eye movement leads to an uncalibrated and therefore unexpected slippage of the image on the retina. The symptoms not only include perceptual illusions such as oscillopsia, but also affect postural balance (8). The impairment of motor control can be attributed to an acute sensory deficiency of visual localization of objects in egocentric coordinates, which is usually calculated from both the position of the target on the retina and the awareness of eye position in the head.

E.G.,♀,60 downbeat nystagmus syndrome

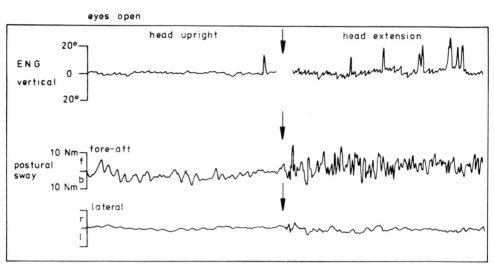

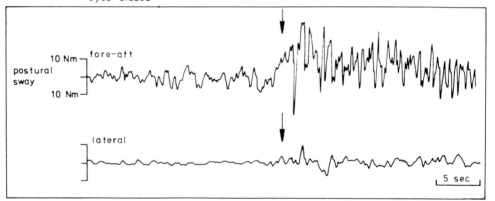

Figure 8. Simultaneous recordings of vertical electronystagmography (ENG) and body sway at upright stance with the head either at normal upright or retroflexion in a 60-year-old female patient suffering from downbeat nystagmus due to an Arnold–Chiari malformation. The vestibulocerebellar lesion causes a pathological postural sway with head extension and eyes closed. With the eyes open visual compensation of postural imbalance is diminished by the concurrent activation of downbeat nystagmus due to head extension.

OPTOKINETIC MOTION SICKNESS: VISUAL PSEUDO-CORIOLIS EFFECT

Motion sickness is a very distressing stimulation vertigo manifested by symptoms including malaise, nausea, and vomiting that cause a performance decrement when the individual is driving a vehicle. Motion sickness is considered to be generated either by unusual and therefore unadapted motion stimulation of one of the "stabilizing" sensory systems or by an intersensory mismatch between the converging inputs and the expected sensory patterns (3,35). The mismatch arises when the multisensory consequences of passive transportation do not match the expected patterns as they have been calibrated by experience from prior active locomotion. In the absence of actual body movements, "pure optokinetic motion sickness" has been reported in persons viewing a tilted swinging room (39) or the moving scene on the screen of a flight simulator (32). This may be explained by visual-vestibular mismatches in cases of surround motion alone, and it has been reported for optokinetic simulator sickness (32) that pilots with real flight experience (and therefore a stored expectation for sensory input patterns due to certain maneuvers) exhibit a higher susceptibility than nonpilots. That vision is a secondary etiological factor in the genesis of motion sickness was concluded from the fact that the incidence rate of blind persons was not significantly different from that of normal subjects (20).

Coriolis effects, which are of particular concern to airplane pilots (36) and typically occur through cross-coupled accelerations when the head, undergoing a rotation about one axis is bent about a second axis, can be mimicked optokinetically (Figure 9). *Visual pseudo-Coriolis effects*, phenomenologically indistinguishable from vestibular Coriolis effects, are elicited by bending the head out of the axis of rotation of a circular visual surround during the illusion of circularvection (13,15). A similar phenomenon can be observed if a subject is simultaneously exposed to a rotation of the visual surround about the line of sight (horizontal axis) during angular acceleration about an earth vertical axis with the head aligned to the Z axis (Figure 9). This effect

VESTIBULAR CORIOLIS EFFECT   VESTIBULAR PURKINJE EFFECT

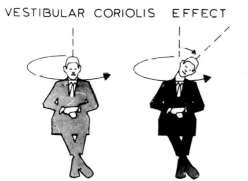 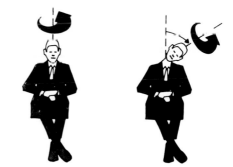

VISUAL PSEUDO-CORIOLIS EFFECT   VISUAL PSEUDO-PURKINJE EFFECT

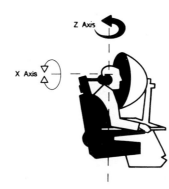

Figure 9. Optokinetic pseudo-Coriolis effect induced by bending the head out of the axis of rotation of the circular visual surround during the illusion of circularvection. Optokinetic pseudo-Purkinje effect induced by simultaneous exposure to a rotation of the visual surrounds about the line of sight and angular acceleration about an earth vertical axis.

can be compared to the Purkinje effect, a tumbling sensation of turning about a tilted axis when the head is bent during a postrotational semicircular canal response. Both the vestibular and the *optokinetically simulated Purkinje effects* are related to Coriolis effects. In visual pseudo-Coriolis effects excitation of semicircular canals, and in visual pseudo-Purkinje effects excitation of the otoliths, are simulated optokinetically, probably on the basis of a visual-vestibular convergence.

According to the mismatch concept, vision has been reported to promote motion sickness during passive transportation if it is at variance with actual body accelerations, whereas sickness is suppressed if vision is in physiological agreement with the simultaneous vestibular input (13,15). This can be practically used to prevent sickness in vehicles by providing ample peripheral vision of the relatively moving surround (Figure 10), as shown in recent car experiments (34) (Figure 11). Conversely, the symptoms are heightened in closed ship cabins, while one is reading, or to a lesser extent while one is sitting in the back set of an automobile. Here, the vestibular signals of accelerations are contradicted by visual information of a seemingly stationary (relative to the subject) environment. When vehicle motion cannot be visually observed, the mismatch can be switched off by eye closure. This also reduces sickness, but not as powerfully as with appropriate visual control.

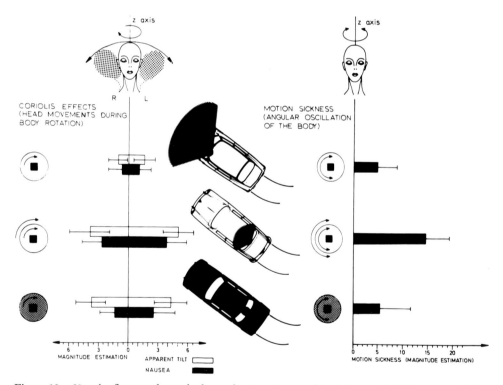

Figure 10. Visual influences during body accelerations in a combined drum and chair system and their effects on vertigo and motion sickness. Left: Magnitude estimations of apparent tilt and nausea induced by Coriolis effects at constant angular velocity of 60 deg/sec. Right: Magnitude estimation of motion sickness induced by 15 min of sinusoidal angular oscillation of the body at 0.02 Hz and peak velocity of 100 deg/sec. The three visual conditions were eyes open (top), rotary chair and visual surrounds mechanically coupled (middle), and eyes open in complete darkness (bottom). Estimations of nausea indicate that the symptom is maximal with conflicting visual-vestibular stimuli (combined movement of chair and drum), when vestibular acceleration is in disagreement with the visual information of no movement.

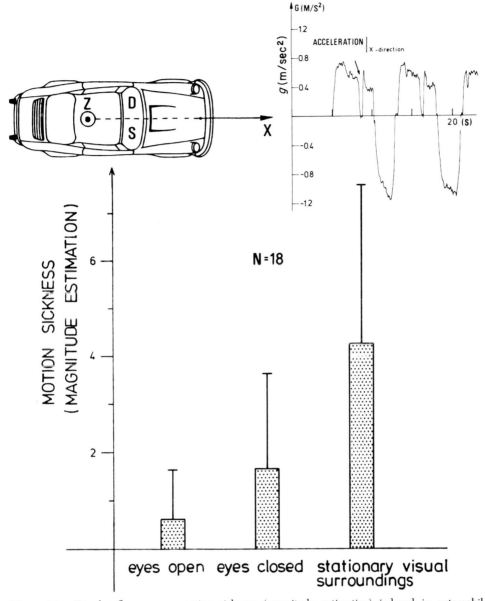

Figure 11. Visual influences on motion sickness (magnitude estimation) induced in automobile passengers by repetitive braking maneuvers (linear accelerations along the horizontal X axis: 0.8 to 1.2 g) under real road conditions (34). The symptom is maximal with conflicting visual-vestibular stimuli. Thus, providing ample peripheral vision of the relatively moving surrounds is the best way to alleviate car sickness physically.

Children below the age of 2 years are highly resistant to motion sickness but thereafter, up to about 12 years of age, reveal a greater susceptibility than adults (33). This has been attributed to a preference for riding in vehicles in the supine position (14) but can be explained more convincingly by the finding that dynamic spatial orientation of young children does not suffer from visual-vestibular mismatches (12).

Anti-motion-sickness drugs, such as the belladonna alkaloid scopolamine (0.6 mg)

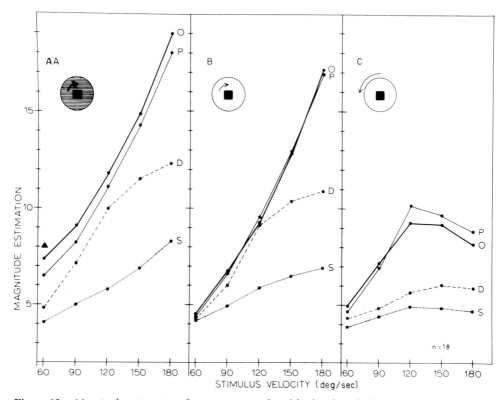

Figure 12. Magnitude estimation of acute nausea induced by bending the head toward the shoulder during (A) chair rotation in the dark (vestibular Coriolis effect), (B) chair rotation in the light (optovestibular Coriolis effects), and (C) pure drum rotation eliciting circularvection (visual pseudo-Coriolis effects). The scalings are presented as means (ordinate) in relation to the angular velocity of chair or drum rotation, respectively (abscissa). Dimenhydrinate and scopolamine reduce nausea under all three stimulus conditions, whereas the placebo effect is rather weak. Key: O, no drug; P, placebo; D, dimenhydrinate; S, scopolamine.

and the antihistamine dimenhydrinate (100 mg), are effective in preventing both vestibular and optokinetic motion sickness (Figure 12) but simultaneously cause remarkable central sedative side effects with performance decrements as documented by psychological efficiency tests (10). In cases of exceptionally strong motion sickness, combinations of either d-amphetamine sulfate and 1-scopolamine hydrobromide (37) or promethazine with d-amphetamine provided far better protection than any single drug (38) without increasing distressing side effects. Different drugs have been selected, e.g., for prophylaxis of space motion sickness in astronauts participating in the Shuttle–Spacelab Program: promethazine (25 mg) + ephedrine (25 mg), oral; scopolamine (0.4 mg) + dexedrine (5 mg), oral; and transdermal therapeutic system (TTS)–scopolamine, which delivers 200 μg priming dose and 10 μg per hour thereafter. The capacity to antagonize acetylcholine by competitive inhibition is the only known similarity among the effectiveness of drugs countering motion sickness. The most probable sites of primary action are the synapses of vestibular nuclei that exhibit a reduced resting discharge and diminished neuronal action to body rotation (23).

ACKNOWLEDGMENT

Research was supported by Deutsche Forschungsgemeinschaft, Br 639/3 "Bewegungskrankheit."

REFERENCES

1. Amblard, B., and Cremieux, J., Rôle de l'information visuelle du movement dans le maintien de l'équilibre. *Agressologie*, 1976, **17**:25–37.

2. Aubert, H., Die Bewegungsempfindung. *Arch. Gesamte Physiol. Menschen Tiere*, 1886, **39**:347–370.

3. Benson, A. J., Possible mechanism of motion and space sickness. In *Proceedings of the European Symposium of Life Sciences Research in Space* (W. R. Burke and T. D. Guyenne, eds.), European Space Agency, Paris, 1977:Sp 130:101–108.

4. Berthoz, A., Pavard, B., and Young, L. R., Perception of linear horizontal self-motion induced by peripheral vision (linearvection). Basic characteristics and visual-vestibular interactions. *Exp. Brain Res.*, 1975, **23**:471–489.

5. Bles, W., Kapteyn, T. S., Brandt, T., and Arnold, F., The mechanism of physiological height vertigo. II. Posturography. *Acta Oto-Laryngol.*, 1980, **89**:534–540.

6. Bles, W., Kapteyn, T. S., and De Wit, G., Effects of visual-vestibular interaction on human posture. *Adv. Oto-Rhino-Laryngol.*, 1977, **22**:111–118.

7. Brandt, T., Arnold, F., Bles, W., and Kapteyn, T. S., The mechanism of physiological height vertigo. I. Theoretical approach and psychophysics. *Acta Oto-Laryngol.*, 1980, **89**:513–523.

8. Brandt, T., and Büchele, W., Ocular myasthenia: Visual disturbance of posture and gait. *Agressologie*, 1979, **20**:195–196.

9. Brandt, T., and Daroff, R. B., The multisensory physiological and pathological vertigo syndromes. *Ann. Neurol.*, 1980, **7**:195–203.

10. Brandt, T., Dichgans, J., and Wagner, W., Drug effectiveness on experimental optokinetic and vestibular motion sickness. *Aerosp. Med.*, 1974, **45**:1291–1297.

11. Brandt, T., Krafczyk, S., and Malsbenden, I., Postural imbalance with head extension: Improvement by training as a model for ataxia therapy. *Ann. N. Y. Acad. Sci.*, 1981, **374**:636–649.

12. Brandt, T., Wenzel, D., and Dichgans, J., Die Entwicklung der visuellen Stabilisation des aufrechten Standes beim Kind: Ein Reifezeichen in der Kinderneurologie. *Arch. Psychiatr. Nervenkr.*, 1976, **223**:1–13.

13. Brandt, T., Wist, E. R., and Dichgans, J., Optisch induzierte Pseudo-Coriolis-Effekte und Circularvektion: Ein Beitrag zur optisch-vestibulären Interaktion. *Arch. Psychiatr. Nervenkr.*, 1971, **214**:365–389.

14. Chinn, H. I., and Smith, P. K., Motion sickness. *Pharmacol. Rev.*, 1955, **7**:33–83.

15. Dichgans, J., and Brandt, T., Visual-vestibular interaction: Effects on self-motion perception and postural control. In: *Handbook of Sensory Physiology* (R. Held, H. W. Leibowitz, and H. L. Teuber, eds.). Springer-Verlag, Berlin and New York, 1978, **8**:755–804.

16. Dichgans, J., Diener, H. C., and Brandt, T., Optokinetic-graviceptive interaction in different head positions. *Acta Oto-Laryngol.*, 1974, **78**:391–398.

17. Dichgans, J., Held, R., Young, L. R., and Brandt, T., Moving visual scenes influence the apparent direction of gravity. *Science*, 1972, **178**:1217–1219.

18. Dichgans, J., Mauritz, K. H., Allum, J. H. J., and Brandt, T., Postural sway in normals and atactic patients: Analysis of the stabilizing and destabilizing effects of vision. *Agressologie*, 1976, **17**:15–24.

19. Fischer, M. H., and Kornmüller, E. E., Optokinetisch ausgelöste Bewegungswahrnehmungen und optokinetischer Nystagmus. *J. Psychol. Neurol.*, 1930, **41**:273–308.

20. Graybiel, A., Susceptibility to acute motion sickness in blind persons. *Aerosp. Med.*, 1970, **41**:650–653.

21. Held, R., Dichgans, J., and Bauer, J., Characteristics of moving visual scenes influencing spatial orientation. *Vision Res.*, 1975, **15**:357–365.

22. Helmholtz, H. von, *Handbuch der physiologischen Optik*. Voss, Leipzig, 1896.

23. Jaju, B. P., Kirsten, E. B., and Wang, S. C., Effects of belladonna alkaloids on the vestibular nucleus of the cat. *Am. J. Physiol.*, 1971, **219**:1248–1255.

24. Kapteyn, T. S., *Het staan van de Mens*. Thesis, Amsterdam, 1973.

25. Kapteyn, T. S., and Bles, W., Circularvection and human posture. Relation between the reactions to various stimuli. *Agressologie*, 1977, **18**:335–339.

26. Kapteyn, T. S., Bles, W., Brandt, T., and Wist, E. R., Visual stabilization of posture: Effect of light intensity and stroboscopic surround illumination. *Agressologie,* 1979, **20**:191–192.

27. Lee, D. N., and Aronson, E., Visual proprioceptive control of standing in human infants. *Percept. Psychophys.,* 1974, **15**:529–532.

28. Leibowitz, H. W., The relation between the rate threshold for the perception of movement and luminance for various durations of exposure. *J. Exp. Psychol.,* 1955, **49**:209–214.

29. Leibowitz, H. W., Rodemer, C. S., and Dichgans, J., The independence of dynamic spatial orientation from luminance and refractive error. *Percept. Psychophys.,* 1979, **25**:75–79.

30. Lestienne, F., Soechting, J. F., and Berthoz, A., Postural readjustments induced by linear motion of visual scenes. *Exp. Brain Res.,* 1977, **28**:363–384.

31. Mach, E., *Grundlinien der Lehre von den Bewegungsempfindungen.* Engelmann, Leipzig, 1875.

31a. Mauritz, K. H., Dichgans, J., and Hufschmidt, A., Quantitative analysis of stance in late cortical cerebellar atrophy of the anterior lobe and other forms of cerebellar ataxia. *Brain,* 1979, **102**:461–482.

32. Miller, J. W., and Goodson, J. E., Motion sickness in a helicopter simulator. *Aerosp. Med.,* 1960, **31**:204–212.

33. Money, K. E., Motion sickness. *Physiol. Rev.,* 1970, **50**:1–39.

34. Probst, T., Krafczyk, S., Büchele, W., and Brandt, T., Visual prevention of motion sickness in cars. *Arch. Psychiatr. Nervenkr.* (in press).

35. Reason, J. T., Motion sickness adaptation: A neural mismatch model. *J. R. Soc. Med.,* 1978, **71**:819–829.

36. Schubert, G., Über die physiologischen Auswirkungen der Corioliskräfte bei Trudelbewegungen des Flugzeuges. *Acta Oto-Laryngol.,* 1931, **16**:39–47.

37. Wood, C. D., and Graybiel, A., Evaluation of sixteen anti-motion sickness drugs under controlled laboratory conditions. *Aerosp. Med.,* 1968, **39**:1341–1344.

38. Wood, C. D., and Graybiel, A., Evaluation of anti-motion sickness drugs: A new effective remedy revealed. *Aerosp. Med.,* 1970, **41**:932–933.

39. Wood, R. W., The "haunted swing" illusion. *Psychol. Rev.,* 1895, **2**:277–278.

40. Young, L. R., Oman, C. M., and Dichgans, J., Influence of head orientation on visually induced pitch and roll sensation. *Aviat. Space Environ. Med.,* 1975, **46**:264–268.

Illusory Movement of Environment during Head Rotation with Normal Eye Movements

DAVID G. COGAN, FRED C. CHU, and DOUGLAS B. REINGOLD

Neuro-ophthalmology Section, Clinical Branch
National Eye Institute, NIH
Bethesda, Maryland

INTRODUCTION

Illusory movement of the environment occurs when there is a mismatch between what the retina tells the brain about the movement of images and what the brain estimates to be the movement of the eyes. Simple illustrations are the illusions that occur with passive manipulation of the eyes, mechanical blockage of ocular movements, and pareses of gaze. In such cases the real and encoded positions of the eyes do not match. The same illusion occurs with inappropriate (caloric) vestibular stimulation.

Much less common and not so easy to explain are the illusions occurring when the eyes make full and appropriate movements. The purpose of this chapter is to describe a patient who complained of an incapacitating illusory movement of the environment to one side despite normal eye movements. The lesion presumably responsible was an intracranial vascular abnormality localized by computerized tomographic (CT) scan in the right parahippocampal region. A patient with a similar symptom was reported by Bender and Feldman (2); she was thought to have a unilateral labyrinthine lesion.

METHODS

The patient was subjected to several conditions of bodily and/or visuoenvironmental rotation. During these maneuvers, the eye movements were recorded by electrooculography (Tables 1 and 2), and the patient's verbal descriptions of motion perception were noted (Tables 3 and 4).

Throughout the testing, the patient was seated on a motorized Bárány chair. He was rotated in darkness to test the vestibuloocular reflex (VOR) and in a vertically

225

NYSTAGMUS AND VERTIGO: CLINICAL
APPROACHES TO THE PATIENT WITH DIZZINESS

TABLE 1
SINUSOIDAL SLOW-PHASE GAIN[a]

Stimulus	Gain
VOR (in darkness)	0.17
OKN	0.75
VVOR	1.00

[a] Peak velocity 60 deg/sec at 0.2 Hz.

TABLE 2
DIRECTION-SPECIFIC SLOW-PHASE GAINS[a,b]

Stimulus	Rightward	Leftward	t test
VOR sine 0.2 Hz	0.08	0.19	
(peak velocity)	(4.94 ± 0.79)	(11.53 ± 2.54)	p < .001
VOR velocity step (15 sec)	0.05	0.22	
(mean velocity)	(2.88 ± 0.52)	(13.33 ± 2.10)	p < .001
OKN velocity step (15 sec)	0.63	0.69	
(mean velocity)	(37.68 ± 3.29)	(41.64 ± 4.52)	ns[c]
VVOR velocity step (15 sec)	0.88	0.89	
(mean velocity)	(52.61 ± 6.98)	(52.23 ± 5.62)	ns[c]

[a] Sixty degrees per second.
[b] Velocities in degrees per second ± standard deviation.
[c] ns, not significant.

TABLE 3
SUBJECTIVE SENSE OF SELF-ROTATION[a,b]

Stimulus	Chair velocity		
	30 deg/sec	60 deg/sec	120 deg/sec
VOR (sine 0.2 Hz)	None	None	Slight
VOR (const. veloc.)	None	None	nd

[a] Tested in the dark.
[b] Abbreviations: const. veloc., constant-velocity rotation in one direction; nd, not done.

striped surround to test the visuovestibuloocular reflex (VVOR). Also, the chair was earth-fixed, and the striped surround was moved as a test for optokinetic nystagmus (OKN). Rotational stimulations were either (a) sinusoidal at 0.2 Hz, 60 deg/sec peak velocity or (b) constant velocity at 60 deg/sec. Other frequencies and amplitudes were tested and gave concordant results.

For the nystagmoid eye movements, the definitions of slow-phase gain depended on the type of stimulation. Gain during sinusoidal rotation was defined as peak slow-phase eye velocity divided by peak chair or stripe stimulus velocity, computed by Fourier analysis. Gain during constant-velocity rotation was defined as mean slow-phase eye velocity (in the epoch following a velocity step) divided by the constant stimulus velocity.

TABLE 4
SUBJECTIVE RATES OF BACKGROUND MOTION[a,b]

Stimulus	Stripe velocity		
	30 deg/sec	60 deg/sec	120 deg/sec
OKN (sine 0.2 Hz)	R = L	R > L	nd
OKN(const. veloc.)	R = L	R = L (*)	nd

Stimulus	Chair velocity		
	30 deg/sec	60 deg/sec	120 deg/sec
VVOR (sine 0.2 Hz)	R = L	R > L	R > L
VVOR (const. veloc.)	R = L	R > L	nd

[a] Tested in a vertically striped surround.

[b] Abbreviations: const. veloc., constant-velocity rotation in one direction; R, rate of apparent background motion rightward; L, rate of apparent background motion leftward; (*), circularvection described; nd, not done.

CASE REPORT

A 48-year-old man consulted his otologist and neurologist because of an illusory movement of the field of vision whenever he moved his head to the left. The field then appeared to "zoom" to the right. He was sufficiently incapacitated that he had to give up working and driving. This symptom appeared abruptly after the patient had been shoveling snow 5 months before our examination. It was accompanied at the outset by a transient period of nausea, vertigo, staggering, and nystagmus. Although these symptoms cleared, the residual illusory movement has persisted for 22 months to date.

In addition to the visual complaint, and presumably related to it, the patient had the phakomatous angiomatosis known as the blue rubber bleb nevus syndrome of Bean (1). The vascular lesions had first appeared in the patient's teen-age years and involved the face, tongue, conjunctiva, lips, and limbs. The lesions bled on mild trauma. Bilateral carotid and vertebral angiograms had been done when the patient was 41 because of mental lapses that were attributed to an automobile accident. The angiograms were reported to have shown abnormal vessels, possibly an angioma, in the right temporal region.

The patient's eye movements were entirely normal by customary clinical tests. He fixated normally; the eyes showed no spontaneous nystagmus; saccadic, pursuit, and optokinetic responses were normal. Rotation in a Bárány chair in the light with the eyes open (a test of VVOR) induced a jerk nystagmus that was normal and symmetric in both horizontal directions (Figure 1). Rotation with the eyes closed or rotation in the dark with the eyes open or closed (tests of VOR) induced no dizziness or other abnormal sensation. As expected, when the patient's head or body was turned to either side, he noted an apparently contraversive movement of the environment. On head motion to the right, this movement was thought to be normal; it caused no untoward symptoms. However, on head motion to the left, the patient estimated a two- to threefold relative increase in the velocity of the background; this was in-

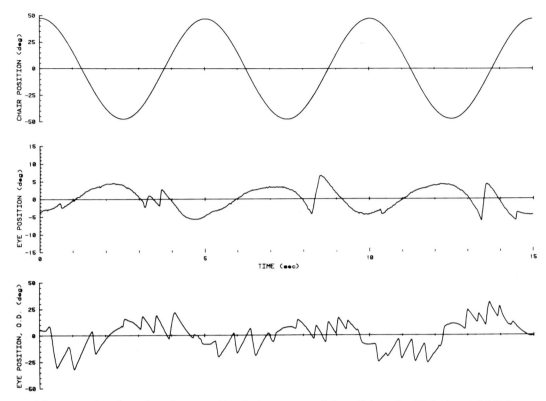

Figure 1. Waveforms for right eye position during two tests of sinusoidal rotation (60 deg/sec at 0.2 Hz). Upward deflections indicate rightward movements. Top curve: Stimulus (chair) velocity. Middle curve: VOR characterized by the relative absence of fast phases and low slow-phase velocity. Bottom curve: VVOR characterized by numerous fast phases and high slow-phase velocity.

capacitating. No abnormal symptoms were induced by vertical movement of the head or eyes.

The eye movement recordings confirmed the normalcy of saccadic, pursuit, optokinetic, and fixational responses. In the dark, however, vestibuloocular gain was reduced to 0.17, with normal subjects of approximately the same age having a gain of 0.67 ± 0.21 (Tables 1 and 2). For chair rotation of less than 120 deg/sec, the patient was unable to tell if he was moving except at the initial accelerations (Tables 3 and 4). The reduction in gain was greater on rotation to the left (with induced slow phases directed rightward). As seen in Table 2, this asymmetry was significant at $p < .001$, whether the VOR was tested sinusoidally for peak velocity gain or with a velocity step for mean velocity gain.

On the other hand, there were no such side-to-side differences for mean slow phase gain of OKN and VVOR that were, of course, recorded in the light (Table 2). Optokinetic after-nystagmus was also symmetrically present in either direction for 5 sec after target motion was extinguished.

Although the patient admitted to circularvection during OKN testing (the feeling that he was moving and the stripes were still), he seemed to have a decreased awareness of it (Tables 3 and 4). It was only with questioning that he would admit to having had the sensation.

The patient reported some subtle, subjective abnormalities during both OKN and VVOR testing that corresponded to his illusion (see Tables 3 and 4). During these tests, the stripes appeared to "zoom" to the right, compared to their "normal" leftward movement. At other times, the sensations were described as a "definite sensation of blurriness," "disorientation," and "slight dizziness," but only as the stripes moved rightward. They usually occurred during sinusoidal stimulation, when the stimulus changed direction periodically every 15 sec. They did not occur during prolonged, constant-velocity rotations in one direction. At no time did we observe abnormal eye movements that corresponded to the reports of asymmetric sensations. The waveforms for VOR and VVOR are depicted in Figure 1.

COMMENT

This patient had an unusually persistent and incapacitating illusion that the environment moved rightward when his head moved leftward. This followed an acute disorder involving the vestibular system. It was a perceptual phenomenon not explained by retinal slippage, since the eye movements were entirely normal during the illusion.

Nevertheless, the gain of VOR when measured in the dark was reduced bilaterally and most markedly on rotation to the left, the side affected by the illusion. Yet the patient did not report asymmetric sensations lateralizing to a particular side if rotated in the dark. In fact, except for the initial acceleration, the patient had difficulty telling if he was moving at all. It appeared that at best he gained few clues from the vestibular system regarding head movement to either side.

When OKN or VVOR was studied, there were no comparable asymmetries in slow-phase gains. Some lateralization might have been anticipated with these tests, since they simulated closely the clinical situations inducing the illusion. Thus, it appeared that visual inputs to the ocular motor system (with respect to OKN and VVOR) could adequately maintain the eyes in the anticipated positions. In particular, the normal VVOR led us to believe that visual inputs compensated functionally for the VOR, which was abnormal when measured in the dark.

Nevertheless, in tests of OKN and VVOR, the patient felt the stripes "zoom" to the right, as compared to their leftward motion. The eye movements, being symmetric, did not account for the unidirectional visual illusion. For the patient to experience that sensation, a directional change in the visual surround was generally necessary. If rotated at constant velocity in one direction, the patient rarely felt uncomfortable or reported that the background "zoomed" in any direction. That the patient had illusions of movement in the light (OKN and VVOR) despite normal eye movements and yet had no lateralizing sensations on rotation in the dark (VOR) despite abnormal slow phase gains seemed a paradox.

The asymmetry of VOR slow-phase gains correlated with the unilateral nature of the illusion. The slow-phase gain was reduced more markedly to the side of the illusion. It would be tempting to suggest, therefore, that the asymmetric vestibular inputs improperly offset the visual signals in the cerebral center for motion perception. Such a simple hypothesis, however, must be questioned, since many persons have asymmetric vestibular responses and yet do not report the same disabling symptom.

Our patient had a unilateral lesion demonstrated by CT scan in the right parahippocampal region. The basis for the lesion was an intracranial complication of the blue rubber bleb nevus syndrome comparable to that reported by Waybright and colleagues (3). Its relationship to the cause of the symptoms is presumptive.

As far as we know, only one other case of a patient with this specific symptom has been reported in the literature (2). That patient had a unilateral lesion, presumably labyrinthine. In neither case, unfortunately, was there sufficient evidence for definitive anatomical localization of the phenomenon. Nevertheless, the specificity of the symptom in the face of normal eye movements, despite its rarity, suggests that it constitutes a definite clinical entity involving visuovestibular interactions. It has remained surprisingly persistent in spite of apparently normal cerebellar functions.

REFERENCES

1. Bean, W. B., *Vascular Spiders and Related Lesions of the Skin.* Thomas, Springfield, Illinois, 1958.
2. Bender, M. B., and Feldman, F., Visual illusions during the head movement in lesions of the brain stem. *Arch. Neurol. (Chicago)*, 1967, **17**:354–364.
3. Waybright, E. A., Selhorst, J. B., Rosenblum, W. L., and Suter, C. G., Blue rubber bleb nevus syndrome with CNS involvement and thrombosis of a vein of Galen malformation. *Ann. Neurol.*, 1978, **3**:464–467.

Quantitative Assessment of Visual-Vestibular Interaction Using Sinusoidal Rotatory Stimuli

ROBERT W. BALOH,[1] ROBERT D. YEE,[2] HERMAN A. JENKINS,[3] and VICENTE HONRUBIA[3]

[1] Department of Neurology, School of Medicine, University of California Los Angeles, Los Angeles, California
[2] Department of Ophthalmology, School of Medicine, University of California Los Angeles, Los Angeles, California
[3] Division of Head and Neck Surgery (Otolaryngology), School of Medicine, University of California Los Angeles, Los Angeles, California

INTRODUCTION

In the last few decades motorized rotatory chairs have been designed to produce angular accelerations that can be precisely controlled. Simultaneously, digital microcomputer techniques have evolved so that nystagmus responses can be accurately measured. As is apparent from other chapters in this volume these advances have led to an increased enthusiasm for the use of rotatory testing in the neurotology clinic. With rotatory testing, multiple graded stimuli can be applied in a relatively short time. An additional advantage is that rotatory testing is less bothersome to patients than caloric testing. Furthermore, unlike caloric testing, a rotatory stimulus is unrelated to physical features of the external ear or temporal bone, so that a more exact relationship between stimulus and response can be determined. These features are particularly important when one is attempting to measure the oculomotor response to combined visual and vestibular stimuli. In this chapter we summarize our experience in using sinusoidal rotatory stimuli for testing patients with focal neurological lesions.

METHODS

We routinely use direct current (dc) electrooculography for clinical recordings. Electrodes are placed at the inner and outer canthi to record horizontal movements and above the eyebrow and below the lower eyelid to record vertical movements of each eye independently. A six-pole, low-pass filter with cutoff frequency of 42 Hz (-3

NYSTAGMUS AND VERTIGO: CLINICAL
APPROACHES TO THE PATIENT WITH DIZZINESS

dB) removes high-frequency noise before the signal enters the analog-to-digital converter. Complete details of the recording system have been reported elsewhere (2).

For rotatory testing the patient is seated in a chair mounted on a motorized rotating table inside a light-tight, electrically shielded room. This rotating table delivers maximum torque of 10 ft lb, which provides a weight-independent maximum acceleration of approximately 140 deg/sec². A cloth drum with one-inch-wide white stripes (15 deg apart) mounted on a black cloth completely surrounds the patient so that the entire visual field is stimulated. An array of three light-emitting diodes (LED's) spaced at center and 15 deg to the right and left is attached to the chair directly in front of the patient. This allows for rapid calibration in any chair position in the light and in the dark. Frequent calibrations are interspersed throughout the testing procedure to correct for any fluctuations in corneoretinal potential. The rotatory chair, optokinetic drum, and calibration lights are all controlled by the same microprocessor that anlyzes the nystagmus response.

For optokinetic nystagmus (OKN) the drum is rotated alone, and the patient is instructed to stare at the stripes directly in front of him and not to follow them as they move around (stare OKN). Visual-vestibular interaction is tested by rotating the chair sinusoidally (a) in the dark (vestibuloocular reflex, or VOR), (b) in the light with the optokinetic drum stationary (visual-vestibuloocular reflex, or VVOR), and (c) in the dark with the center LED lit (VOR with fixation suppression, or VOR-FIX). In the first instance the vestibular system is tested without visual influence, whereas in the second the vestibular and optokinetic systems are stimulated in a synergistic fashion, and in the third the fixation pursuit system is used to suppress vestibular-induced nystagmus. The computer algorithm generates stimulus signals at frequencies of from 0.0125 to 0.2 Hz and peak velocities of 15 to 60 deg/sec. For screening purposes we routinely use 0.05 Hz and peak velocity of 60 deg/sec.

Complete details of the on-line digital computer analysis techniques have been reported elsewhere (1). In brief, the eye position signal (digitized at a rate of 200 samples per second) is differentiated to yield an instantaneous velocity record. Fast components (saccades) are identified on the basis of their characteristic velocity profile and the direction of the stimulus movement. After the fast components are removed, the gaps in the remaining slow eye velocity record are filled by connecting points on each side of the missing segment with a quadratic regression line. A discrete fast Fourier transform analysis is then executed to obtain the dc bias and the gain (peak slow-phase eye velocity/peak stimulus velocity) and phase of the fundamental and first two harmonics. From the plots of slow-phase velocity versus time, the gain in each direction is also calculated separately to evaluate symmetry of response.

Results

normal subjects

A typical normal subject's response to the four sinusoidal rotatory test conditions (0.05 Hz, peak velocity 60 deg/sec) is shown in Figure 1A (left). In this figure slow-phase eye velocity is plotted versus time for two complete cycles of stimulation. The OKN and VVOR gains (peak slow-phase eye velocity/peak drum or chair velocity) are nearly twice that of the VOR. The VOR is completely inhibited with fixation, as shown in the fourth trace of Figure 1A (i.e., the VOR-FIX gain is 0). The mean gain

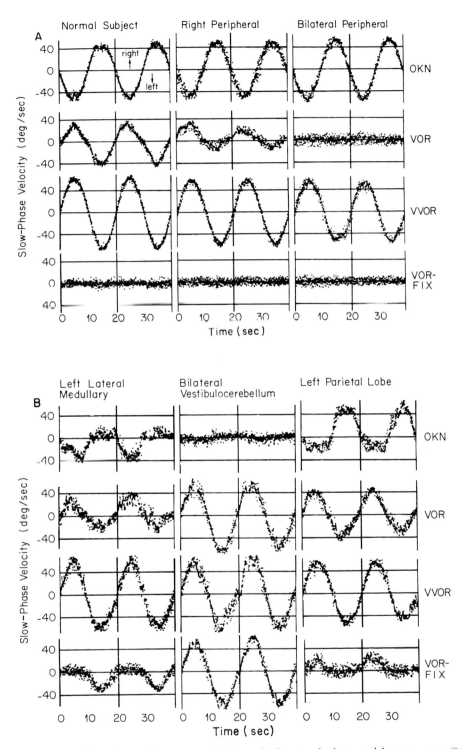

Figure 1. Plots of slow-phase velocity versus time from the four standard sinusoidal rotatory tests (0.05 Hz, peak velocity 60 deg/sec).

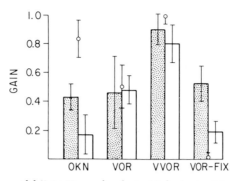

Figure 2.   Summary of sinusoidal (0.05 Hz, peak velocity 60 deg/sec) rotatory test results in six patients with Wallenberg's syndrome (4). Vertical bars with attached lines represent the mean ±1 SD of slow-phase gain toward (stippled bars) and away from (open bars) the side of the lesion. The normal mean ±1 SD is given by the open circles with attached vertical lines.

±1 standard deviation (SD) for similar testing in 20 normal subjects is shown in Figure 2 (open circles with attached vertical lines) (4). Similar values (mean ±1 SD) for both gain and phase measurements over the frequency range of 0.01 to 0.1 Hz (peak velocity 60 deg/sec) are shown in Figure 3 (5). The VOR responses have a progressively decreasing phase lead with increasing frequency, whereas the VVOR and OKN (not shown) responses are in phase over this entire frequency range. The VOR gain increases slightly with increasing frequency, whereas VVOR, OKN, and VOR-FIX gain is unchanged over this low-frequency range.

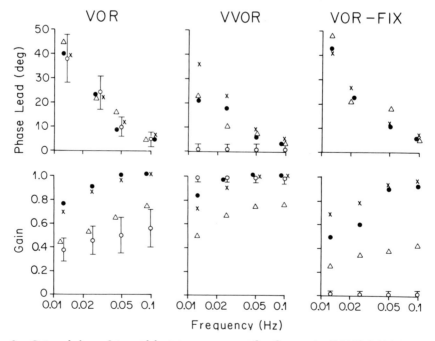

Figure 3.   Gain and phase of sinusoidal rotatory responses at four frequencies (0.0125, 0.025, 0.05, 0.1 Hz, peak velocity 60 deg/sec) in three patients with lesions involving the vestibulocerebellum (5). The normal mean ±1 SD (open circles with attached vertical lines) is given for each frequency. (Most normal subjects do not have measurable VOR-FIX responses at this peak velocity.)

PERIPHERAL VESTIBULAR LESIONS

Patients with unilateral lesions of the labyrinth or eighth nerve have two characteristic abnormalities on VOR testing. They show an asymmetric gain with decreased slow-phase velocity away from the side of the lesion (i.e., with rotation toward the side of the lesion). They also show an advance of the eye velocity record over the stimulus velocity or phase lead greater than that of normal subjects at low frequencies of rotation, 0.05 Hz and lower (7, 8, 10). The asymmetry of response is most pronounced with acute lesions and often disappears as compensation occurs, whereas the increased phase lead at low frequencies remains indefinitely. As a general rule, OKN and visual-vestibular interaction are normal in such patients, although a transient asymmetry of OKN and VVOR responses can occur acutely when there is a strong spontaneous nystagmus.

The patient whose responses are illustrated in Figure 1A (center) underwent a right labyrinthectomy as part of a temporal bone resection for cancer 1 week before testing. At the time of testing he exhibited a low-velocity spontaneous nystagmus to the left with eyes closed and with eyes open in darkness. The gain with rotation toward the side of the lesion was 0.17, whereas that with rotation away from the side of lesion was 0.42 (normal mean ±1 SD = 0.50 ± 0.15). The phase lead at 0.05 Hz was 22 deg (normal mean 10 ± 4 degrees). Gain and phase measurements for OKN, VVOR, and VOR-FIX were normal. Similar patients tested months to years after labyrinthectomy or eighth nerve section often have symmetric VOR gain measurements (8).

With bilateral peripheral vestibular lesions the VOR responses are symmetrically diminished (10). When VOR responses are present, there is an increased phase advance at low frequencies. The gain of OKN responses and that of VVOR responses are approximately the same, usually low normal, and the phase of both is normal. The VOR fixation suppression is also normal. The patient whose responses are illustrated in Figure 1A (right) complained of mild imbalance and oscillopsia after receiving aminoglycoside antibiotics. No detectable VOR response was present at 0.05 Hz, peak velocity 60 deg/sec. The gain of the OKN and VVOR responses for this stimulus was 0.89 and 0.91, respectively (normal OKN and VVOR mean gain ±1 SD = 0.83 ± 0.13 and 0.99 ± 0.05, respectively).

LATERAL MEDULLARY LESIONS

Patients with infarction of the lateral medulla (Wallenberg's syndrome) exhibit prominent oculomotor abnormalities (4). With eyes open in the sitting position there is a tonic pulling of the eyes toward the side of the lesion, resulting in spontaneous nystagmus with fast phase toward the intact side. With eye closure or with eyes open in darkness the spontaneous nystagmus may change direction. This spontaneous nystagmus results in asymmetric visual and vestibular ocular control, as illustrated by the patient responses shown in Figure 1B (left) and average responses of six patients summarized in Figure 2.

The patient whose responses are illustrated in Figure 1B (left) was a 32-year-old man who developed the acute onset of vertigo, nausea, vomiting, dysphagia, and falling to the left. On neurological examination he exhibited spontaneous nystagmus to the right in the light while fixating and to the left in the dark. There was also ipsilateral facial hypalgesia, Horner's syndrome, and extremity ataxia and contralateral extremity hypalgesia. The OKN and VOR responses were asymmetric but in opposite directions, consistent with the changing direction of the patient's spontaneous nystagmus from light to dark. Despite the decreased OKN gain, the VVOR gain was normal in both directions. Fixation suppression of the VOR was impaired in both directions, particularly slow phases toward the side of the lesion. A similar pattern of findings was found in the six patients with Wallenberg's syndrome summarized in Figure 2 (4). In addition to being asymmetric, OKN and VOR-FIX gain measurements were significantly abnormal in both directions, whereas VVOR gain was normal or only slightly decreased. Average VOR responses were normal, with half being greater toward the side of the lesion and the other half greater away from the side of the lesion.

LESIONS OF THE VESTIBULOCEREBELLUM

Patients with lesions involving the vestibulocerebellum are unable to modify vestibular responses with vision (5). This is illustrated by the patient data shown in Figure 1B (center), in which the VOR, VVOR, and VOR-FIX gains are approximately the same (nearly 1) and the OKN gain is markedly decreased in both directions. This patient was a 31-year-old woman who complained only of unsteadiness and oscillopsia. The results of neurological examination were normal except for spontaneous downbeat nystagmus and truncal ataxia. Computerized tomography (CT) scanning and pneumoencephalography documented atrophy of the caudal midline cerebellum and flocculonodular lobe.

Figure 3 summarizes gain and phase measurements for sinusoidal (0.01 to 0.1 Hz, peak velocity 60 deg/sec) vestibular and visual-vestibular testing in three patients with lesions involving the vestibulocerebellum (5). The gain of the VOR, VVOR, and VOR-FIX increased with increasing frequency, whereas the phase lead was inversely related to frequency (similar to VOR responses in normal subjects). Thus, these patients were unable to improve the low-frequency responses of their VOR with vision.

LESIONS OF THE PARIETOOCCIPITAL LOBE

Lesions of the visuomotor pathways in the deep parietal lobe characteristically impair smooth pursuit and optokinetic slow phases toward the side of the lesion (3). The deficit may or may not be associated with a homonymous hemianopsia, depending on whether the geniculocalcarine pathways are involved. The abnormal visual-ocular control does not impair VOR responses but does alter visual-vestibular interaction.

Typical responses to the four sinusoidal rotatory test conditions in a patient with a deep parietal lobe lesion are shown in Figure 1B (right). This 21-year-old man developed bitemporal headaches and slowly progressive right facial and upper extremity weakness. The results of CT scanning were normal, but an angiogram identified a tumor blush in the left parietal region. A left parietal brain biopsy revealed a grade III astrocytoma. The patient did not have a homonymous hemianopsia at the time the test results shown in Figure 1B (right) were obtained. The OKN gain was normal to the right and markedly decreased to the left. The VOR gain was normal in both directions, and the patient was unable to inhibit VOR slow phases to the right with fixation (i.e., the VOR-FIX gain was increased to the right). Although normal in both directions, the VVOR gain was asymmetric with lower gain to the left than to the right.

TABLE 1

Summary of Gain[a] and Phase Abnormalities Found on Sinusoidal Rotatory Testing of Patients with Focal Neurological Lesions

Location of lesion	OKN		VOR		VVOR		VOR-FIX	
	Gain	Phase	Gain	Phase	Gain	Phase	Gain	Phase[b]
Labyrinth or eighth nerve (8,10)								
Unilateral	Normal	Normal	Decreased contralaterally[c] acutely	Increased phase lead	Normal	Normal	Normal	—
Bilateral	Low normal	Normal	Decreased bilaterally	Increased phase lead	Low normal	Normal	Normal	—
Lateral medullary (4)	Decreased bilaterally, ipsilaterally > contralaterally	Normal	Asymmetric variable direction	Increased phase lead	Low normal	Normal	Increased bilaterally, ipsilaterally > contralaterally	—
Bilateral vestibulo-cerebellum (5)	Decreased bilaterally	Normal	Increased bilaterally	Normal	Normal	Increased phase lead	Increased bilaterally	—
Unilateral parietal lobe (3)	Decreased ipsilaterally[c]	Normal	Normal	Normal	Decreased ipsilaterally[c]	Normal	Increased contralaterally[c]	—

[a] Peak slow-phase eye velocity/peak stimulus velocity.
[b] Normal subjects completely inhibit the VOR at this frequency and peak velocity.
[c] Direction of slow-phase eye movement.

SUMMARY

Table 1 summarizes the typical gain and phase abnormalities found in sinusoidal rotatory testing in patients with focal lesions of visual, vestibular, and visual-vestibular pathways. Additional clinical histories and quantitative measurements for individual patients are reported in the references listed for each patient group.

Despite the theoretical advantages suggested in the Introduction, rotatory testing has not been widely accepted for routine clinical evaluation of patients suspected of having a peripheral vestibular lesion, primarily because rotatory stimuli affect both labyrinths simultaneously, whereas with caloric testing it is possible to stimulate one labyrinth selectively. Even with the sophisticated analysis techniques described in this volume the side of a unilateral peripheral vestibular lesion (labyrinth or eighth nerve) cannot be reliably identified with rotatory testing. The degree of asymmetry of rotatory-induced nystagmus seen with partial unilateral lesions is often not outside the normal range, and even with a complete unilateral lesion symmetry returns with compensation (8). An increased phase shift of the VOR at low frequencies of sinusoidal stimulation is a more persistent finding (9), but this indicates only vestibular dysfunction; it does not indicate the side of the lesion or whether it is central or peripheral. For these reasons a standard bithermal caloric test is still an important part of the work-up of a patient suspected of having a unilateral peripheral vestibular lesion.

Sinusoidal rotatory testing is particularly useful for evaluating patients with suspected central nervous system lesions. When combined with quantitative tests of visual-ocular control (1) (saccades, smooth pursuit, and OKN), rotatory testing can often localize the site and extent of the lesion. Lesions in the lateral medulla involving the vestibular nuclei characteristically affect both visual and vestibular ocular responses. Often the OKN gain is greater toward the side of the lesion, whereas the VOR gain is greater away from the side of the lesion. As with peripheral vestibular lesions the VOR may show an increased phase lead at low frequencies. Fixation suppression of the VOR is uniformly impaired, particularly slow phases toward the side of the lesion.

Patients with lesions involving the vestibulocerebellum have severely impaired sinusoidal optokinetic and smooth pursuit responses. The gain of their VOR, VVOR, and VOR-FIX responses are approximately the same (nearly 1), and each of these responses exhibits a low-frequency phase lead characteristic of normal VOR responses. Thus, these patients are unable to improve the low-frequency responses of their VOR with vision. Finally, lesions of the parietal lobe impair ipsilateral visuomotor responses (i.e., smooth pursuit and OKN slow phases) without affecting VOR responses. Fixation suppression of contralateral VOR slow phases is impaired since normally pursuit in one direction is used to inhibit VOR slow phases in the opposite direction (6).

ACKNOWLEDGMENTS

This study was supported by NIH grant NS 09823. The authors thank Susan Sakala and Kathleen Brintnall for technical assistance, Laurn Langhofer for programming assistance, and Karen Einstein for preparing the manuscript.

REFERENCES

1. Baloh, R. W., Honrubia, V., and Sills, A., Eye-tracking and optokinetic nystagmus: Results of quantitative testing in patients with well-defined nervous system lesions. *Ann. Otol., Rhinol., Laryngol.*, 1977, **86**:108–114.

2. Baloh, R. W., Langhofer, L., Honrubia, V., and Yee, R. D., On-line analysis of eye movements using a digital computer. *Aviat. Space Environ. Med.*, 1980, **51**:563–567.

3. Baloh, R. W., Yee, R. D., and Honrubia, V., Optokinetic nystagmus and parietal lobe lesions. *Ann. Neurol.*, 1979, **7**:269–276.

4. Baloh, R. W., Yee, R. D., and Honrubia, V., Eye movements in patients with Wallenberg's syndrome. *Ann. N. Y. Acad. Sci.*, 1981, **374**:600–613.

5. Baloh, R. W., Yee, R. D., Kimm, J., and Honrubia, V., The vestibulo-ocular reflex in patients with lesions involving the vestibulocerebellum. *Exp. Neurol.*, 1981, **72**:141–152.

6. Dichgans, J., von Reutern, G. M., and Rommelt, U., Impaired suppression of vestibular nystagmus by fixation in cerebellar and noncerebellar patients. *A-ch. Psychiatr. Nervenkr.*, 1978, **226**:183–199.

7. Honrubia, V., Baloh, R. W., and Yee, R. D., The differentiation of vestibular syndromes on the basis of vestibulo-ocular reflex measurements. *Am. J. Otolaryngol.*, 1980, **1**:291–301.

8. Jenkins, H. A., Lau, C. G. Y., Baloh, R. W., and Honrubia, V., Implications of Ewald's second law for diagnosis of unilateral labyrinthine paralysis. *Otolaryngol. Head Neck Surg.*, 1979, **87**:459–462.

9. Wolfe, J. W., Engelken, E. J., and Olson, J. E., Low-frequency harmonic acceleration in the evaluation of patients with peripheral labyrinthine disorders. This volume.

10. Yee, R. D., Jenkins, H. A., Baloh, R. W., Honrubia, V., and Lau, C. G. Y., Vestibular-optokinetic interactions in normal subjects and in patients with peripheral vestibular dysfunction. *J. Otolaryngol.*, 1978, **7**:310–319.

Cerebellar Control of Eye Movements

DAVID S. ZEE

Departments of Neurology and Ophthalmology
The Johns Hopkins University School of Medicine
Baltimore, Maryland

INTRODUCTION

A variety of ocular motor abnormalities have been recorded in patients with neurological signs of cerebellar dysfunction, but only some have been convincingly related to isolated cerebellar pathology (Table 1). On the basis of recent physiological and clinical studies, it is now possible to ascribe, at least tentatively, specific ocular motor functions to different portions of the cerebellum and thereby predict the corresponding abnormalities that may arise when these structures are affected by disease.

We recorded and quantitated the eye movement abnormalities in a group of relatives with dominantly inherited cerebellar ataxia (46,47). Recently, one of the patients whom we had investigated died, and postmortem examination of the brain confirmed the restrictive nature of the pathological lesion. The cerebellum was of

TABLE 1
OCULAR MOTOR ABNORMALITIES RELATED TO CEREBELLAR DYSFUNCTION
(4–6, 9, 10, 14–16, 28, 32, 33, 42, 46, 47)

Impaired smooth pursuit and optokinetic nystagmus
Impaired cancellation of the vestibuloocular reflex
Hyperactive vestibuloocular responses
Impaired suppression of caloric-induced nystagmus
Saccadic dysmetria, macrosaccadic oscillations
Square-wave jerks (saccadic fixation instability)
Gaze-paretic nystagmus
Rebound nystagmus
Centripetal nystagmus
Downbeating nystagmus
Positional nystagmus
Postsaccadic drift

241

half-normal size, with striking atrophy restricted primarily to the cerebellar cortex (Figure 1). The deep cerebellar nuclei were largely unaffected, and the brainstem appeared intact.

Individuals in this family showed the following ocular motor abnormalities: (a) inaccurate saccades (dysmetria), especially downward overshoot; (b) impaired smooth tracking either with the head still (smooth pursuit) (Figure 2) or moving (cancellation of the vestibuloocular reflex); (c) inability to hold eccentric positions of gaze (the eyes

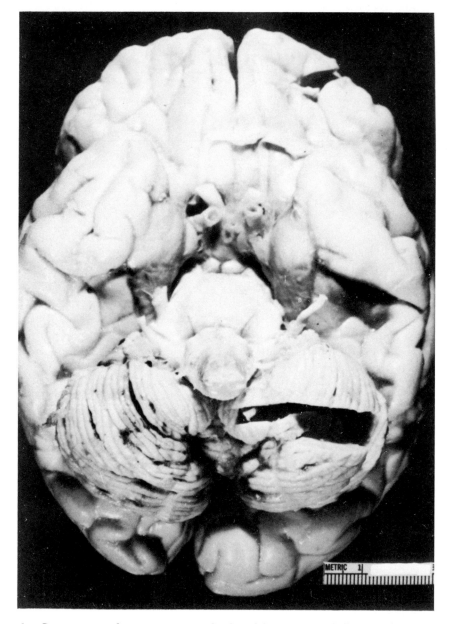

Figure 1. Gross specimen from one patient in a family with hereditary cerebellar ataxia; basal view. Note markedly atrophied cerebellar cortex with normal-sized brainstem.

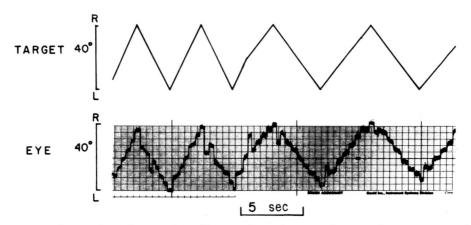

Figure 2. Electrooculographic recording of horizontal smooth pursuit of patient of Figure 1 six months before death. Note impaired pursuit necessitating corrective saccades.

drifted back toward the primary position with an exponentially decaying waveform; repetitive excentering saccades were required to fixate the eccentric target, resulting in the pattern of gaze-paretic nystagmus); (d) rebound nystagmus (when the eyes returned to the primary position after a prolonged attempt at holding gaze, a transient jerk nystagmus occurred with the slow phases in the direction of prior attempted eccentric gaze); (e) downward-beating nystagmus that was accentuated on lateral gaze; (f) increased amplitude or gain (peak eye velocity/peak head velocity) of the vestibuloocular reflex (VOR) measured during rotation of the head in darkness; and (g) postsaccadic drift.

Two portions of the cerebellum appear to be particularly important for ocular motor control, and the neuroophthalmological findings in our patients with cerebellar atrophy can probably be attributed in major part to malfunction in these regions. The dorsal (superior) cerebellar vermis (lobules V, VI, VII), together with the underlying fastigial nuclei, appears to function in the control of saccadic amplitude. On the other hand, the vestibulocerebellum, and especially the flocculus, appears to participate in the generation of a variety of retinal-image-stabilizing reflexes including smooth pursuit, visual modulation of vestibular responses, and holding positions of gaze. Furthermore, both the dorsal vermis and vestibulocerebellum seem to be essential for the elaboration of long-term, plastic, adaptive changes in ocular motor performance. Such a capability is essential to ensure optimal visual performance in the face of naturally occurring diseases and aging that may affect normal eye movement control.

DORSAL CEREBELLAR VERMIS AND FASTIGIAL NUCLEI

The dorsal cerebellar vermis and probably the underlying fastigial nuclei participate in the control of saccades. Experimental stimulation in the vermis elicits saccades (31), single Purkinje cells discharge in relationship to saccades (12,19), and the vermis receives auditory, visual, and extraocular muscle proprioceptive inputs (7,34). Lesions of the vermis cause saccades to be inaccurate but with essentially normal velocities and latencies (2,29).

In monkeys, the saccadic dysmetria resulting from experimental vermal lesions differs from that of complete cerebellar ablation (26). The latter lesion creates an enduring saccadic hypermetria that has two components. First, the rapid, phasic portion of the saccadic eye movement (the saccadic pulse) is too large, which causes the eyes to overshoot the target. This abnormality is called *pulse size dysmetria*. Second, the eyes do not stop abruptly at the end of the saccade but drift on for a few hundred milliseconds as a "glissade." This postsaccadic drift has been attributed to a mismatch between the sizes of the saccadic pulse and the saccadic step. The latter provides the tonic innervation that holds the eye in position at the end of the saccade. Postsaccadic drift thereby reflects *pulse–step match dysmetria*. Thus, totally cerebellectomized monkeys show both components of saccadic dysmetria. Conversely, monkeys with lesions restricted to the dorsal cerebellar vermis and fastigial nuclei show pronounced, enduring saccadic hypermetria (pulse size dysmetria) but without postsaccadic drift. Similarly, less extensive, asymmetric lesions in the dorsal vermis and fastigial nuclei produce mixtures of hyper- and hypometric saccades (44), whereas lesions restricted to the vermis alone cause hypermetric centripetally directed saccades and hypometric centrifugally directed saccades (29). These restricted lesions also have not been reported to produce postsaccadic drift. Thus, it appears that only saccadic pulse size dysmetria is present after removal of the dorsal vermis and underlying fastigial nuclei. As discussed below, postsaccadic drift (pulse–step match dysmetria) alone occurs after bilateral flocculectomy.

It has also been demonstrated that long-term, plastic, adaptive changes in saccadic amplitude depend on the cerebellum. An example of such adaptation is shown by patients who have a partial, unilateral, peripheral ocular muscle palsy but, for reasons of better visual acuity, habitually fixate with their paretic eye (1,13). Such individuals adaptively modify saccadic innervation to compensate for the undershoot and postsaccadic drift created by the palsy. Therefore, saccades made by the palsied eye become nearly normometric. However, because of Herring's law, movements made by the nonparetic eye reflect the changes in saccadic innervation. Thus, when the patient is forced to fixate with the nonparetic eye, it initially shows saccadic dysmetria: saccadic overshoot and postsaccadic drift. These changes, of course, are made to overcome the saccadic hypometria and drift created by the palsy in the other eye. If, however, the patient is forced to use the nonparetic eye continuously (by patching the paretic eye), after a few days, saccades made by the nonparetic eye become normometric, whereas those of the palsied eye again become dysmetric. Thus, saccadic innervation can be appropriately modified in an attempt to meet the ocular motor requirements for optimal visual performance of whichever eye is preferentially used for viewing.

Experimentally, using an alternate patching paradigm, one can show that monkeys also possess the ability to adapt plastically the size of the saccadic pulse and suppress postsaccadic drift in response to experimentally induced ocular muscle weakness (26). However, total cerebellectomy completely abolishes this capability, supporting the hypothesis that the cerebellum is essential for adaptation to or "repair" of saccadic dysmetria. However, removal of the dorsal cerebellar vermis and underlying fastigial nuclei alone abolishes the ability of a monkey with a muscle palsy to modify adaptively the size of the saccadic pulse, but any postsaccadic drift created by the palsy can still be suppressed. These results suggest that the dorsal cerebellar vermis and/or underlying fastigial nuclei are important for long-term, plastic adjustments of saccadic pulse amplitude but not for appropriately matching the size of the saccadic step to the pulse. The latter function appears to be relegated to the flocculus (*vide infra*).

Vestibulocerebellum

The vestibulocerebellum participates in a variety of ocular motor reflexes that function to stabilize images on the retina. The flocculus receives visual, vestibular, and proprioceptive inputs, the latter from both neck and extraocular muscles (20,21). Mossy fiber afferents coding eye position and eye velocity have also been recorded in the flocculus (18,22,25). Single-unit recordings from Purkinje cells in the flocculus reveal a number of neurons that discharge during both smooth pursuit with the head still and cancellation of the VOR when fixating an object rotating with the head (17,22,24). Whether the head is still or moving, these cells discharge in relationship to gaze velocity (the velocity of the eye in space). Such cells appear to be selective for foveal tracking. During optokinetic stimulation, they maintain a steady discharge only with very high stimulus velocities (37), when the pursuit system supplements the contribution of the optokinetic system (which probably saturates at 60 to 90 deg/sec). Other Purkinje cells within the flocculus have been shown to discharge in relation to eye position and/or saccadic eye movements as well as movements of the visual background (17,22,23).

We studied the effects of bilateral and nearly complete flocculectomy in four rhesus monkeys that were trained to fixate and follow targets (45). After floccular ablation, all monkeys had an intact VOR, as measured during head rotation in darkness. Neither the VOR time constant, measured after an impulse of head acceleration, nor the VOR phase, measured during sinusoidal rotation, was significantly affected by the lesion. However, the gain (peak eye velocity/peak head velocity) of the VOR was, on average, slightly increased, although in an individual monkey it could be increased, unchanged, or even slightly decreased.

All monkeys showed a decreased but not absent ability to track targets smoothly [gain (eye velocity/target velocity) about 0.65] with the head still and a comparable defect in the ability to cancel the VOR when fixating a small object rotating with the head. Suppression of caloric-induced nystagmus was also impaired (35). Flocculectomized monkeys also showed an inability to hold eccentric positions of gaze with consequent gaze-paretic nystagmus. The time constant of the exponentially decaying centripetal drift was of the order of several seconds. This finding suggests that an important function of the flocculus is to increase the time constant of the brainstem neural integrator that normally functions to hold positions of gaze.

Flocculectomized monkeys also showed abnormal optokinetic responses, the main finding being a slower rise than normal to maximal eye velocity after a step change in drum velocity. There was also a decrease in the ability to generate nystagmus in response to very high velocity optokinetic stimuli. However, optokinetic after-nystagmus (as measured in complete darkness) was essentially normal. Similar optokinetic responses with a gradual buildup of eye velocity and preservation of optokinetic after-nystagmus have been reported in human patients with presumed vestibulocerebellar lesions (41).

Flocculectomized monkeys showed both rebound and downward-beating nystagmus. The latter was accentuated on lateral gaze. During saccadic eye tracking the lesioned monkeys showed postsaccadic drift (glissades), lasting a few hundred milliseconds. However, the pulse portion of the saccade was accurate, so that significant hyper- or hypometria did not occur.

These findings implicate the flocculus in a variety of retinal-image-stabilizing reflexes. Furthermore, flocculectomy produces an ocular motor syndrome that mimics many of the features shown by patients with cerebellar disease (Table 2) and in particular those individuals with lesions that presumably involve the flocculus (36,40).

The flocculus has also been implicated in long-term, plastic, adaptive changes that ensure that retinal-image-stabilizing reflexes remain appropriate to the visual stimulus. Experimentally, the VOR can be made to seem inappropriate by means of optical devices such as reversing prisms (which cause the seen world to appear to move in the *same* direction as the head) or magnifying (or minifying) spectacles or by coupling image motion in one plane to head rotation in another. In response to such optically imposed retinal-image motion, the amplitude, direction, and phase of the VOR can be adjusted appropriately so that eye movements compensate for any type of image motion that occurs during movements of the head. These changes persist even in the absence of continuous stimulation and are present when the VOR is measured in darkness.

Experimentally, flocculectomy in monkeys (27) and total vestibulocerebellectomy in cats (30) seriously interfere with these VOR adaptative capabilities. However, one type of vestibular adaptation may not depend on the vestibulocerebellum. In the cat, spontaneous nystagmus created by a unilateral, peripheral vestibular lesion is rapidly compensated for (presumably by a rebalancing of the vestibular nuclei) even in the absence of the vestibulocerebellum (11). Of course, other cerebellar structures (for example, the deep nuclei) may still be necessary for this type of adaptation, and we do not yet know the effect of flocculectomy on this type of adaptation in primates. Recently, the adaptive capabilities of the VOR have been tested in human patients with various brainstem and cerebellar lesions using reversing prisms (39). As in experimental animals, human beings with cerebellar lesions show a decreased ability to modify adaptively the gain of the VOR.

Experimental studies have also suggested that monkeys with floccular lesions are unable to adjust the match between the saccadic pulse and step so as to eliminate postsaccadic drift. In the face of a brief period (several hundred milliseconds) of optically imposed, postsaccadic retinal slip, normal monkeys readily learn to program a nearly matching postsaccadic drift of the eyes, which in turn compensates for the artificially induced image movement on the retina. Presumably, this is accomplished by adjusting the match between the saccadic step and pulse. However, flocculectomized monkeys show a strikingly reduced ability to carry out such adaptation (27).

TABLE 2
OCULAR MOTOR SIGNS AFTER FLOCCULECTOMY

Impaired smooth pursuit and cancellation of the VOR (during fixation of a head-fixed target)
Gaze-paretic nystagmus
Rebound nystagmus
Downbeating nystagmus
Postsaccadic drift (glissades)
Impaired suppression of caloric-induced nystagmus
Mildly impaired optokinetic responses

TABLE 3
HYPOTHETICAL SCHEME OF CEREBELLAR CONTROL OF EYE MOVEMENTS

Structure	Function	Disorder
Dorsal vermis and fastigial nuclei	Control saccade amplitude	Saccadic dysmetria
Vestibulocerebellum	Retinal-image stabilization	Impaired tracking (head still or moving)
		Gaze-paretic nystagmus
		Postsaccadic drift (glissades)

CONCLUSIONS

We can not tentatively ascribe specific ocular motor functions to specific portions of the cerebellum and thus infer which structures are malfunctioning in the presence of particular groups of ocular motor signs (Table 3). The dorsal cerebellar vermis and underlying fastigial nuclei appear to function in the control of saccadic amplitude, and the vestibulocerebellum in the control of a number of retinal-image-stabilizing ro flexes including smooth pursuit, visual modulation of the vestibuloocular reflex, and holding positions of gaze. Furthermore, the elaboration of long-term, adaptive changes in ocular motor performance can also be relegated to specific portions of the cerebellum, and the integrity of such structures potentially can be tested by measuring such adaptive capabilities.

Even so, a number of ocular motility disorders that have been attributed to cerebellar lesions in patients do not as yet have an experimental correlate. The nearly *complete* abolition of optokinetic nystagmus and pursuit capability in patients with cerebellar degenerations as well as totally cerebellectomized monkeys is not reproduced by flocculectomy alone (26,38). Perhaps the paraflocculi, cerebellar nodulus, or cerebellar hemispheres also participate in visual tracking (15,31). Furthermore, the pathophysiology of fixation instability, including square-wave jerks, macrosquare-wave jerks, smooth pendular oscillations (3), and various types of continuous saccadic oscillations such as opsoclonus and flutter, is still unclear (8,43). The role that the cerebellum has in the genesis of these abnormalities remains to be discovered.

ACKNOWLEDGMENTS

We thank Vendetta Matthews for editorial assistance. This work was supported by NIH grants EY01849, EY00158, and NS11071.

REFERENCES

1. Abel, L. A., Schmidt, D., Dell'Osso, L. F., and Daroff, R. B., Saccadic system plasticity in humans. *Ann. Neurol.*, 1978, **4**:313–318.
2. Aschoff, J. C., and Cohen, B., Changes in saccadic eye movement produced by cerebellar cortical lesions. *Exp. Neurol.*, 1971, **32**:123–133.
3. Aschoff, J. F., Conrad, B., and Kornhuber, H. H., Acquired pendular nystagmus with oscillopsia in multiple sclerosis. A sign of cerebellar nuclei disease. *J. Neurol., Neurosurg. Psychiatry*, 1974, **37**:570–577.

4. Avanzini, G., Girotti, F., Crenna, P., and Negri, S., Alterations of ocular motility in cerebellar pathology. *Arch. Neurol. (Chicago)*, 1979, **36**:274–280.

5. Baloh, R. W., Jenkins, H. A., Honrubia, V., Yee, R. D., and Lau, C. G. Y., Visual-vestibular interaction and cerebellar atrophy. *Neurology*, 1979, **29**:116–119.

6. Baloh, R. W., Konrad, H. R., and Honrubia, V., Vestibulo-ocular function in patients with cerebellar atrophy. *Neurology*, 1975, **25**:160–168.

7. Batini, C., Extraocular muscle input to the cerebellar cortex. *Prog. Brain Res.* 1979, **50**:315–324.

8. Daroff, R. B., Ocular oscillations. *Ann. Oto-Laryngol.*, 1977, **86**:102–109.

9. Dichgans, J., and Jung, R., Oculomotor abnormalities due to cerebellar lesions. In: *Basic Mechanisms of Ocular Motility and Their Clinical Implications* (G. Lennerstrand and P. Bach-y-Rita, eds.). Pergamon, Oxford, 1975:281–298.

10. Estanol, B., Romero, R., and Corvera, J., Effects of cerebellectomy on eye movements in man. *Arch. Neurol. (Chicago)*, 1979, **36**:281–284.

11. Haddad, G., Friendlich, A., and Robinson, D. A., Compensation of nystagmus after VIII nerve lesions in vestibulo-cerebellectomized cats. *Brain Res.*, 1977, **135**:192–196.

12. Kase, M., Miller, D. C., and Noda, H., Discharges of Purkinje cells and mossy fibers in the cerebellar vermis of the monkey during saccadic eye movements and fixation. *J. Physiol. (London)*, 1980, **300**:539–555.

13. Kommerell, G., Olivier, D., and Theopold, H., Adaptive programming of phasic and tonic components in saccadic eye movements. Investigations in patients with abducens palsy. *Invest. Ophthalmol.*, 1976, **15**:657–660.

14. Larmande, P., and Autret, A., Influence du cervelet sur les mouvements oculaires volontaires. *Rev. Neurol.*, 1980, **136**:259–269.

15. Larmande, P., Delplace, M. P., and Autret, A., Influence du cervelet sur la statique oculaire et les mouvements de poursuite visuelle. *Rev. Neurol.*, 1980, **136**:327–339.

16. Leech, J., Gresty, M., Hess, K., and Rudge, P., Gaze failure, drifting eye movements and centripetal nystagmus in cerebellar disease. *Br. J. Ophthalmol.*, 1977, **61**:774–781.

17. Lisberger, S. G., and Fuchs, A. F., Role of primate flocculus during rapid behavioral modification of vestibulo-ocular reflex. I. Purkinje cell activity during visually guided horizontal smooth pursuit eye movements and passive head rotation. *J. Neurophysiol.*, 1978, **41**:733–763.

18. Lisberger, S. G., and Fuchs, A. F., Role of primate flocculus during rapid behavioral modification of vestibulo-ocular reflex. II. Mossy fiber firing patterns during horizontal head rotation and eye movement. *J. Neurophysiol.*, 1978, **41**:764–777.

19. Llinás, R., and Wolfe, J. W., Functional linkage between the electrical activity in the vermal cerebellar cortex and saccadic eye movements. *Exp. Brain Res.*, 1977, **29**:1–14.

20. Maeda, M., Neck influences on the vestibulo-ocular reflex arc and the vestibulocerebellum. *Prog. Brain Res.* 1979, **50**:551–559.

21. Maekawa, K., Mossy fiber activation of the flocculus from visual and extraocular muscle afferents of rabbits. *Ann. N.Y. Acad. Sci.*, 1981, **374**:476–490.

22. Miles, F. A., Fuller, J. H., Braitman, D. J., and Dow, B. M., Long-term adaptive changes in primate vestibulo-ocular reflex. III. Electrophysiological observations in flocculus of normal monkeys. *J. Neurophysiol.*, 1980, **43**:1437–1476.

23. Noda, H., and Suzuki, D. A., The role of the flocculus of the monkey in saccadic eye movements. *J. Physiol. (London)*, 1979, **294**:317–334.

24. Noda, H., and Suzuki, D. A., The role of the flocculus of the monkey in fixation and smooth pursuit eye movement. *J. Physiol. (London)*, 1979, **294**:335–348.

25. Noda, H., and Suzuki, D. A., Processing of eye movement signals in the flocculus of the monkey. *J. Physiol. (London)*, 1979, **294**:349–364.

26. Optican, L. M., and Robinson, D. A., Cerebellar dependent adaptive control of the primate saccadic system. *J. Neurophysiol.*, 1980, **44**:1058–1076.

27. Optican, L. M., Zee, D. S., Miles, F. A., and Lisberger, S. G., Oculomotor deficits in monkeys with floccular lesions. *Soc. Neurosci. Abst.*, 1980, **6**:474.

28. Precht, W., Cerebellar influences on eye movements. In: *Basic Mechanisms of Ocular Motility and Their Clinical Implications* (G. Lennerstrand and P. Bach-y-Rita, eds.). Pergamon, Oxford, 1975:261–280.

29. Ritchie, L., Effects of cerebellar lesions on saccadic eye movements. *J. Neurophysiol.*, 1976, **39**:1246–1256.

30. Robinson, D. A., Adaptive gain control of vestibulo-ocular reflex by the cerebellum. *J. Neurophysiol.*, 1976, **39**:954–969.

31. Ron, S., and Robinson, D. A., Eye movements evoked by cerebellar stimulation in the alert monkey. *J. Neurophysiol.*, 1973, **36**:1004–1022.

32. Selhorst, J. B., Stark, L., Ochs, A. L., and Hoyt, W. F., Disorders in cerebellar oculomotor control. I. Saccadic overshoot dysmetria, an oculographic, control system and clinico-anatomic analysis. *Brain*, 1976, **99**:497–508.

33. Selhorst, J. B., Stark, L., Ochs, A. L., and Hoyt, W. F., Disorders in cerebellar oculomotor control. II. Macrosaccadic oscillations, an oculographic, control system and clinico-anatomic analysis. *Brain*, 1976, **99**:509–522.

34. Snider, R. S., and Stowell, A., Receiving areas of the tactile, auditory and visual systems in the cerebellum. *J. Neurophysiol.*, 1944, **7**:331–357.

35. Takemori, S., and Cohen, B., Loss of visual suppression of vestibular nystagmus after flocculus lesions. *Brain Res.*, 1974, **72**:213–224.

36. von Reutern, G. M., and Dichgans, J., Augenbewegungsstorungen als cerebellare Symptome bei Kleinhirnbruckenwinkeltumoren *Arch. Psychiatr. Nervenkr.*, 1977, **223**:117–130.

37. Waespe, W., Büttner, U., and Henn, V., Visual-vestibular interaction in the flocculus of alert rhesus monkey. *Ann. N.Y. Acad. Sci.*, 1981, **374**:491–503.

38. Westheimer, G., and Blair, S. M., Functional organization of primate oculomotor system revealed by cerebellectomy. *Exp. Brain Res.*, 1974, **21**:463–472.

39. Yagi, T., Shimizu, M., Sekine, S., Kamio, T., and Suzuki, J. I., A new neurotological test for detecting cerebellar dysfunction. *Ann. N.Y. Acad. Sci.*, 1981, **374**:526–531.

40. Yamazaki, A., and Zee, D. S., Rebound nystagmus: EOG analysis of a case with a floccular tumor. *Br. J. Ophthalmol.*, 1979, **63**:782–786.

41. Yee, R. D., Baloh, R. W., Honrubia, V., Lau, C. G. Y., and Jenkins, H. A., Slow build up of optokinetic nystagmus associated with downbeat nystagmus. *Invest. Ophthalmol.*, 1979, **18**:622–629.

42. Zee, D. S., Leigh, R. J., and Mathieu-Millaire, F., Cerebellar control of ocular gaze stability. *Ann. Neurol.*, 1980, **7**:37–40.

43. Zee, D. S., and Robinson, D. A., A hypothetical explanation of saccadic oscillations. *Ann. Neurol.*, 1979, **5**:405–414.

44. Zee, D. S., and Robinson, D. S., Clinical applications of oculomotor models. In: *Topics in Neuro-ophthalmology* (S. Thompson, ed.). Williams & Wilkins, Baltimore, Maryland, 1979:266–285.

45. Zee, D. S., Yamazaki, A., Butler, P. H., and Gucer, G., Effect of oblation of flocculus and paraflocculus on eye movement in primate. *J. Neurophysiol.*, 1981, **46**:878–899.

46. Zee, D. S., Yee, R. D., Cogan, D. G., Robinson, D. A., and Engel, W. K., Oculomotor abnormalities in hereditary cerebellar ataxia. *Brain*, 1976, **99**:207–234.

47. Ocular motor abnormalities related to lesions in the vestibulocerebellum in primate. In: *Functional Basis of Ocular Motor Disorders* (G. Lennerstrand, D. S. Zee, and E. Keller, eds.). Pergamon Press, New York (in press).

Pathophysiology of Optokinetic Nystagmus

ROBERT D. YEE,[1] ROBERT W. BALOH,[2] VICENTE HONRUBIA,[3] and HERMAN A. JENKINS[3]

[1]Department of Ophthalmology,
School of Medicine, University of California Los Angeles,
Los Angeles, California
[2]Department of Neurology,
School of Medicine, University of California Los Angeles,
Los Angeles, California
[3]Division of Head and Neck Surgery,
School of Medicine, University of California Los Angeles,
Los Angeles, California

INTRODUCTION

Optokinetic nystagmus (OKN) consists of ocular motor responses to the movement of visual targets that occupy large areas in the visual field. The pattern of jerk nystagmus is developed, in which slow components are in the direction of target movement and fast components are in the opposite direction. Optokinetic nystagmus is usually induced by spontaneous movements of the head that produce motion of the visual surround in the opposite direction relative to the eyes. For example, head movement to the right results in motion of the environment to the left. The slow components of OKN track the movement of the visual surround and help to stabilize the position of the eyes relative to the environment. However, in clinical practice OKN is usually produced by movement of vertical stripes or other large patterns on the surface of a hand-held drum or strip of cloth. Optokinetic nystagmus can be a valuable clinical test in detecting and localizing lesions in the ocular motor system. However, careful attention must be given to identifying coexisting defects in the visual pathway, controlling the parameters of the test stimuli, and quantititive analysis of eye movement data. This chapter describes the OKN tests that we have found to be valuable in our laboratory and illustrates the effects of frequently encountered disorders of OKN.

METHODS

Horizontal movements of each eye are recorded with Ag–AgCl (Beckman) electrodes placed at the inner and outer canthi. Electrodes are also placed above and

251

NYSTAGMUS AND VERTIGO: CLINICAL
APPROACHES TO THE PATIENT WITH DIZZINESS

below the eyes to detect vertical eye movements and eyelid artifacts. A reference electrode is placed on the forehead. The dc electrooculography (EOG) system utilizes a differential, armband amplifier and an offset amplifier to achieve an overall amplification of about 300×. Eye movement data are monitored on a polygraph (Grass), recorded on an analog FM tape recorder (Tandberg), and digitized by an on-line LSI-11 (Digital Equipment Corporation) microprocessor. The EOG system has a bandwidth of 0 to 35 Hz ($-$ 3 dB) and an average noise level (root mean square) of 0.11 deg for horizontal, uniocular recordings and can reliably identify eye movements of 0.2 deg. Eye movement data are digitized at 200 samples per second. Fortran programs have been developed (a) to calculate instantaneous eye movement velocity, (b) to identify saccadic eye movements (fast components), (c) to calculate the average slow-component velocity during constant-velocity rotation of the OKN drum, and (d) to calculate slow-component velocity every 50 msec during sinusoidal drum rotation. Details of the recording and analysis systems have been previously described (1).

The subject is seated within a black cloth drum, 1.5 m in diameter. The interior of the drum is decorated with white, vertical stripes, 1.25 cm wide, that are placed every 15 deg. Rotation of the drum stimulates the subject's entire visual field. The subject is instructed to fixate on stripes as they pass directly in front of him. The drum is rotated at constant velocities of 30 and 60 deg/sec and in sinusoidal patterns (0.05 Hz, 30 and 60 deg/sec peak velocity).

RESULTS AND DISCUSSION

FAST COMPONENT

Optokinetic nystagmus consists of saccadic eye movements (fast components) as well as smooth movements (slow components). Therefore, disorders that affect saccades can result in abnormal patterns of OKN. Fast components of OKN have similar velocity–amplitude relationships as voluntary, refixation saccades and fast components of vestibular nystagmus, and they are probably generated by the same burst and tonic neurons in the pontine paramedian reticular formation (PPRF). However, the factors that control the initiation of fast components are not precisely known. In animals and in human beings there is evidence that this initiation during OKN is correlated with the position of the eyes in the orbit at the end of the slow component and the velocity of the slow component (20,21,25). The fast component is not a "resetting" movement that carries the eyes back to the center of the orbit. The fast component might be thought of as an "anticipatory" movement, since it carries the eyes eccentrically in the orbit in the direction of the optokinetic stimulus, as it enters the visual field.

Abnormalities of fast components can be divided among those that primarily decrease velocity, those that delay initiation and decrease amplitude, and those that impair the normal regularity of nystagmus cycles. Fast-component velocity is decreased in ophthalmoplegias that impair the extraocular muscles, peripheral nerves, or supranuclear pathways. Disorders that are commonly encountered include myasthenia gravis, progressive external ophthalmoplegia, dysthyroid ophthalmopathy, third and sixth cranial nerve palsies, internuclear ophthalmoplegia, lesions of the PPRF, and progressive supranuclear palsy. If the yoke muscles, a medial and a lateral rectus muscle, are affected to different degrees, OKN will be disconjugate. In Figure 1 OKN is shown during constant-velocity drum rotation at 30 deg/sec in a patient

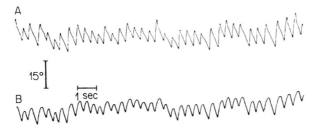

Figure 1.   OKN in patient with left-sided internuclear opthalmoplegia. Drum is rotating at 30 deg/sec to the left. (A) Normal fast and slow components in right eye. (B) Fast components have rounded waveforms and decreased velocities in left eye. Deflections up: right; down: left.

with a lesion in the left medial longitudinal fasciculus, resulting in a left-sided internuclear ophthalmoplegia. During drum rotation to the left, slow components were toward the left and fast components toward the right. Fast components in the right eye (A) were produced by the right lateral rectus and had normally high velocities and slightly peaked waveforms. Fast components in the left eye (B) were produced by the paretic left medial rectus muscle and had abnormally low velocities and slightly rounded waveforms. The nystagmus amplitude was decreased in the left eye due to the decreased amplitude of the fast component, but the slow component velocity was relatively normal. Similar disconjugate OKN has been described in other patients with internuclear ophthalmoplegia(4,29).

The initiation of voluntary saccades and fast components of OKN and vestibular nystagmus is abnormally delayed in certain supranuclear disorders, such as congenital ocular motor apraxia (40) and ataxia telangiectasia (3). This defect results in prolonged latencies of voluntary saccades (time between target movement and the beginning of the saccade) and tonic deviation of the eyes during OKN. Figure 2 demonstrates OKN during sinusoidal drum rotation (0.05 Hz, 60 deg/sec) in a normal subject. The fast components carried the eyes into the side of the orbit opposite to the direction of drum rotation. The average position of the eyes in the orbits was in the direction of the fast component. In Figure 3 OKN and the vestibuloocular response (VOR) during sinusoidal stimulation are shown in a patient with ataxia telangiectasia. The defective initiation of fast components and decreased amplitude of fast components resulted in a tonic deviation of the eyes to the side of the orbit in the

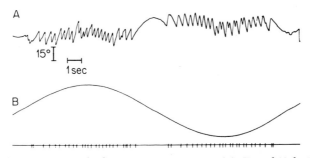

Figure 2.   Sinusoidal OKN in normal subject. Drum is rotating at 0.05 Hz and 60 deg/sec (peak velocity). (A) Eye position; (B) drum velocity; bottom: fast-component identification. Note that fast components carry eyes into side of orbit opposite to direction of drum rotation, and average position of eyes is to side of fast components. Deflections up: right; down: left.

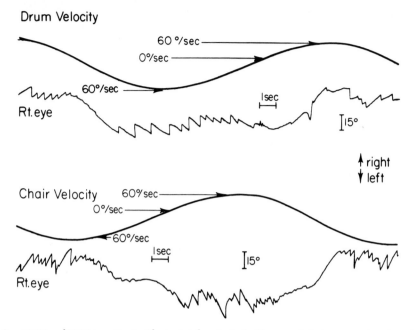

Figure 3.   OKN and VOR in patient with ataxia telangiectasia. Drum and chair are rotating sinusoidally at 0.05 Hz and 60 deg/sec (peak velocity). Note tonic deviation of the eyes to the side of the slow components.

direction of the slow component. Tonic deviation of OKN is also found in disorders that primarily decrease the amplitude of saccades, such as progressive supranuclear palsy (11) and olivopontocerebellar atrophy, and with lesions of the PPRF.

During constant-velocity drum rotation in normal subjects, OKN demonstrates a high degree of regularity of frequency and amplitude, as shown in Figure 4A. Lesions affecting the cerebellar hemispheres often produce saccadic dysmetria (abnormal under- and overshooting of the target) and irregularity of OKN, or dysrhythmia.

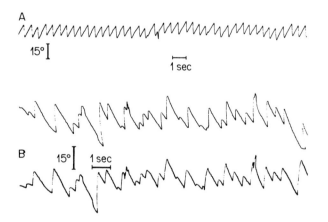

Figure 4.   Constant-velocity OKN in normal subject and patient with cerebellar degeneration. (A) Normal subject. Drum is rotating right at 30 deg/sec. Note uniform amplitude and frequency of OKN. (B) Patient with cerebellar degeneration. Drum is rotating at 30 deg/sec to left. Top: right eye; bottom: left eye. Note great variation of amplitude and frequency. Deflections up: right; down: left.

Optokinetic nystagmus in a patient with an acquired cerebellar degeneration is shown in Figure 4B. Nystagmus cycles of small amplitude were interspersed between cycles of large amplitude, and nystagmus frequency was variable.

SLOW COMPONENT

The slow component of OKN is the smooth movement of the nystagmus cycle that tracks the motion of the optokinetic pattern. Evaluation of the slow component requires careful attention to characteristics of the stimulus, patient factors, and the techniques of quantitative measurement.

Stimulus Characteristics

The slow-component velocity (SCV) of OKN appears to depend on the area of visual field stimulation. Dichgans and co-workers (14) found that SCV did not decrease significantly if the vertical angular size of the stimulus was reduced to 2 deg. However, SCV was reduced significantly when the horizontal angular size was decreased below 60 deg. The correlation of SCV and angular size was most marked at high stimulus velocities, 60 deg/sec and greater. Most laboratories that have reported quantitative studies of OKN have used either large drums that surround the subjects and stimulate the entire visual field or projection systems that stimulate at least 55 deg horizontally of the visual field (10,15,17,19,22–24).

The distance from the surface of the optokinetic stimulus to the eyes appears to be important. Jaglia (24) varied this distance from 0.5 to 2.0 m and found that SCV was greatest at a distance of 1.5 m and decreased at shorter distances. The pattern of the optokinetic stimulus, vertical stripes or randomly spaced dots, does not seem to affect OKN significantly. For example, Cheng and Outerbridge (10) reported that SCV was similar with dots aligned in vertical lines and with dots that were randomly spaced.

Constant-velocity or sinusoidal optokinetic stimulation can be presented. With constant-velocity stimulation, in which there is a step increase in velocity, the dynamic characteristics of buildup of OKN can be studied. The significance of this buildup is discussed in a later section on separation of OKN and pursuit. In addition, optokinetic after-nystagmus (OKAN), the transient persistence of nystagmus after the cessation of stimulation in the dark (9) can be studied. With a constant acceleration of the optokinetic stimulus, as described by Sills and co-workers (30), the optokinetic response at many stimulus velocities can be studied. Sinusoidal stimulation allows one to measure OKN at many velocities and in both horizontal directions during a single test and can decrease the duration of testing. However, the characteristics of buildup and OKAN cannot be studied.

In normal subjects OKN decreases at high stimulus velocities. The most commonly used quantitative parameter of OKN is the SCV. The SCV gain is defined as SCV/velocity of optokinetic stimulus. In normal subjects SCV gain is nearly 1.0 at low stimulus velocities but begins to decrease at velocities greater than about 30 deg/sec (14,19,23,30). It is important to include high stimulus velocities in clinical OKN tests, since OKN gain can be normal at low velocities and abnormal at high velocities. Figures 5 and 6 demonstrate OKN SCV during sinusoidal optokinetic stimulation in a patient with a generalized, cerebellar atrophy syndrome. During drum rotation at 0.2 Hz and 22.6 deg/sec (Figure 5), the patient's OKN gain was 0.88 and was within the normal range for our laboratory. However, during drum rotation at 0.05 Hz and 60

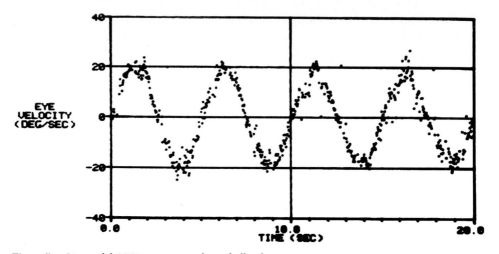

Figure 5.   Sinusoidal OKN in patient with cerebellar degeneration, SCV versus time. Drum is rotating at 0.2 Hz and 22.6 deg/sec (peak velocity). Note high peak SCV.

deg/sec (Figure 6), OKN gain was abnormally low. Figure 7 shows SCV versus drum velocity during three cycles of sinusoidal drum rotation at 60 deg/sec. The SCV closely approximated drum velocity up to about 20 deg/sec but reached a plateau at higher drum velocities.

Patient Factors

In normal subjects OKN appears to decrease with increased age. Therefore, the normal range of OKN should be established within a laboratory for young and elderly groups. In our laboratory the mean SCV gain ±1 standard deviation (SD) during

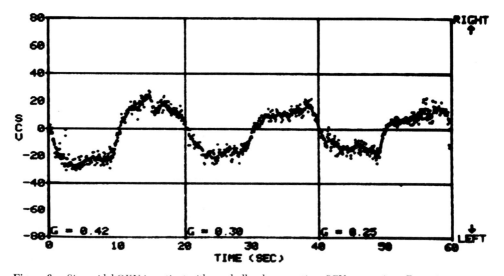

Figure 6.   Sinusoidal OKN in patient with cerebellar degeneration, SCV versus time. Drum is rotating at 0.05 Hz and 60 deg/sec (peak velocity). Note that peak SCV is low compared to peak drum velocity; G is peak SCV gain.

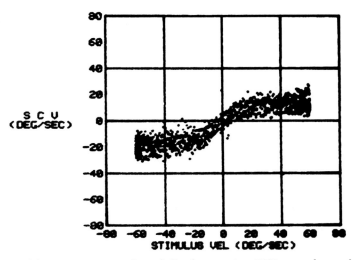

Figure 7.   Sinusoidal OKN in patient with cerebellar degeneration, SCV versus drum velocity. Drum is rotating at 0.05 Hz and 60 deg/sec (peak velocity). Three cycles are overlaid. Velocity + (right); − (left). Note that SCV increases to a peak of only 20 deg/sec.

constant-velocity drum rotation is 0.88 ± 0.05 at 30 deg/sec and 0.79 ± 0.13 at 60 deg/sec for young adults whose ages ranged from 20 to 40 years. There does not appear to be a significant difference in gain in this group during binocular and monocular stimulation. In a group of elderly patients, ranging in age from 50 to 85 years (mean 65 years) [see Spooner et al. (32)], the mean SCV gain was 0.65 ± 0.15 at 30 deg/sec and 0.50 ± 0.09 at 60 deg/sec. The differences between these values in the young adult and elderly groups were statistically significant at the 5% level (Student's *t* test). During sinusoidal drum rotation of 0.05 Hz, the mean SCV in the young adult group was 0.80 ± 0.10 at 30 deg/sec and 0.65 ± 0.16 at 60 deg/sec peak velocity. In an elderly patient group, the mean gain was 0.77 ± 0.21 at 30 deg/sec and 0.52 ± 0.14 at 60 deg/sec. Only the difference in values at 60 deg/sec was significant at the 5% level.

Dichgans and co-workers (14) demonstrated that visual attention to the task of tracking optokinetic stimuli is required for the optimal generation of OKN. Inattention, fatigue, and central nervous system depressants, such as barbiturates, can diminish OKN. Honrubia and co-workers (22) found that differences in the instructions given to subjects can have a marked effect on the SCV and amplitude of OKN. A normal subject was instructed to follow an individual vertical stripe as it entered the visual field until it left at the opposite end of the visual field and then to fixate and follow another stripe as it entered the visual field. The amplitude of this "look" nystagmus was very large (Figure 8A). Figure 9 (top) shows the SCV versus time of each half-cycle of "look" nystagmus to the right and left during sinusoidal drum rotation at 0.05 Hz and 60 deg/sec. The SCV gain was nearly 1.0. In contrast, when the subject was instructed not to follow individual stripes across the visual field, but to attempt to fixate stripes as they passed directly in front of him, the amplitude of this "stare" nystagmus was small and its frequency was very high (Figure 8B). As can be seen in Figure 9 (bottom), the SCV was much lower than that during "look" nystagmus, and the SCV gain was only 0.83.

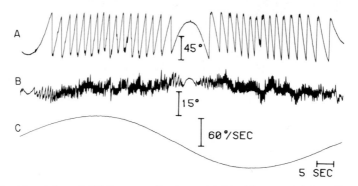

Figure 8. "Look" and "stare" OKN in normal subject. (A) "Look" OKN; (B) "stare" OKN; (C) drum velocity (0.05 Hz, peak velocity 60 deg/sec). Velocity + (right); − (left). Note larger amplitude and lower frequency of "look" OKN.

In our laboratory, instructions for "stare" OKN are routinely used. As discussed in the section on separation of OKN and pursuit, "look" nystagmus probably represents primarily the response of the pursuit tracking system rather than that of the optokinetic system.

Commonly Encountered Clinical Disorders

Visual Defects.   Lesions in the afferent visual pathways, as well as those in the efferent motor pathways, can affect OKN. Several studies that have artificially produced constriction of the peripheral visual fields in normal subjects have demonstrated decreased SCV as the size of the remaining central field was decreased. However, studies in normal subjects may not replicate OKN accurately in subjects with loss of peripheral vision. For example, tubes placed in front of a normal subject's eye (23) restrict stimulation of the peripheral field, but they also limit stimulation of

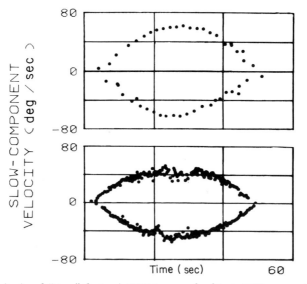

Figure 9. "Look" (top) and "stare" (bottom) OKN in normal subject, SCV versus time. Half-cycles to right and left are overlaid. Note higher peak SCV during "look" OKN.

the central field as the eye moves and its central field approaches the stationary edges of the tube.

We studied OKN in patients with severe loss of peripheral vision, or tunnel vision. Fourteen patients with chronic open-angle glaucoma were studied. Since such patients are usually elderly, each patient was chosen on the basis of having uniocular loss of visual field, so that stimulation of the eye with a full visual field could provide control observations. Visual acuity and the central 5 deg of central field, as determined by Goldmann perimetry with the I-4-e target, were normal in both eyes. In Figure 10 pursuit and OKN are shown during monocular stimulation of the normal eye (A) and the eye with a 5-deg central field (B) in one patient. The pursuit target was an intense, 1-deg diameter, red laser light (helium neon) that was moving in a sinusoidal pattern of 0.2 Hz and 22.5 deg/sec. Pursuit tracking was normal with either eye, but OKN was decreased during stimulation of the eye with tunnel vision. Figure 11 presents SCV versus size of the remaining central field in all of the subjects. The mean SCV ±1 SD for all of the patients during stimulation of the normal eye was lower than that in normal, younger adults. As the size of the central field decreased below 20 deg, SCV progressively decreased. The OKN gains at constant drum velocities of 30 and 60 deg/sec were 0.64 ± 0.04 and 0.42 ± 0.07, respectively, during stimulation of the normal eyes. The gains were 0.38 ± 0.15 and 0.22 ± 0.13 during stimulation of the abnormal eyes at 30 and 60 deg/sec, respectively. These differences were significant at the 5% level (Student's t test for paired observations). Pursuit gains were extremely variable. Some patients could track the laser target equally well with either eye, as in Figure 10. However, some patients appeared to be unable to refixate the smoothly moving target once it passed out of their small central field. As can be seen in Figure 12, in which pursuit gain versus size of the central field is presented, there was no correlation between the size of the field and pursuit gain. During stimulation of the normal eye, the mean pursuit gain for all of the patients was

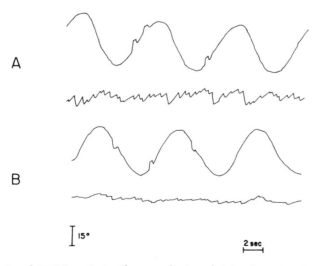

Figure 10.   Pursuit and OKN in patient with monocular tunnel vision. Laser target moving sinusoidally (0.2 Hz, peak velocity 22.5 deg/sec), drum rotating to right at 30 deg/sec. (A) Monocular stimulation of eye with normal visual field. (B) Monocular stimulation of eye with tunnel vision. Deflections up: right; down: left.

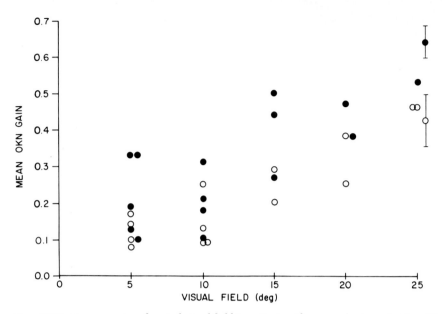

Figure 11.   OKN gain versus size of central visual field in patients with monocular tunnel vision. Closed circle with bars: drum velocity 30 deg/sec, group mean ±1 SD during stimulation of normal eyes. Closed circles: individual patients during stimulation of abnormal eyes. Open circle with bars: drum velocity 60 deg/sec, group mean ±1 SD during stimulation of normal eyes. Open circles: individual patients during stimulation of abnormal eyes.

0.87 ± 0.05 (0.2 Hz, 22.5 deg/sec) and 0.78 ± 0.06 (0.4 Hz, 45 deg/sec). During stimulation of the eyes with tunnel vision, the gains were 0.54 ± 0.31 (0.2 Hz) and 0.46 ± 0.26 (0.4 Hz). The differences were not significant.

The effect of loss of the central visual field, or central scotomas, on OKN is unclear. Some investigators (17,23) have reported increased SCV and others (10,15,17) decreased SCV in subjects with artificially produced and/or naturally occurring central

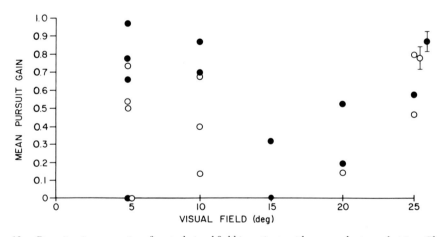

Figure 12.   Pursuit gain versus size of central visual field in patients with monocular tunnel vision. Closed circle with bars: target velocity (0.2 Hz, peak velocity 22.5 deg/sec), group mean ±1 SD during stimulation of normal eyes. Closed circles: individual patients during stimulation of abnormal eyes. Open circle with bars: target velocity (0.4 Hz, peak velocity 45 deg/sec), group mean ±1 SD during stimulation of normal eyes. Open circles: individual patients during stimulation of abnormal eyes.

scotomas. Gresty and Halmagyi (17) reported that occluders placed in front of normal subjects' eyes to produce central scotomas of 13 to 33 deg decreased the SCV. As they pointed out, with this technique subjects could simply fixate the occluders, suppressing OKN. In addition, the position of the scotomas in the visual field would change during movement of the eyes. Several studies have produced artificial central scotomas in normal subjects that maintain stable positions in the subjects' fields by using projection systems to present visual stimuli and negative-feedback systems to monitor eye movements and appropriately change the position of the central scotoma. Using these methods, Cheng and Outerbridge (10) demonstrated that scotomas greater than 5 deg in diameter decreased the SCV, and Dubois and Collewijn (15) found that scotomas greater than 2.5 deg decreased the SCV. Gresty and Halmagyi (17) reported that in three patients with naturally occurring central scotomas of retinal origin, ranging from 12 to 18 deg, the SCV during sinusoidal stimulation was slightly less than that of normal subjects with full visual fields. In contrast, Hood (23) reported that a patient with a unilateral central scotoma of unspecified size had much higher SCV when tracking constant-velocity drum rotations with the scotomatous eye than with the normal eye. Gresty and Halmagyi (17) reported that normal subjects with photo-flash-induced central scotomas of 12 to 33 deg had better OKN during constant velocity drum rotations than normal subjects with intact fields. The latter authors determined that the tracking strategies of subjects can significantly affect OKN. Subject with artificial or naturally occurring scotomas could choose to fixate the scotomas, actively pursue the optokinetic stimuli ("look" nystagmus), or passively track the stimuli ("stare" nystagmus). It is likely that differences in strategies could account for some of the apparent discrepancies in conclusions about the effect of central scotomas and OKN.

We studied OKN in six elderly adult patients with unilateral central scotomas from senile macular degeneration. Visual acuity in the affected eye ranged from 20/70 to 20/400, and the central scotomas varied from 5 to 15 deg in diameter (Goldmann perimetry with I-4-c target). Pursuit and OKN in one such patient are shown in Figure 13. As expected, pursuit was markedly impaired. Mean pursuit gain for the

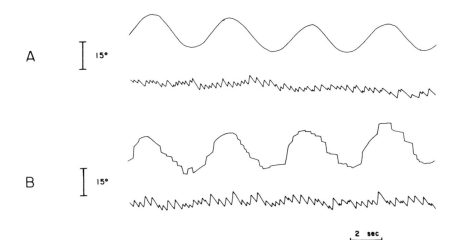

Figure 13.   Pursuit and OKN in patient with monocular central scotoma. Laser target moving sinusoidally (0.2 Hz, peak velocity 22.5 deg/sec), drum rotating to left at 30 deg/sec. (A) Monocular stimulation of normal eye. (B) Monocular stimulation of eye with central scotoma. Deflections up: right; down: left.

group while tracking with the normal eye was 0.84 ± 0.12 (0.2 Hz, 22.5 deg/sec) and was 0.22 ± 0.20 for the group while tracking wit the scotomatous eyes. "Stare" OKN was similar during stimulations of the normal and scotomatous eyes. Optokinetic nystagmus gains during constant-velocity drum rotations at 30 deg/sec were 0.69 ± 0.09 and 0.64 ± 0.17 with stimulation of the normal and scotomatous eyes, respectively. At 60 deg/sec the OKN gains were 0.58 ± 0.11 with the normal eye and 0.40 ± 0.06 with the abnormal eye. These differences were not significant.

Ocular Motor Defects.   Table 1 presents OKN and pursuit in patients with discrete anatomical lesions of the ocular motor pathways who have been studied in our laboratory in the past 5 years. Anatomical localization was based on findings in the neurootological and neuroophthalmic examinations and from radiological tests, such as computerized tomography, cerebral angiography, and pneumoencephalography. Whenever possible, nonocular motor signs and symptoms were stressed in determining anatomical localization. The brainstem was the most frequent location of lesions producing decreased SCV of OKN and pursuit. Pathological processes included infarction, demyelination, intrinsic tumors, and extraaxial tumors. Most lesions affected primarily the pons, but midbrain and medullary lesions also produced impaired OKN and pursuit. Fifty-nine percent of the patients with brainstem lesions had impaired OKN, and 81% had abnormal pursuit.

Lesions in the cerebellum comprised the second largest group affecting smooth tracking. This group included disorders that diffusely damage the cerebellum, such as alcoholic cerebellar degeneration; cerebellar system disorders, such as the familial cerebellar ataxias; familial and nonfamilial spinocerebellar degenerations; olivopontocerebellar degeneration; and localized cerebellar lesions, such as those resulting from tumors, infarctions, and the Arnold–Chiari malformation. With localized and lateralized lesions, OKN and pursuit were usually most impaired during tracking toward the side of the lesion. Of the patients with cerebellar lesions, 75% had abnormal OKN and 94% had abnormal pursuit. Patients with Parkinson's disease, Huntington's chorea, progressive supranuclear palsy, and ataxia telangiectasia were included in the basal ganglia group. However, patients with these disorders have usually had widespread histopathological lesions in the brainstem and cerebellum at autopsy, which could also account for some of the ocular motor abnormalities in these

TABLE 1
OKN AND PURSUIT

Anatomical lesion	OKN		Pursuit		Patients
	Abnormal	Normal	Abnormal	Normal	
Brainstem	74 (59%)	52 (41%)	102 (81%)	24 (19%)	126
Cerebellum	71 (72%)	28 (28%)	93 (94%)	6 (6%)	99
Basal ganglia	21 (58%)	5 (42%)	27 (75%)	9 (25%)	36
Labyrinth, vestibular nerve	4 (1%)	380 (99%)	10 (3%)	374 (97%)	384
Parietal lobe	2 (25%)	6 (75%)	6 (75%)	3 (25%)	8
Other lobes	0 (0%)	5 (100%)	0 (0%)	5 (100%)	5
Cranial n. palsy	0 (0%)	4 (100%)	1 (25%)	3 (75%)	4
Ocular myopathy	2 (8%)	22 (92%)	2 (8%)	22 (92%)	24
					686

syndromes. Fifty-eight percent of these patients had impaired horizontal OKN, and 75% had impaired horizontal pursuit.

In contrast to brainstem, cerebellar, and basal ganglia lesions, lesions limited to the peripheral vestibular system did not usually impair OKN or pursuit. Only 1% of patients with lesions of the labyrinths or vestibular nerves, as verified by findings consistent with canal paresis during bithermal caloric testing (2), had defective OKN, and only 3% had defective pursuit. Vestibular disorders included Ménière's disease, viral labyrinthitis, ischemia of the labyrinths, leutic labyrinthitis, viral neuronitis, acoutic neuroma, and vestibulopathy of unknown cause. All of the patients with impaired OKN or pursuit had had sudden onset of vestibular dysfunction and were studied during the acute phase of their clinical course. Spontaneous vestibular nystagmus was frequently present with fixation and was intense, with the SCV often greater than 10 deg/sec with eyes opened in the dark. We have previously demonstrated that OKN and pursuit systems usually dominate the vestibuloocular system during interactions between these systems, as in antagonistic and synergistic visual-vestibular tests (38). Spontaneous vestibular nystagmus of high velocity is required to affect OKN or pursuit appreciably. In our few patients with defective tracking, OKN and pursuit were usually defective in the direction opposite to that of the slow component of the spontaneous vestibular nystagmus. With lesser degrees of canal paresis and with central compensation for vestibular imbalance, the SCV of vestibular nystagmus decreases, and OKN and pursuit are unaffected.

Since ocular tracking is usually affected by lesions of the brainstem and cerebellum, tests of OKN and pursuit are very helpful in differentiating lesions of the peripheral vestibular system from those affecting the central vestibular pathways. During the past 5 years we have identified 27 patients with an initial clinical diagnosis of a peripheral vestibular disorder who were found to have impaired OKN and/or pursuit and were subsequently demonstrated to have central nervous system lesions. Many other patients with peripheral vestibular lesions were found to have symmetrically, mild to moderately impaired OKN and/or pursuit that could be attributed to visual inattention, advanced age, or the effect of drugs. Careful attention to these patient factors was important in correctly interpreting the significance of OKN and pursuit abnormalities in these patients.

Thirteen patients were studied who had lesions of the cerebral hemispheres localized to one lobe and no evidence of involvement of the brainstem or cerebellum. In most patients cerebral hemisphere lesions result from infarctions and tumors. Simultaneous ischemia of the brainstem and cerebellum or previous ischemic lesions of these areas are often encountered. Ocular motor defects could result from brainstem and cerebellar lesions rather than from cerebral hemisphere lesions in these cases. Cerebral hemisphere tumors are usually large when they come to clinical attention and are associated with edema of the surrounding tissues, which in turn can produce effects in other areas of the brain by herniation and vascular effects. Eight patients with lesions localized to the parietal lobes by neuroradiological tests and neurological examination were studied (five infarctions, three tumors). Abnormal OKN and pursuit were found in only three patients. In these patients pursuit was impaired toward the side of the lesion, and OKN toward that side had nearly normal SCV gain and a gradual buildup of SCV over a period of several to many seconds. These patients are discussed more fully in the section on separation of OKN and pursuit. The ocular motor pathway that is believed to be involved in smooth-tracking eye movements is in the deep white matter of the parietal lobe (internal sagittal stratum). Patients with parietal lobe lesions who have normal smooth tracking or bilaterally defective tracking that can be accounted for by inattention, advanced age, fatigue, or drug effects could have lesions affecting primarily the cortex.

Five patients with localized lesions of the frontal, temporal, and occipital lobes were studied. All of these patients had unilateral lesions. None had significant impairment of OKN or pursuit that could not be accounted for by drug effects or lack of visual attention. Smith (31) reported that pursuit and OKN were normal in patients with unilateral occipital lobe lesions and hemianopsia when the lesions were restricted to that lobe. However, when such lesions extended into the parietal lobe, as in tumors of the parietal and occipital lobes, pursuit and OKN were impaired toward the side of the lesion.

Twenty-eight patients with isolated cranial nerve palsies, affecting the peripheral nerves, and ocular myopathies, such as myasthenia gravis and progressive external ophthalmoplegia, were studied. Most of these patients had slowing or other abnormalities of the fast components of OKN in the affected eyes. However, the SCV was usually normal in the affected and unaffected eyes. In five patients pursuit or OKN smooth movements were impaired when the range of eye movements in both eyes was severely restricted.

SEPARATION OF OKN AND PURSUIT

The smooth movements of OKN and pursuit are induced by smoothly moving targets, whereas refixation saccades are induced by targets moving in rapid, discontinuous movements, as in square-wave patterns. It is possible that OKN and pursuit are produced by the same ocular motor system. Differences in the pattern of eye movements could result simply from differences in stimulus characteristics. Most patients who have impaired OKN demonstrate impairment of pursuit to an approximately equal degree. For example, most of the patients in Table 1 had simultaneous impairment of OKN and pursuit. In Figure 14 pursuit and OKN in a patient with a generalized cerebellar degeneration syndrome are shown. Pursuit and OKN were both impaired and their gains were decreased approximately to the same degree. Clinical observations such as this would substantiate the view that OKN and pursuit are similar eye movements.

An alternative hypothesis was proposed by Ter Braak and co-workers (33–35) on the basis of studies of smooth tracking in animals and in a patient with blindness from bilateral occipital lobe infarctions. They suggested that two anatomically separate smooth-tracking systems exist in human beings and in other primates and animals. One system, termed "passive" OKN by the authors, responds to movement of large objects that are not expected to be of interest to the experimental subject, such as vertical stripes, and uses totally subcortical pathways, since tracking persists after removal of the occipital lobes or cerebral hemispheres. Animals without foveas, such as the rabbit, are thought to have only "passive" OKN smooth tracking. The other system, termed "active" OKN, can track small objects of interest to the experimental subject, such as pictures of rabbits for a dog, and utilizes cortical pathways as indicated by loss of this type of tracking after removal of the occipital lobes or cerebral hemispheres. This second type of tracking is thought to exist in animals with an area centralis or fovea and can be equated with pursuit tracking. Ter Braak and co-workers (34) reported that one patient who was completely blind from histopathologi-

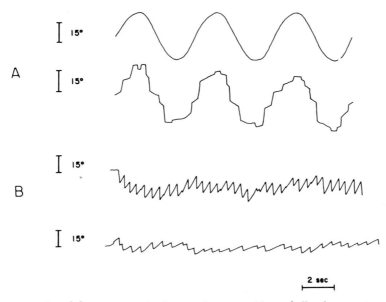

Figure 14. Pursuit and OKN in normal subject and patient with cerebellar degeneration. (A) Pursuit target (0.2 Hz, peak velocity 22.5 deg/sec). Top; normal subject; bottom: patient. (B) Drum (30 deg/sec right). Top: normal subject; bottom: patient. Deflections up: right; down: left.

cally proven, complete infarctions of the occipital lobes responded to stimulation by a full-field OKN drum but could not track small, smoothly moving objects.

During the past several years we have reported studies of OKN and pursuit in patients with discrete, well-defined lesions of the ocular motor system that substantiate the existence of two anatomically separate smooth-tracking systems in human beings. Figure 15 is a diagrammatic representation of pursuit and OKN pathways in human beings that respond to a stimulus moving smoothly to the left. The pursuit pathways are designated by the heavy lines. The afferent pathways consist of the retinogeniculocalcarine projections to both occipital lobes. Ocular motor signals are generated in both occipital lobes, perhaps in the cortex of the visual association areas. Normal pursuit can be produced by only one occipital lobe, since pursuit is normal in patients with unilateral occipital lobe lesions. In tracking a stimulus moving to the left, the motor command from the right occipital lobe decussates in the splenium of the corpus callosum to join the motor command from the left occipital lobe in the internal sagittal stratum of the left parietal lobe. The parietal lobe representation for pursuit is probably ipsilateral. The pursuit motor pathway then descends near the posterior limb of the internal capsule and continues to the PPRF via incompletely delineated pathways in the brainstem tegmentum. An important interaction occurs in the cerebellum, perhaps specifically in the cerebellar flocculus, since pursuit is almost always impaired by lesions in the cerebellum.

The pathways of the subcortical OKN system in Figure 15 are shown by the thin lines and are based on anatomical and neurophysiological studies in animals (8,13,18,26,27). Stimulation of the retina results in activation of the contralateral midbrain nuclei of the accessory optic system via the accessory optic tract. Projections that are presently poorly defined continue to the lower brianstem. These midbrain nuclei probably project to neurons within the nucleus reticularis tegmenti

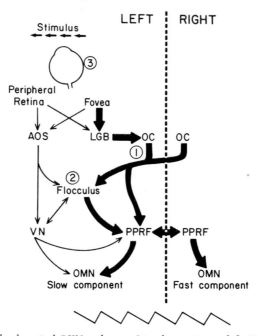

Figure 15. Pursuit and subcortical OKN pathways. Stimulus motion to left. Heavy lines: pursuit pathway; thin lines: subcortical OKN pathway. Abbreviations: LGB, lateral geniculate body; OC, occipital lobe cortex; PPRF, pontine paramedian reticular formation; OMN, ocular motor neurons; AOS, accessory optic system; VN, vestibular nuclei. Below: Jerk nystagmus, slow component to left. Locations: 1, internal sagittal stratum of parietal lobe; 2, cerebellar flocculus; 3, retina.

pontis (NRTP) and dorsal cap of the inferior olive on the same side (7,27). In a recent study, Miyashita and co-workers (27) demonstrated impaired OKN in albino rabbits after ablation of the NRTP. The NRTP sends mossy fibers to the contralateral cerebellar flocculus, and flocculectomy in the rabbit impairs OKN. Climbing fibers from the neurons in the dorsal cap of the inferior olive project to Purkinje cells in the cerebellar flocculus on the opposite side. However, the role of this pathway in the production of OKN is uncertain since lesions in the inferior olive have been found to impair OKN in some studies but have not affected OKN in other studies. Direct pathways from the midbrain relay nuclei of the accessory optic system to the vestibular nuclei may also exist since NRTP and inferior olive lesions do not abolish OKN completely. Participation of the vestibular nuclei in OKN is suggested by the firing of vestibular neurons during OKN in animals and the similarity of OKAN and circularvection during OKN in human beings to postrotatory vestibular nystagmus and subjective sensations of rotation during the vestibuloocular response (9).

Characteristics of subcortical OKN in the rabbit, pursuit in man, and OKN in man are shown in Table 2. Optokinetic nystagmus in the rabbit (12) demonstrates a decrease in SCV gain at stimulus velocities greater than 4 deg/sec and at stimulus frequencies greater than 0.1 to 0.2 Hz. There is a gradual buildup of SCV for several to many seconds, and a transient persistence of nystagmus is present after cessation of stimulation (OKAN). During monocular stimulation, patterns moving in the temporal-to-nasal direction of the visual field are much more effective in producing OKN than patterns moving in the opposite direction (directional selectivity). In

TABLE 2
Smooth-Tracking Characteristics

Characteristic	OKN	OKN (afoveate)	Pursuit
Velocity range	High	Low	High
Frequency range	High	Low	High
Buildup	Rapid	Slow	Rapid
OKAN	+	+	+/−
Circularvection	+		−
Directional selectivity	−	+	−

contrast pursuit gain in man does not decrease until stimulus velocities exceed about 30 deg/sec or stimulus frequencies are greater than about 1.0 Hz (16). A single dot moving repeatedly at constant velocity in one direction, jumping back to the opposite direction, and then moving in the original direction has been shown to produce a nystagmus-like pattern of eye movements, which persists transiently in the dark with termination of stimulation similar to OKAN (28). However, the velocity of pursuit increases immediately to match the stimulus velocity and is not associated with a subjective sensation of self-rotation or directional selectivity.

Optokinetic nystagmus in man has several characteristics that are similar to pursuit. The SCV gain does not decrease significantly until stimulus velocities exceed 20 to 30 deg/sec. Normal subjects in our laboratory maintain a high OKN gain at 0.4 Hz. The SCV increases to maximum levels within one or two beats of OKN, and no directional selectivity is found. We have hypothesized that OKN in normal subjects results from contributions from the cortical pursuit system and the subcortical OKN system. "Look" OKN, in which subjects are instructed to track a single stripe throughout the visual field, probably represents primarily pursuit eye movements. "Stare" OKN, in which SCV gain is lower than that in "look" OKN, probably still results from pursuit and subcortical OKN. The pursuit contribution usually dominates that of subcortical OKN. The subcortical OKN contribution might be identified in patients with lesions of the pursuit pathways that remove the pursuit contribution. In such patients characteristics of subcortical OKN, such as slow buildup of SCV and directional selectivity, could be "uncovered." We predict that smooth-tracking eye movements of such patients would include (a) markedly decreased pursuit gain, (b) normal or nearly normal OKN gain, (c) slow buildup over many seconds of SCV, (d) normal OKAN and circularvection, and (e) directional selectivity. We have demonstrated many of these characteristics in several patients with discrete lesions of the pursuit pathways involving the parietal lobes, cerebellar flocculus, and retina (locaions 1, 2, and 3, respectively, Fig. 15).

We studied three patients with discrete, unilateral lesions of the parietal lobes from an astrocytoma and infarctions (5). Computerized tomography demonstrated that the lesions were relatively small and involved the deep white matter of the parietal lobes. Each patient demonstrated decreased pursuit gain when tracking toward the side of the lesion, normal or nearly normal OKN gain in both directions, and a slow buildup of OKN SCV when tracking toward the side of the lesion. The findings in one patient will be presented in detail. A 21-year-old man developed bitemporal headaches and a slowly progressive right facial and upper extremity weakness over a 1-month period. Neurological examination revealed a fluent aphasia, right central facial weakness, and a right hemiparesis, the arm more involved than the leg. Sensory examination and visual fields were normal. Computerized tomography revealed only slight enlargement of the lateral ventricles. Three-vessel cerebral angiography was unremarkable. During sinusoidal pursuit target motions (0.2 Hz, 22.5 deg/sec and 0.4 Hz, 45 deg/sec), the patient demonstrated normal pursuit when the target moved toward the right but jerky pursuit when the target moved to the left (Figure 16). The gain at 0.2 Hz was 0.98 toward the right and 0.53 to the left. Normal subjects in our laboratory have a mean gain of 0.96 ± 0.04. During 30 deg/sec, constant-velocity drum rotation toward the right, the patient demonstrated a well-formed jerk nystagmus with a mean slow-component velocity of 27.1 deg/sec, representating a gain of 0.90 (Figure 17A). During constant-velocity drum rotation to the left, the SCV increased in the first few seconds to 20 deg/sec and then gradually increased over the next 30 sec to a mean velocity of 27 deg/sec, representing a final gain of 0.90 (Figure 17B). Optokinetic after-nystagmus was present after stimulation in both directions, and circularvection was present during stimulation in both directions. Several months later a mass lesion in the left parietal lobe was demonstrated by computerized tomography and cerebral angiography. A malignant astrocytoma was found at surgery.

We reported slow buildup of OKN and severely impaired pursuit in two patients with downbeating, vertical nystagmus that probably resulted from lesions of the cerebellar flocculus (olivopontocerebellar degeneration and Arnold–Chiari malformation (37). One patient will be discussed in detail. A 59-year-old woman progressively developed over a period of 7 years poor balance, intermittent dizziness, and vertical oscillopsia on lateral gaze. On examination a downbeating, vertical jerk nystagmus with fast components directed downward was found in all directions of gaze but was of greatest amplitude on lateral gaze. This form of vertical nystagmus is of great clinical importance in that it is almost always associated with lesions at the craniocervical junction that affect the cerebellum and lower brainstem. Congenital malformations, such as the Arnold–Chiari malformation and basilar impression, demyelinating lesions, infarctions, and cysts of the fourth ventricle have been associated with downbeating nystagmus. Our patient demonstrated a cerebellar type of ataxia of the legs and slight dysmetria and dysdiadochokinesia of the left hand. Pneumoen-

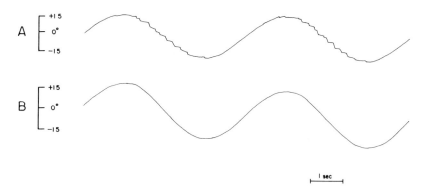

Figure 16.   Pursuit in patient with astrocytoma of left parietal lobe. (A) Eye position; (B) target position (0.2 Hz, peak velocity 22.5 deg/sec). Note impaired pursuit and catch-up saccades to left. Deflections up: right; down: left.

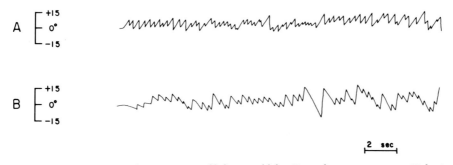

Figure 17.   OKN in patient with astrocytoma of left parietal lobe. Drum begins to rotate at 30 deg/sec at beginning of tracings. Note well-formed OKN and immediate increase in amplitude and velocity to right (A). Note slow buildup of amplitude and velocity to left (B). Deflections up: right; down: left.

cephalography revealed atrophy of the left inferior pons, upper medulla, and midline cerebellum. A clinical diagnosis of olivopontocerebellar degeneration was made. Smooth pursuit was extremely poor, with a gain of 0.17 during target movement to the right and 0.22 to the left at 0.2 Hz (Figure 18A). During 30 deg/sec, constant-velocity drum rotation in both directions, the patient developed a well-formed nystagmus. However, there was a gradual increase in SCV over 20 to 40 sec to nearly normal levels (Figure 18B). The final OKN gain was 0.84 to the right and 0.59 to the left. The patient reported circularvection and demonstrated OKAN. The precise location of lesions in patients with downbeating nystagmus is not known. However, Zee and co-workers (39) have described downbeating nystagmus, severely impaired pursuit, and slow buildup of OKN in monkeys with bilateral lesions of the cerebellar flocculi. Not all patients with downbeating nystagmus have the unique ocular motor syndrome described above. We studied 11 other patients with downbeating nystagmus who have not shown slow buildup of OKN.

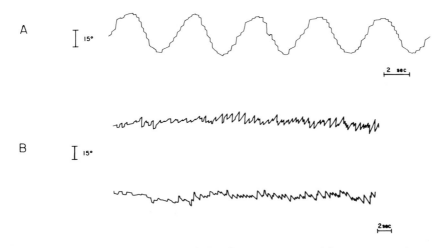

Figure 18.   Pursuit and OKN in patient with downbeating nystagmus. (A) Pursuit target (0.2 Hz, peak velocity 22.5 deg/sec). (B) OKN with drum beginning to rotate at 30 deg/sec at beginning of tracings. Top: right; bottom: left. Note slow buildup of OKN amplitude and velocity in both directions. Deflections up: right; down: left.

We reported severely impaired pursuit, slow buildup of OKN, and directional selectivity of OKN in seven patients with congenital achromatopsia (6,36). Congenital achromatopsia is a rare ocular disorder in which maldevelopment of the cone photoreceptors of the retina results in a distinctive clinical syndrome of poor visual acuity to the level of 20/200 to 20/400, total loss of color vision, central scotoma, nystagmus, and severe photophobia. The ocular motor findings in one patient will be presented in detail. A 12-year-old girl was noted to have oscillation of the eyes in early infancy, which had decreased over the years. She had a younger brother of age 3 who had a horizontal pendular nystagmus and the same clinical syndrome. In the primary position of gaze, there was essentially no nystagmus. However, on lateral gaze a small-amplitude jerk nystagmus with fast components in the direction of gaze was present. Pursuit gain at 0.2 Hz decreased to 0.45 to the right and 0.27 to the left during binocular stimulation. During monocular stimulation (one eye covered) similar impairment of pursuit was found (Figure 19). During 30 deg/sec, constant-velocity drum rotation to the right and left with both eyes opened, OKN was nearly normal (Figure 20). The OKN gain was 0.55 to the right and 0.65 to the left. However, during monocular stimulation the OKN showed a striking asymmetry between the two horizontal directions. During stimulation of the left eye, when the stripes moved from the temporal to the nasal visual field, there was a gradual buildup over 10 sec to a maximum SCV of 15 deg/sec, representing a gain of 0.50. Rotation of the stripes from the nasal to the temporal field resulted in a very poor response, with no buildup and maximum SCV of 2 deg/sec, representing a gain of 0.07. During stimulation of the right eye, the maximum SCV and gain after 17 sec of buildup during stripe movements from the temporal to nasal field were 13 deg/sec and 0.43, respectively. During rotation in the opposite direction, there was no buildup, the maximum SCV was 3 deg/sec, and the gain was 0.10. Circularvection and OKAN were present during or after binocular stimulation in both directions and monocular stimulation in the temporal-to-nasal direction. Abnormalities in the number and/or morphology of retinal cone photoreceptors have been reported in congenital achromatopsia. How-

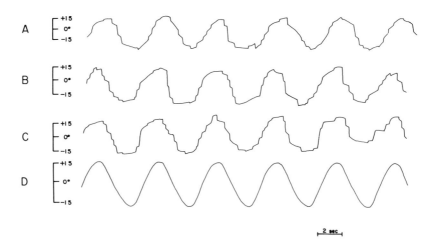

Figure 19. Pursuit in patient with congenital achromatopsia. Target moving sinusoidally (0.2 Hz, peak velocity 22.5 deg/sec). (A) Both eyes stimulated; (B) left eye stimulated; (c) right eye stimulated; (D) target position. Deflections up: right; down: left.

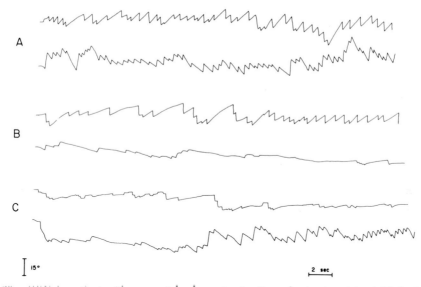

Figure 20. OKN in patient with congenital achromatopsia. Drum begins to rotate at 30 deg/sec at beginning of tracings. Top of each set: drum to right; bottom of each set. drum to left. (A) Binocular stimulation; (B) left eye stimulation; (C) right eye stimulation. Note slow buildup of well-formed OKN only during drum rotation in temporal-to-nasal direction of visual field during monocular stimulation (B, top; C, bottom). Deflections up: right; down: left

ever, whether other lesions in the visual and ocular motor pathways are present is not known.

OKN–PURSUIT INTERACTION TESTS

Tracking of objects in the natural environment produces stimulation of pursuit and OKN systems, since objects are often moving against a stationary, visual background. For example, if the eyes pursue an object that is moving smoothly to the right, the visual background moves to the left relative to the eyes. Therefore, the pursuit and optokinetic stimuli are in opposite directions. A demonstration of modification of pursuit by simultaneous optokinetic stimulation would offer further evidence for a separation of pursuit and OKN systems. We have begun to study tracking of pursuit targets against stationary and moving optokinetic backgrounds in normal subjects and patients. The paradigm consists of tracking the laser target that is moving in constant-velocity, triangular-wave ramps of 1 to 60 deg/sec against (a) a featureless, white screen, (b) the stationary OKN drum, and (c) the drum rotating at constant velocities of 30 and 60 deg/sec. The pursuit gain is calculated. Subjects are instructed to track the laser target carefully during all of the tests.

Figure 21 presents OKN–pursuit interaction tests in a normal subject who had an OKN gain of 0.93 at 30 deg/sec. On line A the subject was tracking the laser target moving at constant velocities of 30 deg/sec. Pursuit gain was 0.93. On line B pursuit was significantly degraded during tracking of the laser target on the surface of the satationary drum. The pursuit gain was 0.76. During pursuit to the right the optokinetic background appears to move toward the left, and during pursuit to the left it moves to the right relative to the eyes. On line C the drum was rotating to the right at 30 deg/sec. When the pursuit and OKN stimuli were moving in the same direction

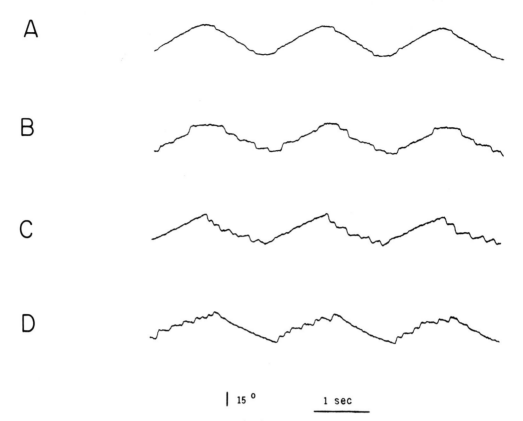

Figure 21.   OKN–Pursuit interaction in normal subject. Target ramps of 30 deg/sec. (A) Target against featureless screen (pursuit gain 0.93); (B) target against stationary drum; (C) target against drum moving 30 deg/sec right; (D) target against drum moving 30 deg/sec left. Note impaired pursuit against stationary drum, improvement of pursuit when target and drum move in same direction, and impairment of pursuit when target and drum move in opposite directions. Deflections up: right; down: left.

(right), the eyes were able to track the laser target almost perfectly. However, when the stimuli moved in opposite directions (left), tracking was markedly impaired, with many of the smooth eye movements in the direction opposite to movement of the laser target. A similar marked degradation of pursuit during antagonistic pursuit and OKN stimulations is seen on line D, in which the drum was rotating to the left.

The synergistic and antagonistic effects of pursuit and OKN are less evident in subjects with high pursuit gain while tracking against the screen. The results shown in Figure 22, line A, are for another normal subject tracking against the featureless screen. The pursuit gain was 0.97 at 30 deg/sec. The OKN gain at 30 deg/sec was 0.91. In the following lines there is much less effect of the OKN stimulus on tracking. It appears that tracking against antagonistic optokinetic stimuli is a difficult task for the pursuit system. OKN–Pursuit interaction tests could be helpful in identifying mild defects in the pursuit system. Although the difference in pursuit gains was small in the two subjects illustrated above (0.93 and 0.97), the difference in the degree of OKN–pursuit interaction was marked.

We have not found the measurement of OKAN and circularvection to be clinically helpful in assessing the subcortical OKN system. Although patients with impaired OKN usually have little or no OKAN, many normal subjects with high OKN gain also

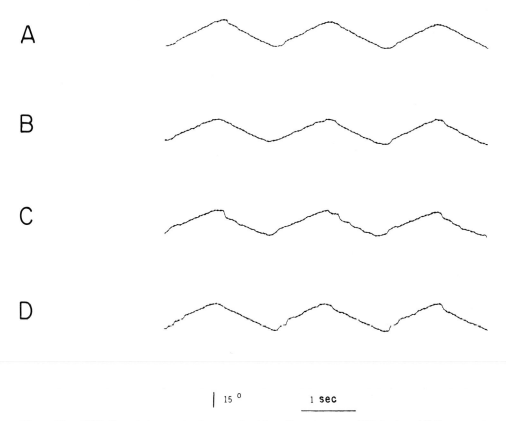

| 15 °   1 sec

Figure 22. OKN–Pursuit interaction in normal subject. Target ramps of 30 deg/sec. (A) Target against screen (pursuit gain 0.97); (B) target against stationary drum; (C) target against drum moving 30 deg/sec right; (D) target against drum moving 30 deg/sec left. Note that effect on pursuit is much less than in previous patient (Figure 21) with lower pursuit gain. Deflections up: right; down: left.

have little or no OKAN. Patients with essentially no OKN or pursuit can appreciate circularvection. However, we have observed that the duration of OKAN can be markedly prolonged in patients with spontaneous vestibular nystagmus when the slow components of the OKAN and vestibular nystagmus are in the same direction. For example, OKAN is often absent when OKAN and the spontaneous nystagmus are in opposite directions but lasts for 20 sec or more when they are in the same direction, even if the SCV of the vestibular nystagmus in the dark is less than 5 deg/sec. OKN–Pursuit interaction tests might offer an opportunity to assess quantitatively the function of the subcortical OKN system by measuring the effects of optokinetic stimulation on pursuit tracking.

REFERENCES

1. Baloh, R. W., Langhofer, L., Honrubia, V., and Yee, R. D., On-line analysis of eye movements using a digital computer. *Aviat. Space Environ. Med.* 1980, **51**:563–567.
2. Baloh, R. W., Solingen, L. D., Sills, A., and Honrubia, V., Caloric testing. I. Effect of different conditions of ocular fixation. *Ann. Otol., Rhinol. Laryngol.*, 1977, **86**(Suppl. 43):1–6.
3. Baloh, R. W., Yee, R. D., and Boder, E., Ataxia-telangiectasia, quantitative analysis of eye movements in six cases. *Neurology*, 1978, **28**:1099–1104.

4. Baloh, R. W., Yee, R. D., and Honrubia, V., Internuclear ophthalmoplegia. II. Pursuit, optokinetic responses and vestibulo-ocular reflex. *Arch. Neurol. (Chicago).* 1978, **35**:490–493.

5. Baloh, R. W., Yee, R. D., and Honrubia, V., Optokinetic nystagmus and parietal lobe lesions. *Ann. Neurol.*, 1980, **7**:269–276.

6. Baloh, R. W., Yee, R. D., and Honrubia, V., Optokinetic asymmetry in patients with maldeveloped foveas. *Brain Res.*, 1980, **186**:211–216.

7. Barmack, N. H., Immediate and sustained influences of visual olivocerebellar activity on eye movement. In: *Posture and Movement* (R. Talbott and D. Humphrey, eds.). Raven, New York, 1979:123–167.

8. Brandth, S. E., and Karten, A. J., Direct accessory optic projections to the vestibulo-cerebellum: A possible channel for oculomotor control systems. *Exp. Brain Res.*, 1977, **28**:73–84.

9. Brandt, T., Dichgans, J., and Büchele, W., Motion habituation: Inverted self-motion perception and optokinetic after-nystagmus. *Exp. Brain Res.*, 1974, **21**:337–352.

10. Cheng, M., and Outerbridge, J. S., Optokinetic nystagmus during selective retinal stimulation. *Exp. Brain Res.*, 1975, **23**:129–139.

11. Chu, F. C., Rheingold, D. B., Cogan, D. G., and Williams, A. C., The eye movement disorders of progressive supranuclear palsy. *Ophthalmology*, 1979, **86**:422–428.

12. Collewijn, H., Optokinetic eye movements in the rabbit: Input-output relations. *Vision Res.*, 1969, **9**:117–132.

13. Collewijn, H., Direction-selective units in the rabbit's nucleus of the optic tract. *Brain Res.*, 1975, **100**:489–508.

14. Dichgans, J., Nauck, B., and Wolpert, E., The influence of attention, vigilance and stimulus area on optokinetic and vestibular nystagmus and voluntary saccades. In: *The Oculomotor System and Brain Functions* (V. Zikmund, ed.). Butterworth, London, 1973:279–294.

15. Dubois, M. F. W., and Collewijn, H., Optokinetic reactions in man elicited by localized retinal motion stimuli. *Vision Res.*, 1979, **19**:1105–1115.

16. Fender, D. H., and Nye, P. W., An investigation of the mechanisms of eye movements. *Kybernetick*, 1962, **1**:81–88.

17. Gresty, M., and Halmagyi, M., Following eye movements in the absence of central vision. *Acta Oto-Laryngol.*, 1979, **87**:477–483.

18. Hoffman, K. P., and Schoppman, A., Retinal input to direction sensitive cells in the nucleus tractus opticus of the cat. *Brain Res.*, 1975, **99**:359–366.

19. Holm-Jensen, S., and Peitersen, E., The significance of the target frequency and the target speed in optokinetic nystagmus (OKN). *Acta Oto-Laryngol.*, 1979, **88**:110–116.

20. Honrubia, V., Baloh, R. W., Lau, C. G. Y., and Sills, A. W., The pattern of eye movements during physiologic vestibular nystagmus in man. *Trans. Am. Acad. Ophthalmol. Otolaryngol.*, 1977, **84**:339–347.

21. Honrubia, V., Baloh, R. W., Yee, R. D., and Jenkins, H. A., Identification of the location of vestibular lesions on the basis of vestibulo-ocular reflex measurements. *Am. J. Otolaryngol.*, 1980, **1**:291–301.

22. Honrubia, V., Downey, W. L., Mitchell, D. P., and Ward, P. H., Experimental studies on optokinetic nystagmus. II. Normal humans. *Acta Oto-Laryngol.*, 1968, **65**:441–448.

23. Hood, J. D., Observations upon the role of the peripheral retina in the execution of eye movements. *J. Otolaryngol.*, 1975, **37**:65–73.

24. Jaglia, F., Effect of the distance of optokinetic stimuli from the eyes on certain parameters of the optokinetic nystagmus. *Physiol. Bohemoslov.*, 1978, **27**:359–365.

25. Lau, C. G. Y., Honrubia, V., and Baloh, R. W., The pattern of eye movement trajectories during physiological nystagmus in humans. *Proc. Extraordinary Meet., Bárány Soc., 6th, 1977;*

26. Maekawa, K., and Takeda. T., Electrophysiological identification of the climbing and mossy fiber pathways from the rabbit's retina to the contra-lateral cerebellar flocculus. *Brain Res.*, 1976, **109**:169–174.

27. Miyashita, Y., Ito, M., Jastreboff, P., Maekawa, K., and Nagao, S., Effect upon eye movements of rabbits induced by severance of mossy fiber visual pathway to the cerebellar flocculus. *Brain Res.*, 1980, **198**:210–215.

28. Muratore, R., and Zee, D. S., Pursuit after-nystagmus. *Vision Res.*, 1979, **19**:1057–1059.

29. Pola, J., and Robinson, D. A., An explanation of eye movements seen in internuclear ophthalmoplegia. *Arch. Neurol. (Chicago)*, 1976, **82**:223–231.

30. Sills, A. W., Honrubia, V., Konrad, H. R., and Baloh, R. W., A rapid optokinetic nystagmus test: Comparison with standard testing. *Trans. Am. Acad. Ophthalmol. Otolaryngol.*, 1976, **82**:223–231.

31. Smith, J. L., Homonymous hemianopsia. A review of one hundred cases. *Am. J. Ophthalmol.*, 1962, **54**:616–623.

32. Spooner, J. W., Sakala, S. M., and Baloh, R. W., Effect of aging on eye tracking. *Arch. Neurol. (Chicago)*, 1980, **37**:575–576.

33. Ter Braak, J. W. G., Untersuchen über optokinetischen Nystagmus. *Arch. Neerl. Physiol.*, 1936, **21**:309–376.

34. Ter Braak, J. W. G., Schenk, V. W. D., and Van Vliet, A. G. M., Visual reactions in a case of long-standing cortical blindness. *J. Neurol., Neurosurg. Psychiatr.*, 1971, **34**:140–147.

35. Ter Braak, J. W. G., and Van Vliet, A. G. M., Subcortical optokinetic nystagmus in the monkey. *Psychiatr., Neurol., Neurochir.*, 1963, **66**:277–283.

36. Yee, R. D., Baloh, R. W., and Honrubia, V., Eye movement abnormalities in congenital achromatopsia. *Ophthalmology*, 1981, **88**:1010–1018.

37. Yee, R. D., Baloh, R. W., Honrubia, V., Lau, C., and Jenkins, H. A., Slow build-up of optokinetic nystagmus associated with downbeat nystagmus. *Invest. Ophthalmol. Visual Sci.*, 1979, **18**:211–216, 1980.

38. Yee, R. D., Jenkins, H. A., Baloh, R. W., Honrubia, V., and Lau, C., Vestibular-optokinetic interactions in normal subjects and patients with peripheral vestibular dysfunction. *J. Otolaryngol.*, 1978, **7**:310–319.

39. Zee, D. S., Yamazaki, A., and Gucer, G., Ocular abnormalities in trained monkeys with floccular lesions. *Soc. Neurosci. Abstr.*, 1978, **4**:168.

40. Zee, D. S., Yee, R. D., and Singer, H. S., Congenital ocular motor apraxia. *Brain.* 1977, **100**:581–599.

FREE COMMUNICATIONS

Optokinetic Pattern Asymmetry in Patients with Cerebral Lesions

KIMITAKA KAGA and JUN-ICHI SUZUKI

Department of Otolaryngology
Teikyo University School of Medicine
Itabashi-ku
Tokyo, Japan

INTRODUCTION

Optokinetic nystagmus (OKN) is caused by a function of the visual-oculomotor system, which favors the subject's recognition of moving targets. This horizontal nystagmus, which consists of a slow phase in the direction of the target and a fast phase in the opposite direction, is primarily a kind of reflex in the oculomotor system (13,14) but is also strongly influenced by the will and state of alertness. Definite disturbances in OKN responses usually indicate lesions within the visual or oculomotor systems.

Since asymmetry of OKN responses suggests lateralization of lesions in the nervous pathway, OKN testing is useful as a diagnostic tool for detecting disorders:

1. In peripheral diseases, a unilateral decrease in slow-phase velocity occurs transiently when the optokinetic stimulus moves contralaterally to an acute labyrinthine lesion; this induces spontaneous nystagmus in the direction of the stimulus (1,2,5,17,19).

2. Focal lateralized lesions of the brainstem and cerebellum cause impaired OKN when the stimulus moves toward the damaged side (1,2,5,15,19).

3. Cortical or subcortical parietooccipital lesions impair OKN when the stimulus moves toward the damaged hemisphere (3,4,7,9,15,16). However, its pathophysiology is still not clear. Temporal lobe lesions do not impair OKN, but the influence of frontal lobe lesions is controversial (3,4,7,8,10,11).

Studies of patients with unilateral lesions of the cerebral cortex have provided various arguments for the existence of two distinct mechanisms for the slow and fast phases of OKN with centers in the frontal, parietal, and occipital cortices, respectively. However, which components of OKN are affected by lateralized cortical lesions is still controversial.

NYSTAGMUS AND VERTIGO: CLINICAL
APPROACHES TO THE PATIENT WITH DIZZINESS

The optokinetic test is not sufficiently standardized to allow comparisons to be made among different laboratories. However, it is evident that more information is needed in anatomically verified cases of cerebral lesions in order to resolve the significance of an asymmetric OKN sign.

The optokinetic pattern test (OKP test) is one of the most convenient methods for detecting slow-phase and fast-phase asymmetry of OKN (17,19). The purpose of this chapter is to report briefly on the OKN asymmetry, as determined by the OKP test, of 19 patients with cerebral lesions caused by cerebrovascular accidents and anatomically verified by computerized tomography (CT) scan.

MATERIALS AND METHODS

The subjects of the study to be described here were 19 patients with left hemisphere damage caused by cerebrovascular accidents. The patients with frontal, parietal, and occipital lesions numbered 5 each, and those with temporal lobe lesions accounted for the remaining 4. The size and the depth of cerebral lesions were observed by CT scans of the brain. Because these patients had consulted our speech clinic for problems in speech, reading, writing, and hearing, their lesions were presumed to be limited to the left hemisphere.

The procedure of the OKP test is explained by J. Suzuki in another chapter in this volume (18). In this test, the eye-speed recording is condensed by slowing the flow speed of the chart and can then be visualized as a pattern that simply indicates four important characteristics of the responses: (a) the direction of OKN, (b) the amplitude of OKN, (c) the frequency of OKN, and (d) the increase in slow-phase eye speed with the increase in the speed of optokinetic stimulus.

The OKP obtained by counterclockwise rotation of the drum is called right OKP, and that obtained by clockwise rotation is called left OKP, since the quick phase of induced nystagmus is directed to the right in the former and to the left in the latter. The slow-phase intensity is shown in the direction opposite to the fast phase.

RESULTS

NORMAL FINDINGS IN THE OKP TEST

The direction of the quick phase of OKN in normal subjects is the opposite of the drum rotation(Figure 1A). No remarkable directional differences between rotation to the right and to the left are seen. Directional difference or amplitude change, if any, must be caused by a directional preponderance of the optokinetic reaction. Thus, it is necessary to compare the patterns through both rotations.

The slow-phase eye speed in normal subjects increases along with the increase in drum speed up to about 90 deg/sec. The maximum slow-phase eye speed is usually not much more or less than 100 deg/sec. The middle portion of the OKP response is different in each individual, and even in normal subjects it can be flat, convex, or concave. There may be a slight variation between right and left OKP's in normal subjects (Figure 1B).

The frequency of induced nystagmus is expressed in the OKP as density changes. The middle parts of the OKP usually have the highest density in normal subjects, nystagmic beats being about four per second. A lower or sometimes higher density than this in the central portions of the response usually indicates an abnormal response.

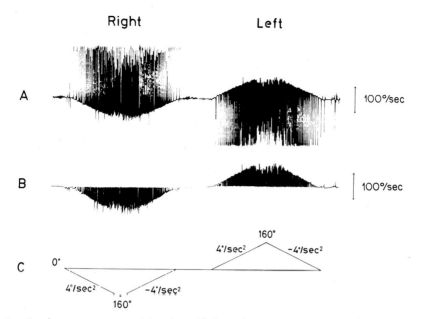

Figure 1. Optokinetic pattern test. (A) Right and left OKP's in a normal patient. (B) Slow-phase changes shown by clipping normal OKP's of A on the baseline. (C) Explanation of drum velocity change.

ABNORMAL OKP's IN CLINICAL CASES

Optokinetic patterns and lesions of the cerebrum in typical cases that showed a marked asymmetry are illustrated in Figures 2, 3, and 4.

Frontal Lobe Lesions

The asymmetry of patients 1, 2, and 3 is characterized by the fact that the right OKP had a lower density (frequency) and a moderately depressed slow-phase eye speed, especially during high-speed drum rotation, but less than the left OKP (Figure 2). Computerized tomography scans of these three patients showed lesions of the third frontal and precentral gyrus. It should be noted that the principal lesions of these three patients were in the motor cortices.

Temporal Lobe Lesions

The OKP's of four patients with temporal lobe lesions were studied. Although the CT scans revealed severe damage of the temporal lobes in each case, there was no marked difference between the right and left OKP's, or there was little impairment of the slow-phase eye speed and density.

Parietal Lobe Lesions

As shown in Figure 3, all OKP's of three patients with parietal lobe lesions showed remarkable asymmetry. In patients 1 and 2, the slow-phase eye speed of the right OKP was markedly and constantly impaired at all speeds of drum rotation, whereas those of the left OKP's were also impaired but not more than those of the right. In addition, the amplitude of the right OKP in patient 1 was smaller than half that of the left OKP, and the densities of both OKP's in patients 1 and 2 were lower than those of

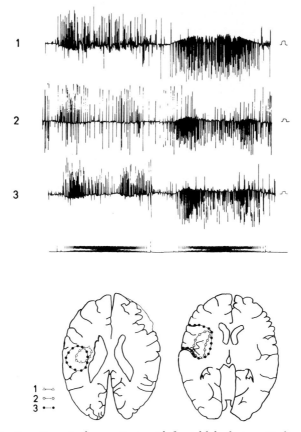

Figure 2. Optokinetic patterns in three patients with frontal lobe lesions. Outlines of their lesions are shown above two illustrations of brain CT scans.

the controls. In patient 3, only a decrease in the amplitude of the OKP but a slight impairment of slow-phase eye speed and density between the right and left OKP's were found. Computerized tomography scans of these three patients revealed deep cortical lesions in the inferior parietal lobe. These lesions were localized in the association cortices.

Occipital Lobe Lesions

In patients 1, 2, and 3, slow-phase eye speed of the right OKP was markedly and constantly impaired at all drum rotation speeds (Figure 4). The amplitude of the right OKP was less than half that of the left OKP. The density in each direction was slightly impaired in patients 1 and 2 but not in patient 3. Computerized tomography scans revealed deep cortical lesions of the occipital lobe in patients 1 and 2 but, in patient 3, only a lesion of the visual radiation. These lesions were localized in the visual radiation and visual cortices.

DISCUSSION

In order to obtain more information concerning optokinetic asymmetry occurring with lateralized cerebral lesions, we attempted an analysis of OKP tests in patients

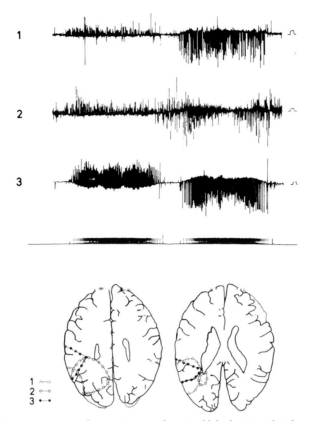

Figure 3. Optokinetic patterns in three patients with parietal lobe lesions. Sketches of their CT scans are illustrated.

with cerebrovascular accidents. The present results of parietal lesions support, in part, previous findings (3,4,7,9,15,16) that deep parietal lesions elicit marked asymmetry of OKN and that the amplitude and frequency of nystagmus elicited by stripes moving toward the affected side of the parietal lobe are smaller than those elicited by stripes toward the intact side. Our cases of parietal lesions showed that OKP's consisted of an ipsilateral slow-phase deficit and small amplitude of the contralateral fast phase of OKN when the drum is moved toward the damaged hemisphere. However, we should emphasize that a contralateral slow-phase decline was also found.

Our patients with occipital lobe lesions showed almost the same asymmetry of OKP. These results suggest that the parietal and occipital lobe lesions affect both directions of OKN but impair remarkably ipsilateral slow phase of OKN in comparison with contralateral slow phase. In the patients with frontal lobe lesions, there was such an asymmetry of OKP that the density of the OKP was sparse when the drum was moved toward the damaged hemisphere, and the slow phase was depressed during high-speed drum rotation. However, in the patients with temporal lobe lesions, normal OKP's could be generated, despite the extensive and deep damage.

Optokinetic nystagmus consists of a slow phase and a fast phase. Which of these phases is impaired in patients with parietal lobe lesions is a key to revealing some roles of the cerebral cortex in OKN reflex. There are two major hypotheses concern-

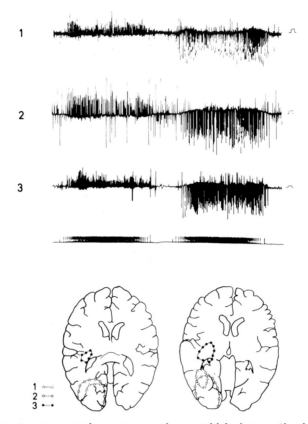

Figure 4. Optokinetic patterns in three patients with occipital lobe lesions. Sketches of their CT scans are illustrated.

ing OKN asymmetry in the cerebral cortex. The first was proposed by Dix and Hood (8) and Gay and colleagues (10). They believe that two distinct mechanisms exist for the slow and fast components of OKN, with centers in the frontal and occipital cortex, respectively, and for a cortical association pathway between the two centers. Gay and co-workers stated that the slow phase is initiated by the occipital lobe contralateral to the direction of the eye movement and that the fast phase is initiated by the frontal lobe contralateral to the direction of the eye movement. They also inferred that deep parietal lobe lesions cause a loss or decrease of the fast phase of OKN when the movement of the stripes is toward the side of the lesion, because the connections to the frontal lobe from both occipital lobes are via pathways lying deep in the parietal lobe. However, we cannot evaluate their hypothesis because they did not show actual recordings of OKN in patients with various cerebral lesions.

The second hypothesis was proposed by Cords (6) and Baloh and colleagues (3). According to Cords, there must be an efferent optomotor lesion to account for the asymmetric response, and the most likely site is in the internal and external sagittal strata of the middle and posterior third of the optic radiations, or deep in the parietal lobe. Recently, Baloh (3) quantitatively recorded OKN in patients with parietal lobe lesions and found that the ipsilateral slow-phase OKN deficit seen in such cases resulted from damage to the foveal pursuit pathway. Although he did not describe the effect of other cerebral lobe lesions except parietal lobe lesions on OKN, he supported Cords's slow-component hypothesis and proposed a clearer hypothesis: "Corticofugal fibers, which run from the parietoccipital association areas to the horizontal gaze center of the ipsilateral brainstem pass parallel beneath the optic radiations in the parietal lobe. Parietal lobe lesions can selectively involve these corticofugal fibers or, more commonly, can damage both fugal and petal fibers, producing a combined homonymous hemianopia."

There have been many reports of OKN asymmetry in patients with cerebral lesions. Only deep parietal lobe lesions were demonstrated to produce asymmetric horizontal OKN (3,4,7,9,15,16). On the other hand, Penfield (12) found that electrical stimulation in the parietal lobe of patients might at times result in a sense of rotation or bodily displacement, and his impression was that such a phenomenon, the same as a vertiginous sensation, was apt to appear as the result of stimulation or discharge in the posterior medial portion of the parietal lobe. These classical reports of parietal lobe lesions and electrical stimulation in patients imply the possibility that the parietal lobe is a sensory-motor association cortex for OKN. However, whether the parietal lobe is an area responsible only for producing OKN in cerebral cortices is an important issue.

Our data provide evidence that not only the parietal lobe but also the occipital lobe has a main function in eliciting the ipsilateral slow phase of OKN to the direction of the drum rotation. Then, a parietooccipital association area may possibly be considered a center of OKN. However, this area also has a small function in eliciting the contralateral slow phase. On the other hand, a role of the frontal lobe in producing OKN cannot be ruled out because such lesions impair the ipsilateral OKN during high-speed drum rotation; however, this function is not yet clear.

The OKP test is a pattern recognition test for observing OKN but is convenient to use as a routine test for detecting any asymmetry of OKN in cerebral lesions.

REFERENCES

1. Baloh, R. W., and Honrubia, V., *Clinical Neurophysiology of the Vestibular System.* Davis, Philadelphia, Pennsylvania, 1979.
2. Baloh, R. W., Honrubia, V., and Sills, A., Eye-tracking and optokinetic nystagmus quantitative testing in patients with well-defined nervous system lesions. *Ann. Otol., Rhinol., Laryngol.*, 1977, **86**:108–114.
3. Baloh, R. W., Yee, R. D., and Honrubia, V., Optokinetic nystagmus and parietal lesions. *Ann. Neurol.*, 1980, **7**:269–276.
4. Carmichael, E. A., Dix, M. R., and Hallpike, C. S., Lesions of the cerebral hemispheres and their effects upon optokinetic and caloric nystagmus. *Brain*, 1954, **77**:345–372.
5. Coats, A. C., Central and peripheral optokinetic asymmetry. *Ann. Otol., Rhinol., Laryngol.*, 1968, **77**:938–948.
6. Cords, R., Optisch-motorisches Feld und optisch-motorische Bahn. *Albrecht von Graefes Arch. Ophthalmol.*, 1926, **117**:58–113.
7. Davidoff, R. A., Atkin, A., Anderson, P. J., and Bender, M., Optokinetic nystagmus and cerebral disease. *Arch. Neurol. (Chicago)*, 1966, **14**:73–81.
8. Dix, M. R., and Hood, J. D., Further observation upon the neurological mechanism of optokinetic nystagmus. *Acta Oto-Laryngol.*, 1971, **71**:217–226.
9. Fox, J. C., and Holmes, G., Optic nystagmus and its value in the localization of cerebral lesions. *Brain*, 1926, **49**:333–371.
10. Gay, A. J., Newman, N. M., Keltner, J. L., and Stroud, M. H., eds., *Eye Movement Disorders.* Mosby, St. Louis, Missouri, 1974.

11. Hoyt, W. F., and Daroff, R. B., Supranuclear disorders of ocular control systems in man. In: *The Control of Eye Movements* (P. Bach-y-Rita, C. C. Collins, and J. E. Hyde, eds.). Academic Press, New York, 1971:175–235.

12. Penfield, W., Vestibular sensation and the cerebral cortex. *Ann. Otol., Rhinol., Laryngol.*, 1957, **66**:691–698.

13. Raphan, R., and Cohen, B., Brain stem mechanisms for rapid and slow eye movements. *Annu. Rev. Physiol.*, 1978, **40**:527–552.

14. Shimazu, H., Excitatory and inhibitory premotor neurons related to horizontal vestibular nystagmus. In: *Integration in the Nervous System* (H. Asanuma and V. J. Wilson, eds.). Igaku-Shoin, Tokyo, 1979:123–142.

15. Smith, J. L., *Optokinetic Nystagmus*. Thomas, Springfield, Illinois, 1963.

16. Smith, J. L., and Cogan, D. G., Optokinetic nystagmus: A test for parietal lobe lesions. *Am. J. Ophthalmol.*, 1959, **48**:187–193.

17. Suzuki, J., Examination of optokinetic nystagmus. In: *Neuro-otological Examination* (T. Uemura, J. Suzuki, J. Hozawa, and S. M. Highstein, eds.). Igaku-Shoin, Tokyo, 1977:106–119.

18. Suzuki, J., A report from Japan on the routine clinical evaluation of patients with vestibular disorders. This volume.

19. Suzuki, J., and Komatsuzaki, A., Clinical application of optokinetic nystagmus. *Acta Oto-Laryngol.*, 1962, **54**:49–55.

The Transitions between Saccades and Smooth Eye Movements

DOUGLAS B. REINGOLD

Eye Movement Laboratory
Neuro-Ophthalmology Section
Clinical Branch, National Eye Institute, NIH
Bethesda, Maryland

INTRODUCTION

Saccadic eye movements are usually studied with the head fixed and targets motionless. But voluntary eye movements are normally accompanied by movements of the head, and what we are looking from or toward may also be moving. Therefore, immediately preceding and following saccades there is sometimes a smooth eye movement. We have examined the transition between smooth eye movements and saccades. If saccades are simply superimposed on smooth movements, we would expect the transition between the movements to be abrupt. If, however, the transition is gradual, and smooth eye movements are attenuated before saccades, this would express an interaction between the movements. We have constructed an experimental paradigm for studying these transitions.

METHODS

To study the transition between smooth and saccadic eye movements, we designed two types of experiments, one using multiple targets in the "target array" experiments and the other using a single target in the "target jump" experiments.

TARGET ARRAY EXPERIMENTS

We chose to use an array of targets that remained illuminated throughout an experiment. We reasoned that the jumping target customarily used in testing saccades would be unsatisfactory for our purposes. When a target jumps while being pursued, its image disappears from the fovea in the several hundred milliseconds immediately preceding and coinciding with saccades. In interpreting the results of such an experiment, it is difficult to distinguish whether an alteration of smooth eye movements immediately preceding and following saccades is due to the saccade or is instead due to the disappearance of the target from the fovea (10).

NYSTAGMUS AND VERTIGO: CLINICAL
APPROACHES TO THE PATIENT WITH DIZZINESS

These experiments tested whether the transitions were abrupt or gradual and whether these depended on the type of the preceding smooth eye movements: those generated as visual pursuit or those as vestibular slow phase. In the former, the target array slowly moved; in the latter, the targets were fixed, while the patient was rotated *en bloc* past the targets.

The paradigm we constructed for the first experiments is illustrated in Figure 1. We projected an array of Landolt rings at eye level, 20 deg apart. The gap in each ring subtended 4 min of arc and was pseudorandomly oriented upward or downward. To study the transitions between pursuit eye movements and saccades, the target array was rotated in the horizontal plane, at constant velocity or sinusoidally. The constant-velocity motion was 30 or 60 deg/sec for 5 sec, followed by constant acceleration for 1 sec to constant velocity in the other direction, and then repeated. The sinusoidal motion was 30, 60, or 120 deg/sec peak velocity at 0.2 Hz. As targets moved past, subjects were asked to look from target to target and to follow closely enough to discern their orientations.

To study the transitions between visuovestibular ocular reflex slow-phase eye movements and saccades, the targets were motionless and the subject was rotated horizontally past them with waveforms identical to the pursuit case. Again, the subjects were asked to gaze at each target closely enough to determine its orientation and to look from target to target at will.

TARGET JUMP EXPERIMENTS

We attempted to replicate the studies of Jurgens and Becker (6), which suggested that pursuit is suppressed in the vicinity of saccades. For these experiments we used, as they did, a single target which moved in "ramp–step–ramp" movements, i.e., which jumped during constant-speed motion. Our target moved in a 60 deg/sec

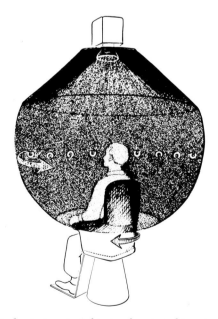

Figure 1.   Setup for first set of experiments. Subject and projected target array. Subject or target array is rotated to study the transition between saccades and smooth eye movements. Stimulus and recording methods have been described by Reingold *et al.* (14).

ramp, between 30 deg left and 30 deg right, reversing direction with constant acceleration in 0.25 sec. Upon these ramps were superimposed steps of 20 deg, either a backward step each time the target reached straight ahead, or a step at random times. The horizontal movements of either eye were studied in two subjects using electrooculography.

RESULTS

TARGET ARRAY EXPERIMENTS

To introduce saccade position and velocity waveforms, Figure 2 shows a profile of 20-deg saccades obtained by averaging 12 rightward saccades made by one subject's

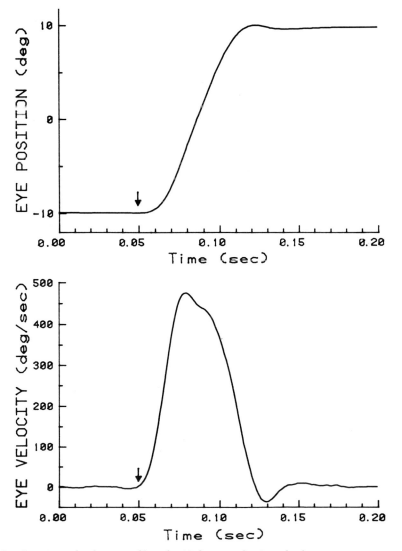

Figure 2.   Position and velocity profiles of a 20-deg saccade. Saccades between two targets separated horizontally by 20 deg were recorded in a normal subject by infrared oculography. Twelve rightward saccades made by the right eye were selected which had similar amplitudes and durations, and the 12 were aligned on their beginnings and averaged.

right eye, aligned on their inceptions. The right eye is initially fixed on a target 10 deg to the left of straight ahead. At the time indicated by the arrow, the eye initiates a rapid horizontal movement to the right and fixes again at the new position. The upper curve illustrates the horizontal eye position over time, and the lower illustrates the eye velocity over time. The eye velocity, initially zero, peaks and returns to zero.

Figure 3 shows schematically the effect of target motion on the position profile. In Figure 3A, the targets are stationary, as in the previous figure. The positions of the two stationary targets in the horizontal plane are indicated by the two dashed lines. The lower dashed line represents the position of the left target, and the upper, that of the right. The distance between the two targets is represented by the vertical separation between the two lines. If a saccade is made from the left to the right target at the time indicated by the arrow, the eye position over time will again resemble the curve shown.

The eye movement trajectory that results when the two targets maintain a constant separation but are moving leftward is shown schematically in Figure 3B. Now the saccade is immediately preceded and followed by a pursuit movement. The distance between the two targets is again represented by the vertical separation of the dashed lines. Similar curves would illustrate the case in which the head is moving to the right past the targets, rather than the targets moving to the left past the head.

In Figures 4 and 5, the subject is fixed and the targets are rotating. Velocity waveforms for a typical subject during two cycles of tracking the target array are shown in Figure 4. Target peak velocity here is 60 deg/sec. A given target in the array moves about 95 deg, so the tracking consists of pursuit of one target, execution of a 20-deg saccade to the adjacent target, pursuit of that target, and so on. Of note are the relatively sharp transitions between the saccades and pursuit movements. In the transition from pursuit to saccades, the pursuit is not attenuated prior to 20 msec before a saccade.

To get a closeup view of eye velocity immediately before and after saccades, we averaged for each subject the velocity records, aligning them on saccade initiations and terminations, determined under visual inspection as the point of departure of the

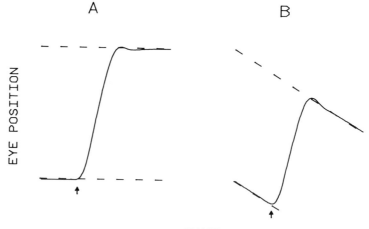

Figure 3. Position profiles for saccades between fixed and moving targets. (A) As in Figure 2; (B) schematically shows position profile between moving targets.

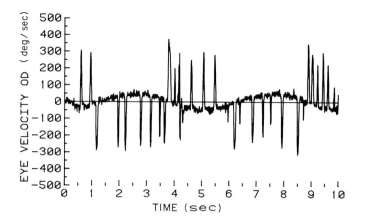

Figure 4. Position and velocity of eye movements during tracking of moving target array.

acceleration from baseline. Figure 5 shows the average saccade initiations and terminations during tracking of the target array moving in 60 deg/sec ramps. The first two curves show the beginnings and endings of rightward saccades; the second two curves, leftward saccades. The passage through zero velocity without change in acceleration and the lack of attenuation of pursuit velocity in the period before saccades are noteworthy.

In Figures 6 and 7 the targets are fixed and the subject is rotating. As in the previous case, in the transition between the smooth (visual-vestibular ocular) eye movement and saccade, the saccade begins abruptly without previous attenuation of the smooth movement, the transition being less than 20 msec.

TARGET JUMP EXPERIMENTS

In the second set of experiments we used a jumping target, as had Jurgens and Becker (6), and obtained results reminiscent of theirs, as shown in Figure 8. In these transitions between smooth eye movements and saccades, the eye movement slows. It is of interest that the subject does not reduce the latency from target jump to saccade. To get a closer look at these movements we isolated the segments of data

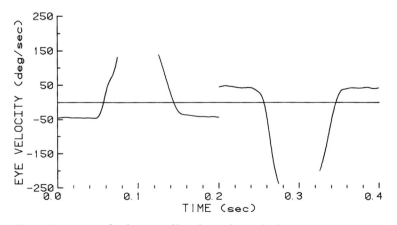

Figure 5. Averaged velocity profiles of saccades made during array tracking.

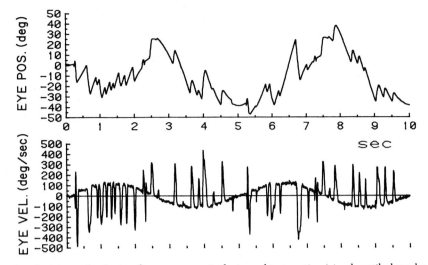

Figure 6.   Position and velocity of eye movements during subject motion (visual-vestibuloocular reflex) with refixations guided to discrete visual targets.

containing saccades. Figure 9 shows four such segments. The segments were selected to display the usual case in which the transition from smooth eye movement to saccade is associated with slowing or "suppression" of pursuit. Occasionally such slowing was not observed, and such saccades were excluded from the figure. Each column refers to a 0.5-sec "window" of data. The top and second rows show target and right eye trajectory, respectively, and the bottom row shows corresponding eye velocity. Such graphs show more clearly the time course of the transition from pursuit to saccades in this case.

To determine the effect of anticipation in these results, we programmed the target steps to occur at random times. Typical results are shown in Figure 10. The suppression of smooth eye movements before saccades is seen less often, in contrast to the findings when target jumps occur at predictable times.

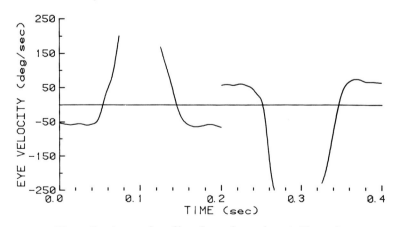

Figure 7.   Averaged profiles of saccades made as in Figure 6.

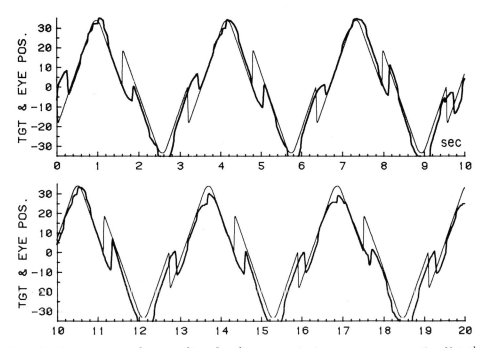

Figure 8. Eye movements during tracking of single target moving in ramp step ramp motion. Note the attenuation of pursuit before saccades.

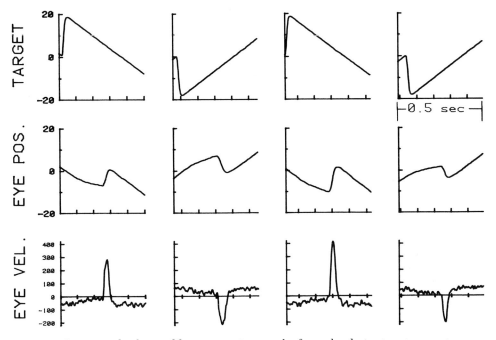

Figure 9. Position and velocity of four consecutive records of saccades during target ramp–step–ramp motion.

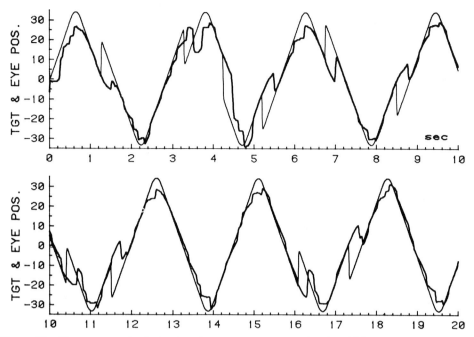

Figure 10. Eye movements during target ramp–step–ramp motion in which target steps were randomized.

Discussion

Traditionally, slow eye movements were thought of as responses to "velocity" stimuli, continuous motion of the head or a visual target. Rapid eye movements, on the other hand, were thought of as responses to "position" disparity, the angle between the line of sight and the direction of a visual target, of intended gaze, or of new visual surroundings coming into view as the head or surroundings moves. Consequently, studies of saccadic eye movements were almost exclusively conducted when isolating the influence of this presumed position variable.

However, velocity inputs do have profound effects on saccades, as has been demonstrated by several investigators. Atkin (1) showed that head movement affects the velocity of saccades additively, and Morasso and colleagues (11) showed that the effect arose in the vestibular end organs. Nauck and colleagues (12) and Dichgans and colleagues (4,5), however, showed that the slowness of quick phases of vestibular nystagmus compared with saccades was due not to the opposing slow phase but to the darkness during vestibular testing. Jurgens and colleagues (8) tested the additivity of vestibular influences on saccades and vestibular quick phases and found that the slow-phase velocity did not have an independent effect on quick-phase velocity but did affect the velocity of saccades made during head movement (7).

In addition to such studies on the effects of vestibular stimuli on saccades, several investigators probed the effects of moving visual stimuli on saccades. Mackensen and Schumacher (9) found the trajectories of quick phases of optokinetic nystagmus to be similar to the trajectories of voluntary saccades and to be independent of drum speed. Rashbass (13) and Zuber (17) showed that target velocity influences saccade amplitude. Robinson (15), Atkin (2), and Barmack (3) showed abrupt transitions between saccades and pursuit movements. Schilling (16) found that in response to ramp–step–ramp stimuli, saccade amplitude and peak velocity decreased for negative initial pursuit velocity, increasing only slightly for positive initial pursuit velocity. Dichgans (5) used a paradigm of moving two targets that had a fixed separation while subjects made saccades between them. Saccade velocities were higher even though they were opposite to the preceding pursuit movements.

Jurgens and Becker (6) asked whether pursuit continues during saccades. They measured a transient decrease in pursuit velocity in the 80 msec preceding and following saccades, and the magnitude of the reduction increased with the angle of the stimulus step to a maximum of 30%. They proposed a strategy whereby pursuit is switched off during saccades.

These authors also reported on the interaction of vestibular inputs and saccades and found contrasting results. Unfortunately, the two experiments were conducted quite differently. Different stimuli (jumping target versus stationary array) were used, and different waveforms (constant-velocity ramps versus sinusoids) were employed. There was thus some doubt as to whether a difference in the mode of interaction of saccades with slow movements of different origins was real. Therefore, in our experiments we sought to provide a straightforward determination of whether smooth eye movements influenced saccades differently depending on whether they were of vestibular or of visual origin. Relations among the parameters describing the resulting saccades showed no dramatic differences for the different testing situations other than that which was predicted on the basis of saccades being smaller when the target moves toward the eyes than when the target is moving away from the eyes, all else being equal. Conspicuous, however, was the lack of slowing of pursuit associated with saccades when the target array was used and its presence when a single target making a ramp–step–ramp was employed. We are not impressed by any difference between the way that vestibular and pursuit eye movements interact with saccades.

CONCLUSION

We have seen that, with a target array, smooth eye movements persist up to within a few tens of milliseconds of a saccade, regardless of whether a vestibular signal is present (from rotation of the subject). However, when targets execute steps during ramp motions, especially when at predictable positions, there is a consistent tendency for the resulting pursuit movement to be attenuated over 100 msec before saccades. This phenomenon may result from target disappearance from the fovea, target displacement, or anticipation of forthcoming saccades.

REFERENCES

1. Atkin, A., Effect of head movement on gaze movement velocity. *Physiologist*, 1964, **7**:82.
2. Atkin, A., Shifting fixation to another pursuit target: Selective and anticipatory control of ocular pursuit initiation. *Exp. Neurol.*, 1969, **23**:157–173.
3. Barmack, N. H., Modification of eye movements by instantaneous changes in the velocity of visual targets. *Vision Res.*, 1970, **10**:1431–1441.
4. Dichgans, J., Nauck, B., and Brooks, B., Saccadic eye movements directed to a visible target and intended saccades in the dark and with eyes closed. Their relations to quick phases of optokinetic and vestibular nystagmus. *Pfluegers Arch.*, 1969, **312**:R143–R144.
5. Dichgans, J., Nauck, B., and Wolpert, E., The influence of attention, vigilance and stimulus area on

optokinetic and vestibular nystagmus and voluntary saccades. In: *The Oculomotor System and Brain Functions* (V. Zikmund, ed.). Butterworth, London, 1973:281–294.

6. Jurgens, R., and Becker, W., Is there linear addition of saccades and pursuit movements? In: *Basic Mechanisms of Ocular Motility and their Clinical Implications* (G. Lennerstrand and P. Bach-y-Rita, eds.). Pergamon, Oxford, New York, 1975:525–529.

7. Jurgens, R., and Becker, W., A computer program library for detecting and analyzing eye movements. *BIOSIGMA, International Conference on Signals and Images in Medicine and Biology*, Section C VIIA. Physiologie Sensorielle, Paris, 1978.

8. Jurgens, R., Becker, W., and Rieger, P., The programming of the fast eye movements during natural vestibular stimulation—two types of interaction. In: *IFAC Symposium on Control Mechanisms in Bio- and Ecosystems. Visual and Vestibular Control of Movements*. Leipzig, 1977:3:120–129.

9. Mackensen, G., and Schumacher, J., Die Geschwindigkeit der raschen Phasen des optokinetische Nystagmus. *Albrecht von Graefes Arch. Ophthalmol.*, 1960, **162**:400–415.

10. Mitrani, L., and Dimitrov, G., Pursuit eye movements of a disappearing moving target. *Vision Res.*, 1978, **18**:537–539.

11. Morasso, P., Bizzi, E., and Dichgans, J., Adjustment of saccade characteristics during head movements. *Exp. Brain Res.*, 1973, **16**:492–500.

12. Nauck, B., Dichgans, J., and Jung, R., Different peak-velocities of rapid phases in optokinetic and vestibular nystagmus. *Pfluegers Arch.*, **312**:R142.

13. Rashbass, C., The relationship between saccadic and smooth tracking eye movements. *J. Physiol. (London)*, 1961, **159**:326–338.

14. Reingold, D. B., Chu, F. C., Cogan, D. G., Leighton, S. B., and McMinn, W. O., A computerized testing facility for clinical study of versional eye movement control. In: *Computers in Ophthalmology* (R. H. Greenfield and A. Colenbrander, eds.). IEEE, New York, 1979:220–222.

15. Robinson, D. A., The mechanics of human smooth pursuit eye movement. *J. Physiol. (London)*, 1965, **180**:569–591.

16. Schilling, R. J., *The Dynamics of the Saccadic Trajectory of the Human Eye with Nonzero Initial Pursuit Velocities*. MSEE Thesis, University of California, Berkeley, 1970.

17. Zuber, B., *Physiological Control of Eye Movements in Humans*. Ph.D. Thesis, Massachusetts Institute of Technology, Cambridge, 1965.

Author Index

Numbers in parentheses are reference numbers and indicate that an author's work is referred to, although the name is not cited in the text. Numbers in italics show the page on which the complete reference is listed.

A

Abel, L. A., 244(1), *247*
Adam, J., 187(20), *189*
Adams, R. D., 180(37), *190*
Allum, J. H. J., 89(6), *94*, 179(1,7), 180(7), 183(1), 184(1), *189*, 213(18), 216(18), *223*
Amblard, B., 211(1), *223*
Anderson, D. J., 191(5), 192(1,4), 202(2), *204*
Anderson, H., 148(1), *155*
Anderson, P. J., 279(7), 283(7), 285(7), *285*
Andres, R. O., 191(5), 192(3,4), 193(3), *204*
Anzaldi, E., 89(1), *94*
Arnold, F., 214(5,7), 215(5,7), *223*
Aronson, E., 216(27), *224*
Aschoff, J. C., 243(2), *247*
Aschoff, J. F., 247(3), *247*
Atkin, A., 279(7), 283(7), 285(7), *285*, 294, *295*
Aubert, H., 211(2), 214(2), *223*
Autret, A., 241 (14,15), 247(15), *248*
Avanzini, G., 241(4), *248*

B

Babin, R. W., 39(2), *46*
Baloh, R. W., *56*, 57(1), 62(3), 72(2,4,10), 75(19), *77*, *78*, 95(2), 103(1,2), *105*, 107(1), 109(1), *113*, 143(1), *144*, 232(2), 234 (4,5), 235(4,7,8,10), 236(4,5), 238(8), *238*, 239, 241(5,6), 245(41), *248*, *249*, 252(1,20,21,25), 253(3,4), 255(30), 257(32), 263(2,38), 267(5), 268(37), 270(6,36), *273*, *274*, *275*, 279(1–3), 283(3), 284, 285(3), *285*

Bárány, R., 35, *36*
Barber, U. O., 143(2), *144*
Barnack, N. II., 19, *22*, 266(7), *274*, 294, *295*
Barr, B., 148(1), *155*
Barr, C. C., 96(3), *105*
Batini, C., 243(7), *248*
Bauer, J., 210(21), *223*
Bean, W. B., 227, *230*
Becker, W., 288, 291, 294(7,8), *295*, *296*
Bender, M. B., 128(11), *134*, 225, 230(2), *230*, 279(7), 283(7), 285(7), *285*
Bensel, C. K., 179(2), *189*
Benson, A. J., 120(1), *122*, 211(3), 218(3), *223*
Berlin, C. I., 148(2), *155*
Bernstein, N., 180, *189*
Berthoz, A., 168(15), 172(15), *178*, 179(19), *189*, 210(4,30), 216(4), *223*, *224*
Bizzi, E., 294(11), *296*
Black, F. O., 93(14), *94*, 95(13), 104(13), *105*, 107(9), 109(9), 113(9,11), *113*, 171(1), 173(1,21), 174(21), 177(21), *177*, *178*
Blair, S. M., 117(2), *122*, 247(38), *249*
Blanks, R. H. I., 8(4), *22*
Bles, W., 214(5,7), 215(5,7), 216(6,25,26), *223*, *224*
Blom, S., *155*
Blum, E., 193(8), 196, *204*
Bock, O., 82, *94*
Boder, E., 253(3), *273*
Borg, E., 147(4), 148(3), *155*
Braitman, D. J., 248(22), *248*
Brandt, T., 118(3), *123*, 179(7), 180(7), *189*, 207(9), 208(9), 209, 210(15–17), 211(15), 212(11), 213(11,18), 214(5,7), 215(5,7),

216(12,18,26), 217(8), 219(13,15),
220(13,15,34), 221(12,34), 222(10), *223*,
224, 255(9), 266(9), *274*
Brandth, S. E., 265(8), *274*
Briggs, P. A. N., 111(2), *113*
Brockman, S. J., 31(10), *37*
Brooks, B., 294(4), *295*
Büchele, W., 217(8), 220(34), 221(34), *223*,
224, 255(9), 266(9), *274*
Büdingen, H. J., 179(1), 183(1), 184(1), *189*
Büttner, U., 75(5), 76(5), *77*, 116(4–6),
118(4,5,26), 119(5), *123*
Buettner, U. W., 75, 76, *77*, 116(5,6),
118(4,5), 119(5), *123*
Buizza, A., 89(3), 91(3), 93(10), *94*
Burke, D., 183(4), *189*
Butler, P. H., 245(45), *249*

C

Cabiati, C., 87(4), *94*
Carhart, R., 147(5), 148(13), *155*
Carmichael, E. A., 279(4), 283(4), 285(4), *285*
Chan, C. W. Y., 186(5), 187(5), *189*
Cheng, M., 255(10), 260(10), 261, *274*
Chinn, H. I., 221(14), *223*
Chu, F. C., 254(11), *274*, 288(14), *296*
Chun, K. S., 101(4), *105*
Coats, A. C., 279(5), *285*
Cogan, D. G., 254(11), *274*, 279(16), 283(16),
286(16), *286*, 288(14), *296*
Cohen, B., 118(7), 120(23), *123*, 128(11),
131(14), *134*, 243(2), 245(35), *247*, *249*,
279(13), *286*
Collewijn, H., 255(15), 260(15), 261, 265(13),
266(12), *274*
Collins, W. E., 117(8), *123*
Conrad, B., 247(3), *247*
Cooke, J. D., 186, *190*
Cordo, P. J., 171(16), *178*
Cords, R., 284, *285*
Corvera, J., 241(10), *248*
Cramer, R. L., 95(5), 96, *105*
Cremieux, J., 211(1), *223*
Crenna, P., 241(4), *248*
Curthoys, I. S., 13(2), *22*

D

Daroff, R. B., 207(9), 208(9), *223*, 244(1),
247(8), *247*, *248*
Daroff, R. R., 279(11), *286*
Davidoff, R. A., 279(7), 283(7), 285(7), *285*
Davies, W. D. T., 108(3), 111(3), *113*
Davis, K. R., 40(1), *46*
Dechesne, C., 21(3), *22*

Dell Osso, L. F., 244(1), *247*
Delpace, M. P., 241(15), 247(15), *248*
Dennett, D., 120(23), *123*
DeWit, G., 179(6), *189*, 216(6), *223*
Dichgans, J., 118(3,9), 122(10), *123*,
179(7,16,21,22), 180(7,21), 181(21),
182(16), 183(22), *189*, *190*, 209, 210(15–
17,21,29,40), 211(15), 213(18,31),
216(12,18), 217(12), 219(13,15),
220(13,15), 221(12), 222(10), *223*, *224*,
238(6), *239*, 241(9), 246(36), *248*, *249*,
255(9), 257(14), 266(9), *274*,
294(4,5,11,12), *295*, *295*, *296*
Diener, H. C., 210(16), *223*
Dietz, V., 171(9), *178*, 186(8), *189*
Dimitrov, G., 287(19), *296*
Dirks, D., 147(10), *155*
Dix, R., 36, *36*
Dix, M. R., 279(4,8), 283(4), 284, 285(4), *285*
Djupesland, G., 147(6), *155*
Dolan, K. D., 39(2), *46*
Dorland, P., 39(7), *47*
Dotti, D., 89(5), *94*
Dow, B. M., 248(22), *248*
Downey, W. L., 255(22), 257(22), *274*
Draganova, N., 193(6), *204*
Dubois, M. F. W., 255(15), 260(15), 261, *274*
Dufor, M., 39(7), *47*
Dunev, S., 193(6), *204*
Dunn, R. F., 107(7), *113*
Duysens, J., 167(3), *177*
Dzendolet, E., 179(2), *189*

E

Eklund, G., 183(4), *189*
Engel, W. K., 241(46), *249*
Engelken, E. J., 72(23), *78*, 95(14), 96(6),
99(15), *105*, 107(10), 109(10), *113*, 238(9),
239
Estanol, B., 241(10), *248*
Estes, M. S., 8(4), *22*
Evarts, E. V., 183(9), 188, *189*

F

Feinmesser, M., 149(16), *155*
Feldman, A. G., 180(13), *189*
Feldman, F., 225, 230(2), *230*
Fender, D. H. 267 (16), *274*
Fernandez, C., 8(5,11), *22*, 58(6), 61, *78*,
116(11–13), 121(14), *123*
Ferrendelli, J. A., 180(38), *190*
Finley, C., 115(17), 118(17), *123*
Fischer, M. H., 109(19), 216(19), *223*
Flock, A., 5(6,32), 21(7), *22*, *23*

Flock, B., 5(6), *22*

Forssberg, H., 167(4), *178*

Fowler, E., 147(7), *155*

Fox, J. C., 279(9), 283(9), 285(9), *285*

Fregly, A. R., 166, *178*

Friendlich, A., 246(11), *248*

Fuchs, A. F., 245(17,18), *248*

Fukuda, T., 130(1,2), 131 (1,2), 132(1), 133(1), *134*

Fuller, J. H., 245(22), *248*

Furman, J. M., 102, *105*, 107(5), 108, 109(6), 110, *113*

Futaki, T., 130(3), 133(3), *134*

G

Gacek, R. R., 7(8,10), 8(29), 21(9), *22, 23, 36, 37*

Galambos, R., 149(14), *155*

Gantchev, G., 193(6,7), *204*

Gavin, M., 117(2), *122*

Gay, A. J., 143(3), *144*, 279(10), *284, 285*

Gelfand, J. M., 183(11), *189*

Ghez, C., 183, 187, *189*

Gilman, S., 147(10), *155*

Girotti, F., 241(4), *248*

Godfrey, K. R., 111(2), *113*

Goldberg, J. M., 8(5,11), 21(12), *22*, 58(6), 61, *78*, 116(11-13), 121(14), *123*

Goodhill, V., 26, 31(5,6,8-10), 32, 34, *37, 56*

Goodson, J. E., 219(32), *224*

Graf, W., 118(9), *123*

Graybiel, A., 166, *178*, 219(20), 222(37,38), *223, 224*

Gresty, M., 241(16), *248*, 255(17), 260(17), 261, *274*

Grillner S., 167(4,6), *178*

Grimm, R. J., 176(17), *178*, 183, *190*

Groen, J. J., 57(22), 60(22), *78*, 118(15,24), *123*

Gucer, G., 249(45), *249*, 269(39), *275*

Gurfinkel, V. S., 171(7), *178*, 179(14,15), 180, 183(11,15), *189*

Gussen, R., 39(4), 42(4), *46*

H

Haddad, G., 246(11), *248*

Hallpike, C. S., 36, *36*, 57(1,8), *78*, 279(4), 283(4), 285(4), *285*

Halmagyi, M., 255(17), 260(17), 261, *274*

Hamilton, A. E., 149(17), *155*

Hanafee, W. N., 39(3,4,6), 42(4), *46, 47*

Hantz, I., 31(10), *37*

Harris, I., 31(10), *37*

Hatam, A., 39(5), *46*

Held, R., 210(17,21), *223*

Helmholtz, H. von, 209(22), *223*

Henn, V., 75(5), 76(5), 77, 115, 116(6), 117(18,19), 118(17,26,27), 119(25,28-30), 120(20,23,31), *123, 124*, 245(37), *249*

Henriksson, N. G., 57(9), *78*

Hess, K., 241(16), *248*

Hibi, T., 129(16), 132(16), *134*

Highstein, S. M., 18(13), *22*, 128(17), *134*

Hillman, D. E., 3(19), *22*

Hillyard, S. A., 149(14), *155*

Hoffman, K. P., 265(18), *274*

Holmes, G., 279(9), 283(9), 285(9), *285*

Holm-Jensen, S., 255(19), *274*

Homick, J. L., 192(1), *204*

Honrubia, V., *56*, 62(3), 72(2,4,10), 75(19), 77, 78, 86, 89(11), *94*, 95(2), 103(1,2), *105*, 107(1,7), 109(1), *113*, 143(1), *144*, 232(2), 234(4,5), 235(4,7,8,10), 236(4,5), 238(8), *238, 239*, 241(5,6), 245(41), *248, 249*, 252(1,20,21,25), 253(4), 255(22,30), 257, 263(2,38), 267(5), 268(37), 270(6,36), *273, 274, 275*, 279(1-3), 283(3), *284(3)*, 285(3), *285*

Hood, J. D., 57(8), *78*, 255(23), 257(23), 260(23), 261, *274, 284, 285*

Hore, J. 187, 188, *190*

Hoyt, W. F., 241(32,33), *249*, 279(11), *286*

Hozawa, J., 128(17), *134*

Hufschmidt, A., 179(16,21), 180(21), 181(21), 182(16), *189*, 213(31), *224*

Hufschmidt, M., 179(16), 182(16), *189*

Hughes, D. W., 130(4), 133(4), *134*

Hulk, J., 57(11), 60(11), *78*

I

Isoviita, V., 119(39), *124*

Ito, M., 14(15), 18(14), *22*, 265(27), 267(27), *274*

J

Jacoby, C. C., 39(2), *46*

Jaeger, J., 117(18,19), 120(20), *123*

Jaglia, F., 255, *274*

Jaju, B. P., 222(23), *223*

Janetta, P. J., 148(2), *155*

Jastreboff P., 265(27), 267(27), *274*

Jenkins, H. A., 72(10), *78*, 235(8,10), *239*, 241(5), 249(41), *248, 249*, 252(21), 263(38), 268(37), *274, 275*

Jerger, J., 147(8), *155*

Jewett, D. L., 149(9), *155*

Jones, G. M., 95(8), *105*

Jones, K. W., 192(1), *204*

Jongkees, L. B. W., 57(11,22), 60(11,22), 78, 118(24), *123*
Jung, R., 241(9), *248*, 294(12), *296*
Jurgens, R., 288, 291, 294(7), 295, *296*

K

Kaga, K., 130(5), 132(5), *134*
Kamio, T., 246(39), *249*
Kaplan, H., 147(10), *155*
Kapteyn, T. S., 214(5,7,24), 215(5,7), 216(6,25,26), *223*, *224*
Karten, A. J., 265(8), *274*
Kase, M., 243(12), *248*
Keller, E. L., 118(21), *123*
Keltner, J. L., 143(3), *144*, 279(10), *285*
Kiang, N. Y. S., 8(29), *23*
Kim, Y. S., 72(10), *78*
Kimm, J., 234(5), 236(5), *239*
Kirikae, I., 127, 128(7), 130(6), *134*
Kirsten, E. B., 222(23), *223*
Kitahara, M., 130(3), 133(3), *134*
Kline, D. G., 148(2), *155*
Klinke, R., 21(16), *22*
Knapp, H., 138(4), *144*
Koenig, E., 118(3), *123*
Komatsuzaki, A., 129(12), *134*, 279(19), 280(19), *286*
Kommerell, G., 244(13), *248*
Konrad, H. R., 72(2), 77, 103(1), *105*, 241(6), *248*, 255(30), *275*
Kornhuber, H. H., 143(5), *144*, 247(3), *247*
Kornmüller, E. E., 209(19), 216(19), *223*
Kos, C. M., 72(23), *78*, 95(14), 96(16), 99(15), *105*
Koschitzky, H. V., 82(2), *94*
Kots, Y. M., 180(13), *189*
Krafczyk, S., 212(11), 213(11), 220(34), 221(34), *223*
Krausz, H. I., 149(14), *155*
Kunley, W., 89(11), *94*
Kurdziel, S., 148(11), *155*

L

Lang, W., 120(20), *123*
Langhofer, L., 62(3), 77, 232(2), *239*, 252(1), *273*
Larmande, P., 241(14,15), 247(15), *248*
Lau, C. G. Y., 72(10), *78*, 235(8,10), 238(8), *239*, 241(5), 245(41), *248*, *249*, 252(20,25), 263(38), 268(37), *274*, *275*
Lee, D. N., 179(17), *189*, 216(27), *224*
Lee, R. G., 187(18), *189*
Leech, J., 248(16), *248*
Leibowitz, H. W., 210(29), 214(28), *224*

Leigh, R. J., 241(42), *249*
Leighton, S. B., 288(14), *296*
Lestienne, F., 179(19), *189*, 210(30), *224*
Lindeman, H. H. 6(17), *22*
Lipshits, M. J., 171(7), *178*, 179(15), 183(15), *189*
Lisberger, S. G., 245 (17,18), 246(27), *248*
Lishman, J. R., 179(17), *189*
Llinás, R., 243(19), *248*
Lombardi, R., 89(5), *94*
Lorente de Nó. R., 57(12), 76, *78*
Lowe-Bell, S. S., 148(2), *155*
Lundquist, P. G., 5(32), *23*
Lyon, M., 21(9), *22*

M

Mach, E., 209(31), *224*
MacKay, W. A., 176, *178*
Mackensen, G., 294, *296*
McLaren, J. W., 3(19), *22*
McMinn, W. O., 288(14), *296*
Maeda, M., 132(15), *134*, 245(20), *248*
Maekawa, K., 245(21), *248*, 265(26,27), 266(27), *274*
Malcolm, R., 5(18), 21(18), *22*
Malsbenden, I., 212(11), 213(11), *223*
Mancall, E. L., 180(37), *190*
Mancuso, A., 39(6), *47*
Marco, L. A., 15(33), *23*
Margolis, R., 148(15), *155*
Markham, C. H., 8(4), 13(2), *22*
Marsden, C. D., 187(20), *189*
Mathieu-Millaire, F., 241(42), *249*
Mathog, R. H., 72, *78*
Matsuo, V., 118(7), *123*
Mauritz, K. H., 171(9), *178*, 179(16,21,22), 180(7,21), 181(21), 182(16), 183, *189*, *190*, 213(18,31a), 216(18), *223*, *224*
Melvill-Jones, G., 186(5), 187(5), *189*
Merton, P. A., 187(20), *189*
Metzger, J., 39(7), *47*
Meyer, M., 193(8), 196, *204*
Michaels, D. L., 89(6), *94*
Miles, F. A., 245(22), 246(27), *248*
Miles, T. S., 120(20), *123*
Miller, D. C., 243(12), *248*
Miller, J. B., 8(29), *23*
Miller, J. W., 219(32), *224*
Milsum, J. H., 58(16), 59(16), *78*, 95(8), *105*
Mira, E., 89(1,3), 91(3), 93(7), *94*
Mitchell, D. P., 255(22), 257(22), *274*
Mitrani, L., 287(10), *296*
Miyashita, Y., 265(27), 266, *274*
Miyata, H., 132(15), *134*
Moller, A., 39(5), *46*

Money, K. E., 221(33), *224*
Morasso, P., 294, *296*
Morgenstein, K. M., 36, *37*
Mori, S., 179(15), 183(15), *189*
Morimoto, M., 127, 130(3), 133(3), *134*
Morton, H. B., 187(20), *189*
Mowrer, O. H., 117(22), *123*
Muratore, R., 267(28), *274*
Murphy, J. T., 176, *178*
Murray, E., 5(6), *22*

N

Nadol, J. B., 30(12), *37*
Nagao, S., 265(27), 267(27), *274*
Nashner, L. M., 168(15), 170(14,18,19),
    171(1,10,12-14,16), 172(15), 173(1),
    176(11,17), *177, 178*, 179(23,24,28), 180,
    183(25,26), 185(24), 186(26), 188(27),
    190, 198, *204*
Nauok, B., 255(14), 257(14), *274*, 294(4,5)
    295(5), *295, 296*
Negri, S., 241(1), *248*
New, P. F. J., 40(1), *46*
Newman, N. M., 143(3), *144*, 279(10), *285*
Noda, H., 243(12), 245(23-25), *248*
Noffsinger, D., 147(12), 148(11,13), *155*
Nye, P. W., 267(16), *274*

O

Ochs, A. L., 241(32,33), *249*
Ojemann, R. J., 40(1), *46*
O'Leary, D. P., 86, 93(14), *94*, 95(13),
    104(13), *105*, 107(5,7,9), 108(5),
    109(5,6,9), 110(5), 113(9,11), *113*,
    173(21), 174(21), 177(21), *177, 178*
Olivecrona, H., 39(5), *46*
Oliver, D., 244(13), *248*
Olsen, W., 147(12), 148(11,13), *155*
Olson, J. E., 95(14), 99(15), *105*, 107(10),
    109(10), *113*, 238(9), *239*
Oman, C. M., 57(24), 60(24), 75(24), *78*,
    89(9), *94*, 210(40), *224*
Oosterveld, W. J., 138(6), *139*
Optican, L. M., 243(26), 244(26), 246(27),
    247(26), *248*
Oscarsson, O., 183(30), *190*
Outerbridge, J. S., 255(10), 260(10), 261, *274*

P

Pal'Tsev, Y. J., 180(13), *189*
Parker, S. W., 40(1), *46*
Pastormerlo, M., 87(4), *94*
Pavard, B., 210(4), 216(4), 221(34), *223*

Pearson, K. G., 167(3), *177*
Peitersen, E., 255(20), *274*
Penfield, W., 285, *286*
Pertuiset, B., 39(7), *47*
Phillips, C. G., 183(31), *190*
Picton, T. W., 149(14), *155*
Pola, J., 253(29), *274*
Popelka, G., 148(15), *155*
Popov, K. E., 171(7), *178*, 179(15), 183(15),
    189
Popov, V., 193(7), *204*
Precht, W., 13(22), 14(23), *22*, 76, *78*, 103,
    105, 241(28), *248*
Probst, T., 220(34), *224*

R

Rademakers, W. J. A. C., 138(6), 139, *144*
Rand, R. W., 39(4), 40(1), 42(4), *46*
Raphan, R., 279(13), *286*
Raphan, T., 118(7), 120(23), *123*
Rashbass, C., 294(13), *296*
Rasmussen, A. T., 6(20), *22*
Rasmussen, G. L., 7(10), *22*
Reason, J. T., 218(35), *224*
Reingold, D. B., 254(11), *274*, 288, *296*
Rieger, P., 294(8), *296*
Ritchie, L., 243(29), 244(29), *248*
Roberson, G. H., 40(1), *46*
Robinson, D. A., 57(18), 58(20), *78*, 96(3),
    101(4,10-12), *105*, 108(8), 111(8), *113*,
    241(46), 243(26,31), 244(26,44),
    246(11,30), 247(26,31,43), 253(29), *248,
    249*, 253(29), *274*, 294, *296*
Rodemer, C. S., 210(29), *224*
Romberg, M. H., *178*
Romero, R., 241(10), *248*
Rommelt, U., 122(10), *123*, 238(6), *239*
Ron, S., 243(31), 247(31), *249*
Rosenblum, W. L., 230(3), *230*
Rossignol, S., 167(4), *178*
Rossiter, V. S., 149(18), *155*
Rudge, P., 241(16), *248*
Russell, I. J., 21(7), *22*

S

Sakala, S. M., 257(32), *275*
Sakata, E., 128(9), *134*
Sala, O., 21(21), *22*
Sans, A., 21(3), *22*
Schenk, V. W. D., 264(34), *274*
Schilling, R. J., 295, *296*
Schmid, R., 85(16), 89(3,5), 91(3), 93(7,10), *94*
Schmidt, C. L., 21(16), *22*, 118(9), *123*
Schmidt, D., 244(1), *247*

Schmitt, C., 179(22), 183(22), 185(32), *190*
Schoppman, A., 265(18), *274*
Schubert, G., 219(36), *224*
Schubiger, O., 40(8), *47*
Schuknecht, H. F., 36, 37, *56*
Schultheis, L. W., 96(3), *103*
Schumacher, J., 294, *296*
Sekine, S., 246(39), *249*
Selhorst, J. B., 230(3), *230*, 241(32,33), *249*
Semplici, P., 89(3), 91(3), *94*
Seung, H. I., 36, 37
Sheena, D., 87(15), *94*
Shik, M. L., 183(11), *189*
Shimazu, H., 13(22), 14(23), *22*, 76, 78, 279(14), *286*
Shimizu, M., 246(39), *249*
Shinoda, Y., 183, 187, *189*
Sills, A. W., 72(4), 75(19), *77*, *78*, 89(11), *94*, 95(2), 103(2), *105*, 232(1), *238*, 252(20), 255, 263(2), *273*, *274*, *275*, 279(2), *285*
Silverskiöld, B. P., 180(33,34), *190*
Singer, H. S., 253(40), *275*
Skavenski, A. A., 58(20), *78*
Smith, J. L., 264, *275*, 279(15,16), 283(15,16), 285(15,16), *286*
Smith, P. K., 221(14), *223*
Snider, R. S., 243(34), *249*
Soechting, J. F., 179(19), *189*, 210(30), *224*
Sohmer, H., 149(16), *155*
Solingen, L. D., 263(2), *273*
Spoendlin, H. H., 4(24), 5(25), 6(25), *22*
Spooner, J. W., 257, *275*
Stark, L., 241(32,33), *249*
Starr, A., 149(17), *155*
Stefanelli, M., 93(7), *94*
Steinhausen, W., 57(21), *78*
Sterkers, J. M., 39(7), *47*
Stockard, J. J., 149(18), *155*
Stockwell, C. W., 143(2), *144*
Stowell, A., 243(34), *249*
Stroud, M. H., 143(3), *144*, 279(10), *285*
Suter, C. G., 230(3), *230*
Suzuki, D. A., 245(23,24,25), *248*
Suzuki, J. I., 128(7,11,17), 129(12), 130(4,5), 132(5), 133(4,10), *134*, 246(39), *249*, 279(17,19), 280(17-19), *286*
Suzuki, T., 129(16), 132(16), 133(16), *134*
Szabo, G., 149(16), *155*

T

Taborikova, H., 184, 185(35), *190*
Takeda, T., 265(26), *274*
Takemori, S., 131(13,14), *134*, 245(35), *249*
Tanji, J., 183(9), 188, *189*
Tareras, J. M., 40(1), *46*
Tarlov, E., 17(26), *22*

Tatton, W. G., 187(18), *189*
Ter Braak, J. W. G., 264, *275*
Theopold, H., 244(13), *248*
Thomas, D. P., 179(36), *190*
Tokita, T., 129, 132(16), 133, *134*
Tokumasu, K., 128(7), *134*
Tole, J. R., 89(6,9,12), *94*
Tomita' T., 129(16), 132(16), 133(16), *134*
Tomovie, R., 83(13), *94*
Trincker, D., 5(27,28), *23*
Tsetlin, M. L., 183(11), *189*
Tuma, G., 170(19), *178*

U

Uemura, T., 128(17), *134*
Umeda, Y., 130(18), *134*
Uyeda, R., 130, *134*

V

Valavanis, A., 40(8), *47*
Valvassori, G. E., 39, *47*
Van Egmond, A. A. J., 57(22), 60(22), *78*, 118(24), *123*
Van Vliet, A. G. M., 264(34,35), *274*
Victor, M., 180(37, 38), *190*
Vilis, T., 186, 187, 188, *190*
von Reutern, G. M., 122(10), *123*, 238(6), 239, 246(36), *249*

W

Waespe, B., 119(25), *123*
Waespe, W., 115, 116(4), 118(26,27), 119(25,28-30), 120(20), *123*, *124*, 245(37), *249*
Wagner, W., 222(10), *223*
Wall, C. III, 93, *94*, 95(13), 104(13), *105*, 107(9), 109(9), 113(9,11), *113*, 171(1), 173(1,21), 174, 177(21), *177*, *178*
Walsh, B. T., 8(29), *23*
Wang, S. C., 222(23), *223*
Ward, P. H., 255(22), 257(22), *274*
Warr, W. B., 21(30), *23*
Watt, D. G. D., 186(5), 187(5), *189*
Waybright, E. A., 230(3), *230*
Wedenberg, E., 148(1), *155*
Weiss, A. D., 40(1), *46*
Wellauer, J., 40(8), *47*
Wenzel, D., 216(12), 217(12), 221(12), *223*
Werness, S., 202(2), *204*
Wersäll, J., 4(31), 5(32), *22*, *23*
Westheimer, G., 247(38), *249*
Whitney, R. J., 179(36), *190*
Wiley, T., 148(15), *155*
Williams, A. C., 254(11), *274*

Williston, J. S., 149(9), *155*
Wilson, V. J., 15(33), *23*, 176, *178*
Wist, E. R., 216(26), 219(13), 220(13), *223*, *224*
Wolfe, J. W., 72, *78*, 95(14), 96(6,16), 99(15), *103*, 107(5,10), 108(5), 109(5,6,10), 110(5), *113*, 238(9), *239*, 243(19), *248*
Wolpert, E., 255(14), 257(14), *274*, 294(5), 295(5), *295*
Wood, C. D., 219(39), *224*
Wood, R. W., 222(37,38), *224*
Woolacott, M., 170(18,19), *178*
Wylie, R. M., 15(33), *23*

Y

Yagi, T., 130(4), 133(4), *134*, 246(39), *249*
Yamazaki, A., 245(45), 246(40), *249*, 269(39), *275*
Yee, R. D., 62(3), *77*, 232(2), 234(4,5), 235(4,7,10), 236(4,5), *239*, 241(5,46),

245(41), *248*, *249*, 252(1,21), 253(3,4,40), 263(38), 267(5), 268(37), 270(6,36), *273*, *274*, *275*, 279(3), 283(3), 284(3), 285(3), *285*
Yoshida, M., 14(15), *22*
Young, L. R., 57(24), 60(24), 75(24), *78*, 87(15), 89(9,12), *94*, 115(17), 118(17), 120(31), *123*, *124*, 210(4,17,40), 216(4), *223*, *224*

Z

Zakrisson, J., *155*
Zambarbieri, D., 85, 93(10), *94*
Zangemeister, W. H., 82(2), *94*
Zanibelli, A., 89(3), 91(3), *94*
Zee, D. S., 122(32), *124*, 241(42,46), 244(44), 245(45), 246(27,40), 247(43), *249*, 253(40), 267(28), 269, *274*, *275*
Ziedes des Plantes, B. E., 42(10), *47*
Zuber, B., 294, *296*

Subject Index

A

Acoustic impedance, 146-147, 154
Acoustic neuromas, 39, 49, 51, 61, 99, 103
Acoustic reflex, 147, 154
Adaptation, 74, 75
Arnold-Chiari malformation, 268
Ataxia, 179, 180, 199
Auditory brainstem response, 148, 149-152
Auditory tests, 145-155

B

Bleb nevus syndrome, 227, 230

C

Caloric tests, 61, 72, 73, 82, 83, 95, 103, 140
Cerebellar ataxia, 241
Cerebellar atrophy, 213
Cerebellar control, 243-244
Cerebellar lesions, 138, 176, 180-189, 262, 263
Cogan's syndrome, 157-160
Computer analyses, *see also* Fourier analysis, 96, 108, 109, 146, 154, 232
Coriolis effect, 219

D

Dizziness, 25-27, 30, 49-56

E

Electronystagmography, 135, 138
Equilibrium control, 165-177
Europe, vestibular research in, 135-144
Ewald's second law of labyrinthine function, 61, 72

E

Eye movements (ocular motor), 81-94, 142
recording, 87

F

Fourier analysis, 59, 62, 63, 72-74, 76, 193
Frenzel glasses, 128

H

Head rotation, 225-229

J

Japan, vestibular research in, 127-133

L

Labyrinthectomy, 121, 235
Labyrinthine lesions, 50, 51, 52, 57-76, 96, 97, 98, 101, 103, 104, 182, 225-230

M

Ménière's disease, 30, 50, 52, 62, 65, 66, 98, 99, 133, 263
Motion sickness, 117, 218-222

N

Nystagmus, *see also* Optokinetic nystagmus, 25, 27, 35, 36, 54, 55, 56, 62, 82, 86, 89, 90, 91, 108-113, 115, 117, 118, 120, 138-143, 207, 227, 232

O

Ocular motor defects, 216, 262, 264, 265
Optokinetic nystagmus, 118, 129, 142, 226, 227, 229, 251-273

Optokinetic stimulation, 118, 210, 216, 220, 232–238
Otological tests, 27, 29, 30, 31

P

Pendular test, 86, 142
Pendulum model of vestibular function, 57, 74
Postrotatory nystagmus, 74, 75
Postural imbalance (sway), 179–189, 191–203
  case histories, 199, 200, 201, 202, 203
  tests, 191, 192
Pursuit tests, 271, 272
  components, 252, 253, 255
  effect of age, 256, 257
  recording, 251, 252

R

Radiology, 39–44
Rotatory tests, 82, 83, 103, 115–120, 132, 140, 231–238

S

Saccades, 87, 89, 96, 143, 287–296
Semicircular canals, 42, 90, 95
Slow component in eye movement, 57, 63, 67
Spinocerebellar atrophy, 182, 183
Stretch reflexes, 184–188, 200

T

Tumors, 40, 44

U

Unilateral labyrinthine paralysis, 61, 65, 72, 76

V

Vertigo, 25, 26, 27, 35, 49, 50, 52, 136, 207, 214, 227
Vestibular functions, 107–113
Vestibular lesions, 50, 51, 173, 174, 175, 176, 238
Vestibular nerve responses, 57–75
  impulse acceleration, 59, 70, 74
Vestibular neurons, 3–9, 12, 17, 19, 21, 99, 121
Vestibular nuclei, 9, 11–16, 57, 61, 75, 76, 116
Vestibular optic responses, 17, 18, 19, 227, 228, 229, 232–238
Vestibular pathways
  vestibulocerebellar, 12, 13, 51, 180, 245, 246
  vestibulospinal, 15, 17
Vestibular research in Europe, 135–144
  in Japan, 127–133
Vestibular testing, 19, 57–76, 119
  rotatory, 57, 61, 63, 65, 73, 74, 138
Vestibuloocular reflexes, 57, 60, 61, 74–76, 83, 86, 90, 92, 93, 95, 101, 103, 109, 110, 115, 174, 177, 225
  ampullofugal and ampullopetal responses, 60, 61, 63–74
  eighth nerve response, 59, 60, 75
  primary afferent neurons, 57, 60, 75
  semicircular canals, 60
Visual defects, effects of, 258, 260, 261
Visual-vestibular stimulation, 119, 207
Visuovestibuloocular reflex, 226

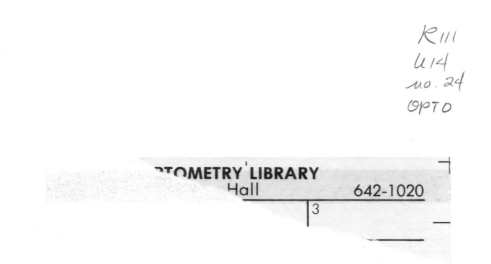